THE TORTOISE DIET

THE TORTOISE DIET

Patricia S. Church RN, BSN

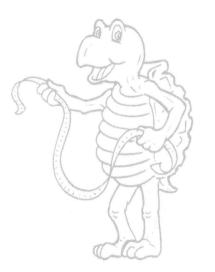

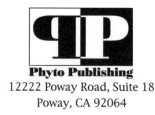

Phyto Publishing

12222 Poway Road, Suite 18
Poway, CA 92064

Please consult your doctor before beginning this or any
other diet or exercise program. After evaluation, your
doctor may want to modify the nutritional or exercise
recommendations contained in this book to fit any special
conditions or needs you may have.

All efforts have been made to insure the accuracy of the
information contained in this book. The author expressly
disclaims responsibility for any adverse effects arising
from the use of the information described herein.

ISBN 0-9773538-0-X

Printed in United States of America
c 10 9 8 7 6 5 4 3 2 1
p 10 9 8 7 6 5 4 3 2 1

This book is intended to encourage and inspire all of my fellow lifetime "dieters" who have tried and failed so many times before. Believe in yourself. Visualize yourself as being healthy, strong, and in control of your own destiny.

In loving memory of my sister Susan.

ACKNOWLEDGMENTS

When, for the first time in my life, I began to really be successful at losing body fat, I knew I had to write a book to tell others what I was learning. Starting to write down what I was learning was the easy part! I had no idea whatsoever what a huge project it would be to bring to fruition the book you are now holding. I definitely need to say a big heartfelt thank you to the following people:

My family and friends

* To my sister, Diane Rafferty, for helping me edit an initial very rough draft by cutting about half of the exclamation points (my excitement was really showing in the early days!)

* To my brother, Alan Stordal, for his unrestrained enthusiasm and support for my project! That meant a lot as I was struggling to get my ideas into print.

* To my mother and father, Ralph and Shirley Stordal, for taste-testing recipes, talking constantly to their friends about the book (for at least a year before it was out!) and for walking those pounds off!

* To my husband Charlie. For every recipe my mother and father tried, Charlie had to taste five additional recipes, at least! Thank you for your constant encouragement and love.

* Thank you to all my friends who helped with my book in so many ways big and small.

The professionals

*To Penny C. Sansevieri, an accomplished author, and also my book publicist. Penny's Learning Annex class inspired me to believe that I could really write a book! (www.authormarketingexperts.com)

* To Jeniffer Thompson, my editor and web site designer, who cried when she first read my rough draft because she knew someone very close to her who was in serious need of a really workable weight loss program. I couldn't have made a better choice for my editor and web designer. (www.monkeycmedia.com)

* To Thomas K. Mathews, the wonderfully creative artist and author who is responsible for the cover design, creative book design, and cartoon illustrations throughout the book. You really made the book come alive! (www.thomaskmatthews.com)

CONTENTS

THE OLD FABLE OF THE TORTOISE AND THE HARE WAS, AS YOU MAY REMEMBER, ABOUT A RACE.

The Hare was much quicker than the Tortoise, and he immediately jumped off the starting line to take a big lead. The Tortoise could have become discouraged, but he ignored the Hare and just kept plodding along. Unfortunately for the Hare, the race was filled with many challenges. Because he had very little patience, he ended up scurrying around in circles, so much so that he completely tired himself out. At this point, of course, the slow and steady Tortoise passed him and won the race.

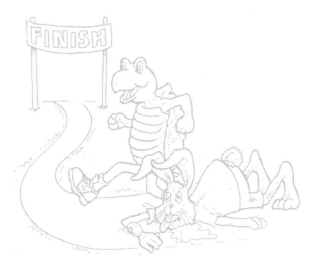

INTRODUCTION

I'm confident the book you are holding will change your life! I sincerely believe this, because my own life has changed in ways I could not have imagined possible three years ago. What you will be reading is quite different from many other currently popular diet books. I'm not a famous personality, and I'm not a doctor. However, unlike the people writing diet books who have never had a pound to lose in their lives, I am a person who used to have a serious weight problem. I'm thrilled to report those days are gone for me! In fact, by practicing the principles I will soon explain, I was able to lose 120 pounds! Even better, I am now able to maintain that weight loss, without starvation and while enjoying my life. For someone like me, a semi-professional dieter for most of my life, this is AMAZING!

Because significant weight loss is a very personal and life-changing journey, I feel strongly that I am a true weight loss "expert." I have struggled to learn to make new and better decisions as I faced the daily challenges of weight loss. I have genuinely walked the walk, and now I'm ready to talk the talk! In the following pages I will teach you what I've learned about how to personalize your own weight loss plan and begin to change poor health habits into the twenty-five good health habits necessary for successful and permanent weight loss. This is information I want to share with you, because I know how hard it is to lose weight and keep it off.

Let me begin by introducing myself. My name is Patty. I'm 5'1½" tall (I always have to add the half inch!). I am a Registered Nurse with a bachelor's degree and I've spent a total of twelve years working in Intensive Care Units taking care of critically ill patients. Many of the patients I've cared for in the hospital were suffering from serious illnesses that resulted from years of living an unhealthy, sedentary and overweight lifestyle. I certainly should have known better than to let myself get so heavy, but knowing and doing are two different things. As a result, I "woke up" and discovered myself at age 45 weighing 248 pounds! I had struggled with being "pudgy" since childhood, and had been up and down all over the scale many times in my life, but this was the horrifying topper.

I was in trouble! I was already one year post-hysterectomy related to a uterine fibroid tumor, and at yet another medical check up, my doctor scared me by telling me that he had found some other pre-cancerous cells. My blood pressure was too high, my cholesterol was too high, and I had problems with my skin, not to mention always being fatigued, stressed out and unhappy. As the stark reality hit, I began to consciously imagine my future. I envisioned myself at age 55 ... age 65 ... age 75. What would my life be like? On a daily basis I had seen how frightening and debilitating the diseases related to obesity could be. Despite my medical knowledge, my life was out of control. I knew that unless I changed my ways, I could anticipate an old age filled with nothing but medical problems, pain and unhappiness.

As I examined my situation, I began to contemplate once again the prospect of losing weight. My chances for success didn't seem good. After all, much of the first forty-five years of my life were spent endlessly repeating a predictable cycle of "dieting." Usually it would begin when I found myself unable to zip up some pants that used to fit me just fine, or when I realized that a social event or vacation was fast approaching. Panic stricken, I would, one more time, gather up all my willpower and vow to lose weight. After following some sort of starvation-type plan for a while, I usually managed to lose a few pounds. It was always tough going, however, because I felt irritable and hungry most of the time.

Inevitably, the weight loss would slow down and discouragement would then set in. When I couldn't stand it any longer, I would just "blow my diet." Once that happened, it was all over. The pounds came rebounding back, and always a few more for good measure.

This miserable cycle of dieting and the inevitable discouragement that followed affected more than just my body, it made me feel bad about myself. I believed that I wasn't very strong and my weakness prevented me from accomplishing what I wanted in life. I felt like I was trapped deep inside some kind of "fat suit." I knew none of the crazy diets worked, but I continued to fantasize about somehow finding a way to unzip that "fat suit" and crawl out. If I could do that, maybe the real me buried inside could emerge, and I could finally step into the life I dreamed of. If it were possible to magically lose weight like that, what would my life really be like? Would I make a job change to explore my dream career? Would I have the courage to seek out social situations that had always sounded fun? Most importantly, would the "real me" that I imagined was being held prisoner somewhere under there be a happier and more fulfilled person?

From somewhere deep down inside of my being, I decided this time was going to be different. I finally understood that this was MY ONLY LIFE, and I had squandered the minutes and days away. Seeing that awful number on the scale caused me to finally make the decision to figure out, once and for all, how to lose weight and keep it off.

It was pretty obvious that my overweight condition had not just "happened." I made many choices each and every day that brought me to my current state. I began to realize that to prevent the bleak future I envisioned, it was time to deliberately make new kinds of choices. I knew I had some work ahead of me.

Once I understood the path I would have to take, I mapped out a strategy, made a couple of important commitments to myself, and began. First I told myself I was worth the effort, so this time my experience, as I slowly lost weight, was different. I began to learn things that really worked, I felt strangely calm and centered, and in control of my own destiny. "If it's to be ... it's up to me" became a very real concept for me.

As time progressed, my weight loss became a phenomenon, and a subject of great interest to everyone I met. Every day there were eager questions: "Are you cutting out carbs?" "Did you have the gastric bypass surgery?" "Are you taking some kind of a new pill?" WHAT ARE YOU DOING TO LOSE WEIGHT? I found myself at a loss to explain my weight loss in the proverbial twenty-five words or less. It was much more complicated than that. I was reading everything I could get my hands on about nutrition and exercise. I kept a journal in which I documented the effects that various dietary and exercise practices had on my body. Slowly, I discovered what worked, and just as importantly, what didn't. In looking back at the mountain of information I had in my journals, it was evident there were some core health habit changes that had contributed to my success. The real surprise came when I realized that the new habits I developed weren't a huge struggle like diets had always been in the past. I wasn't too hungry! I ate real food that I enjoyed. I went out to dinner. I went on vacation. In other words, I lived my life while continuing to lose weight. In addition to that, the health benefits I enjoyed ran the gamut from having a clearer complexion to not getting my usual winter session of bronchitis and multiple colds.

My weight loss wasn't as rapid as those other popular diets promise. Far from a simple unzipping, escaping from inside that "fat suit" was more like a slow un-peeling of many layers. It took me almost three years to lose 120 pounds and reach my target weight. During my weight loss, as I plodded along, the old story of the "Tortoise and the Hare" kept coming to mind. I really started to identify with that Tortoise. Now you know how the book got its funny name!

Are you ready to think of weight loss in a new way? Are you ready to judge your success, not by how quickly you lose weight, but by how effectively you can keep that weight off for the rest of your life? Are you ready to make this profound change in your approach to weight loss? If so, think of your self, like I did, as a Tortoise beginning a long and steady race. Use this book as your own personal training manual to begin your weight-loss journey, a journey to win the race to lose!

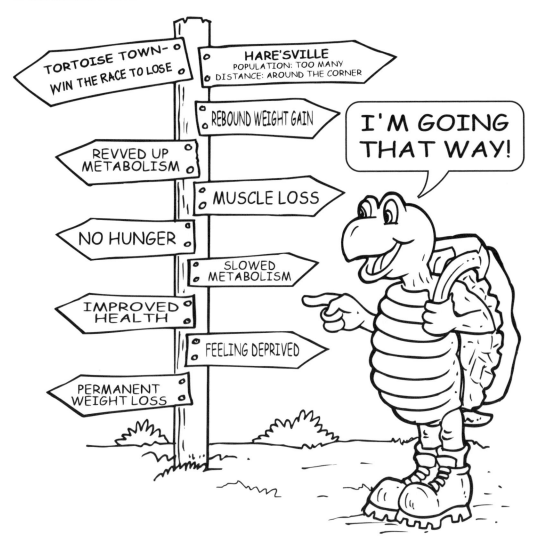

CHAPTER ONE
COMMITMENTS

THE TWO COMMITMENTS

One of the first things I decided to do early on was to keep an informal journal, recording some of my thoughts, the various things I was doing to lose weight, and the knowledge I was acquiring. Three years later, the book you are holding now has literally emerged from the pages of that journal. As I reviewed my notes, it became clear there were two very important commitments I had made that formed the basis of my success. As you begin, these same commitments are also important for you.

The first commitment I made was to value my health.

When I first began my weight loss, I got the idea to fill two huge suitcases with enough books that when I put them on the scale they weighed 120 pounds. They were so heavy I could hardly lift them, much less lug them around! It was shocking to see what huge demands I was placing on every system in my body by carrying around so much excess weight. Even if you only need to lose ten pounds this is an eye opening little experiment. Try it for yourself. Pack a suitcase (or two) with enough clothes or books so they weigh approximately the number of pounds you need to lose. Pick the suitcases up and carry them around. If you have only ten or twenty pounds to lose, you're probably saying "not a problem." Before you get too confident, though, take the suitcase and go up and down the stairs a few times. How are you feeling now? You'll be as shocked as I was, I'm sure.

It's only possible to live a sedentary life and eat junky foods for so many years before the consequences eventually catch up to you. Beyond the sheer physical discomforts that come from carrying around excess body weight, there are very serious health concerns that are directly correlated to obesity:

1. High Blood Pressure

This increases the resistance against which your heart must pump blood, which causes your heart to work extra hard-60 seconds x 60 minutes x 24 hours x 365 days, every year of your life.

2. Elevated "LDL" Cholesterol

This is the BAD cholesterol, the one that makes your blood sticky, which leads to a build up of deposits (plaque) in your blood vessels. Similar to a hose that has gotten full of some kind of gunk, causing the flow of water to slow to a trickle, these plaque deposits can eventually harden and cause the inside of the artery to become so small that blood cannot flow to the area beyond the blockage. When the blockage becomes large enough, the areas beyond the blockage will not receive enough oxygen and nutrition to function effectively, causing tissue to die. Some people experience pain in their legs, arms, and chest when they exert themselves. This may be an indicator that their circulation is impaired. It is not uncommon, however, for people to suffer from heart attacks or strokes with no prior warning, both of which can result in large areas of tissue death.

3. Diabetes

This disease has many severe health consequences, including skin ulcerations, heart disease, blindness, and nerve damage, not to mention the daily multiple measurements of blood sugar and insulin injections that may be required.

4. Cancer

Many studies closely link excess body fat with the development of several types of cancer, particularly cancers of the breast, prostate, and colon.

5. Osteoarthritis

Excess weight puts excess strain on hip, knee and ankle joints, which may degrade joints and cause painful debilitation.

6. Sleep Disturbances

Getting a good night's rest may be difficult for people who have gastric reflux and sore joints. Large breasts and abdomens can also make finding a comfortable sleep position difficult. A more serious obesity-related sleep disturbance is Sleep Apnea, a condition that causes a person to actually stop breathing for periods of time during the night. Besides a chronic lack of adequate oxygen caused by many repeated cycles of apnea throughout the night, the person suffering from this condition exists in a chronic state of sleep deprivation. They are never able to get enough sleep, and the sleep they do get is disrupted so often that they never get the deep restorative REM sleep we all require.

You may already know about these health consequences related to obesity. Due to my nursing experience, I certainly did. Despite all I knew, I still ended up weighing 248 pounds! Knowing the long-term physical consequences of obesity should scare us all into changing our ways, but knowing and believing these things to be true doesn't automatically motivate us to do something about it. If you do believe your suitcase full of fat may lead to serious health consequences, and if you do value your health as a top priority, making the commitment to get rid of the excess baggage may not only change your life, it may truly save your life!

The second commitment I made was to achieve permanent weight loss.

I decided to once and for all STOP the ridiculous cycle of "dieting." I had to fight my instinctive desire to look for the easy way. There are literally hundreds of "hare-brained" quick weight loss diets out there, all of which make the claim that losing weight with their program is easy. My goal, however, was not just to quickly lose 10 pounds to fit into a dress for a special event, and not care much if I gained the weight back. This time I wanted to learn once and for all how to eat, exercise, and live my life in such a way that I could lose weight permanently. I was done losing and re-losing the same weight over and over again.

Because I had made the commitments to value my health and to achieve permanent weight loss, it was obvious that for any plan to help me achieve these goals, it would have to be one that I could live with for the rest of my life. Taking this long-term and change-your-life approach was uncharted territory for me. I am convinced, however, that these commitments formed the foundation of my success.

IF IT'S TO BE ... IT'S UP TO ME

As I reviewed my journal of the foods I ate, it became clear that restaurant meals, fast food, and other convenience snack foods appeared quite regularly on the pages! Those high-calorie foods were quick and convenient, but eating them too often was a problem for both my health and my weight. It wasn't just the foods I was eating, because they were only a visible symptom of the real underlying problem. I had to figure out the reasons why I reached for junky foods so often.

Part of the reason I was eating poorly was that most of my days were jam-packed with activities. Invariably, I ended up feeling stressed out after trying to cram 25 hours worth of activities into the mere 24 hours available. I felt tangled up and bogged down with responsibilities, which can leave anyone frazzled and exhausted. Being the boss, the mom, the teacher, the breadwinner, or however many "hats" must be worn each day can be overwhelming. Many times I would arrive home after a long day with my physical and emotional energy level so low, all I could manage was to inhale some comforting and fattening dinner and then plop onto the couch. Relaxing and eating something fattening was my "reward" for working hard all day.

To have the time and energy to take control of my health and weight loss, in addition to all the usual activities that filled each day, I had to make some changes. First, I had to learn to prioritize all my daily activities. Which ones were really necessary? Which ones did I value or enjoy? These kinds of activities were kept as top priority. On the other hand, there were plenty of low-priority activities I could happily "dropkick" out of my schedule. If I squandered my time and energy on unimportant things, the things that were really important, like meeting my goals for health and weight loss, could never get done. As I reorganized my daily activities, I realized some things were out of my control, but one of the things that I COULD control was what types of food and how much of it I ate each day. Remember, the way you personally spend your time, day after day is your real life ... the only one you've got!

"If I squandered my time and energy on unimportant things, the things that were really important, like meeting my goals for health and weight loss, could never get done."

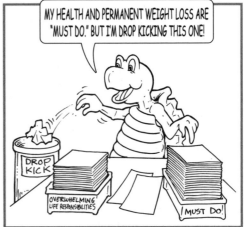

3

A JOURNEY OF A 1000 MILES BEGINS WITH A SINGLE BAD HABIT

A wise person once said: "A journey of a thousand miles begins with a single step." I've changed the saying somewhat for the title of this section. It now indicates that a good first step toward successful weight loss is to identify a poor health habit, and then develop a strategy to change it into a good health habit. Losing a significant amount of weight is a big task, much like a journey of a thousand miles or moving a mountain.

If your job was to move a mountain, how would you best approach the challenge? You might begin by thinking very hard about trying to move it all at once. This approach would, of course, be doomed to failure as mountains are simply too large. You might, instead, look at that big mountain to be moved, decide that the job is entirely too difficult, and give up.

Although either of these approaches will fail, they are the courses of action many people choose when faced with a huge challenge. The third possibility, and your best option for success, is to approach the overwhelming task of moving the mountain by breaking it down into smaller, more manageable chunks. You might, for example, first get some good help and develop some knowledge about how best to approach the job with the right techniques and equipment. With the right people and tools, you could begin moving that mountain of dirt, one shovelful at a time. In this way, over a period of time, the mountain can be moved.

> Change very rarely happens all at once in our lives. In reality, big, sweeping changes happen as a result of a whole series of small but consistent steps, and small changes for the better happen when we develop good habits.

What is a habit anyway? My definition of a habit is a behavior you repeat so often that it becomes second nature and is done without conscious thought. Many times a behavior starts off being difficult and feeling "weird," but becomes easier and feels more natural with time and repetition. I promise that you can learn to replace bad habits with good ones, and those new habits will come to feel as easy and natural as the bad habits once did. Good habits are also every bit as easy to practice on a daily basis. You can begin to nurture behaviors that will allow you to succeed! You will get to the point where you feel good about making healthy decisions without even thinking about them. You will feel more powerful and self-confident ... and in control of your life and your destiny.

Throughout this book I'll give examples of specific poor habits that should be abandoned, and good habits that should replace them. Let me give you the first example right now. A bad habit many overweight people have is waiting to eat until they are far too hungry. It is virtually impossible to eat sensibly when you are starving! When you start to feel ravenous, it is astounding how fast you can eat a thousand fat-filled calories without stopping to look up. I know because I have done it!

How could this bad habit be changed fairly painlessly? How about taking some food with you when you leave the house? Throw some almonds, a barbecued chicken breast sandwich, an apple, or maybe even your entire food supply for the day into your purse, your briefcase, or a little cooler you take in the car.

This way you'll always be prepared when hunger strikes. What if you did this every day, knew exactly what you were going to take with you, and you got to the point that it became a habit? If you can consistently pack a lunch (pretty easy, really!), you will have formed a very good new habit that will prevent you from becoming out-of-control hungry ever again. Think about it, if you leave the house with no food and no clear idea of where you're going to get your next meal, that next meal will likely be a double cheeseburger with fries! If you leave the house with some healthy food that's easy to pack, easy to eat, and is something you really enjoy, you will be less likely to make poor food choices. This one simple new habit will start you on the road to successful weight loss.

It's a big project to change habits so deeply ingrained, and you may find that some are more difficult to tackle than others. What does it take to change a poor health habit into a good one? The answer is commitment and time. It's been said that it takes twenty-one days to change a behavior. I think this is probably true if you've had your old behavior for about twenty-one days! But I'm talking about eating and exercise habits you may have had for 10, 20, or even 30 years! But I'll bet by the time you pack a lunch for yourself every day for six months it will feel easy and natural. You'll likely never go back to grabbing a fast food lunch because you're ravenously hungry. In six months packing a lunch will have become a new and improved habit!

By chipping away at bad habits, one at a time, you'll soon see a noticeable difference in your life. While your present behaviors may be familiar and comfortable, they are preventing you from living the healthy life you desire. If you make the commitment to begin your "journey of a thousand miles," and do it one step at a time, you will succeed.

Changing Habits Is The Key To Success!

GOING PUBLIC

If you've made the commitment to improve your health and achieve permanent weight loss, and you want it bad enough to make the effort to learn new habits, it's time to "go public." Telling other people about your commitment to change your life and begin the Tortoise Diet may be a little scary. After all, you may have repeated that yo-yo cycle of losing some weight before, only to gain it back again. This time, though, it's different. You're not on a "diet" in the normal sense of the word. You are committing to a slow and steady process of working hard to change your life by developing new health habits. This is not an overnight process. Because it's going to take awhile, you'll need some help and support from the people who care about you and want you to succeed.

Making yourself accountable to someone else will greatly increase the chances that you will follow through with your commitments. When we make appointments to exercise with friends, for example, we feel obligated to show up so they won't be left stranded and alone. If we tell our friends and family that we're changing our eating habits to focus on eating healthy foods for long term health and weight loss, they may help us reach that goal. My favorite example of this in my own life is a friend who bought me a Christmas gift. The gift was a set of four candles, each smelling like a wonderful dessert! He knew I had been working very hard to lose weight, so he didn't want to bring me candy and have me ruin everything that I'd worked so hard to achieve. HOW SWEET! The only way he could give me this support and encouragement was because I had "gone public" with my plans for changing my life. His gift made me feel great! I felt really motivated to continue in my efforts because, after all, he was rooting for me. That's better than candy any day!

"Making yourself accountable to someone else
will greatly increase the chances that you
will follow through with your
commitments."

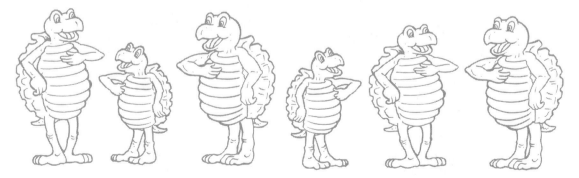

CHAPTER TWO
GOOD FOODS AND NOT SO GOOD FOODS

LEARNING THE BASICS OF HEALTHY NUTRITION

Nutrition is a large and complicated science. Because there are so many "experts" out there, each with their own nutritional theories, navigating your way through this huge maze of confusing, sometimes contradictory nutritional information can be difficult. To make it easier, we're going to focus on learning which foods provide the high-quality energy our bodies require. Let's start with the basics - protein, carbohydrates, and fats. Each of these nutrient groups is essential, performing critical functions in the body. Similar to a high-performance automobile, however, the proper mixture of the highest-quality fuel will keep your "engine" purring along at top efficiency, while poor quality fuel may cause a "breakdown."

MORE BANG FOR YOUR CALORIE BUCK

The combination of protein, carbohydrates, and fat you put into your body can be either nutrient-dense or calorie-dense. Foods are considered nutrient-dense if they pack a lot of nutrition into a relatively small amount of calories. That's a good thing for anyone who wants to lose weight. On the other hand, calorie-dense foods pack a lot of calories into a relatively small amount of food. You guessed it ... that's not such a good thing. These foods contribute less to good health and nutrition and more to expanding your waistline. Calorie-dense foods should be enjoyed sparingly, while nutrient-dense foods should be enjoyed liberally every day.

The real beauty of eating foods that are nutrient dense, like vegetables, fruits, whole-grains and legumes, is you can pile food high on your plate, eat until you feel satisfied, and still not have eaten too many calories. For example, did you know that an entire cantaloupe contains only 120 calories? If you decided to eat a whole cantaloupe, a very nutrient-dense food filled with vitamins and disease-preventing phytonutrients, and you gave your stomach ten or twenty minutes to tell your brain that some good food had arrived, you would probably feel full. Don't worry, you'll be able to eat much more than just a cantaloupe on the Tortoise Diet! But I hope the point is clear, that the fiber, water and nutrition from such a food helps you feel full.

FOR THE SAME CALORIES I'LL TAKE THIS MEAL!

For that same 120 calories, you could enjoy only a very small portion of foods like cinnamon rolls, candy bars, cakes, or a steak ... certainly not nearly enough to provide you much in the way of either satisfaction or nutrition. We eat these foods because they taste rich and good, usually because they are high in fat and/or sugar. The problem is they can really pack the excess pounds on our frames. By eating too many calorie-dense foods, far too many calories will be taken in before you feel full and satisfied. These types of foods are best reserved for the small, tasty "bites" that we savor and enjoy, but do not subsist on every day.

All foods contain calories, and they do count, but there's no need to feel hungry all the time. The healthy eating habits I have learned, and are taught in the Tortoise Diet, are those that must be maintained for a lifetime. You won't be asked to "starve," and none of the calorie-dense foods you enjoy are considered off limits. You will, however, be encouraged to include more nutrient-dense foods in your daily meals. Maybe you don't venture into the produce section of your grocery store too often, but I will guarantee that the person who successfully loses weight and keeps it off spends a lot of time there. You may be surprised at how good these healthy foods will taste, once you've given them a chance. I never used to like things like broccoli, Brussels sprouts, squash, lentils, or even oatmeal. Now they are the foods that keep me going with lots of energy and keep me zipping up my small-sized jeans!

THE SIMPLE AND THE COMPLEX, THE STORY OF CARBS

Many "fad" diets promote the idea that carbohydrate foods are bad for us, and are to blame for us being fat. So, are they good or are they bad? The answer is that they are not only good, but they are absolutely necessary for successful and permanent weight loss.

What exactly are "carbs", and what do they do? Carbohydrates provide four calories per gram. They provide glucose, which is the essential fuel that the body prefers and continuously requires. These foods also contain many vitamins, minerals and phytonutrients that contribute to good health and disease prevention.

Naturally occurring simple carbohydrates, those found in foods like milk, fruit, honey, molasses, beets and cane, are easily digested and broken down into glucose. Complex carbohydrate foods contain longer chains of glucose molecules, which are then bundled up in a fiber and water "package." Digestion of these foods is much slower because the links in the chain, as well as the package itself, must first be broken apart before the glucose can be used. When eaten in their whole-foods form, with as little refining and processing as possible, the fiber these complex carbohydrate foods contain is the dieter's friend. For this reason, eating complex carbohydrate foods that contain fiber is an integral part of the Tortoise Diet.

> **Fiber is beneficial for the following reasons:**
> **1.** It causes digestion to be slowed, so blood sugar levels remain stable. This keeps fuel for the brain and other tissues of the body available for a longer period of time. Because of this, the calories are used up for fuel and are not stored as fat.
> **2.** Bulk is added to the stomach contents. This increases the sensation of "fullness," so overeating is less likely.
> **3.** Fiber continues to absorb water in the bowel, which keeps us feeling full even longer.
> **4.** The absorption of water also helps keep the bowels functioning better so there is less time for toxins to remain in the body. This helps to prevent constipation, hemorrhoids and diverticulitis, and may also be a key to lowering the risk of colon cancer.
> **5.** Soluble fiber, found in oatmeal, apple peel, oranges, carrots and legumes, binds with the bad (LDL) cholesterol in the body, helping to decrease the risk of cardiac disease.

If fiber is the dieter's friend, refined sugars and flours should be considered the dieter's foe. White sugar and white flour are the carbohydrates found most often in packaged and/or baked goods. Because they are so highly processed, they no longer contain the fiber and nutrition they started with. Because of this, they are digested almost immediately, causing a large amount of glucose to be quickly dumped into the bloodstream. Glucose is your body's primary fuel, so you might

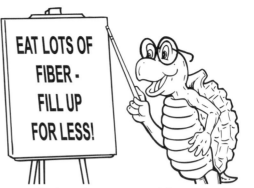

think that getting a full tank would be good. For weight loss, however, it is the worst thing you can do. When glucose enters your bloodstream quickly, blood sugar levels rise sharply. Because not all of that excess flood of energy can be used up for the body's current needs, some of it will likely be stored as fat. After that, when the blood sugar plummets, you'll soon feel hungry again and it's likely you'll eat more sugar and white flour! Obviously, this is a vicious cycle that many people struggling with their weight repeat over and over.

When you begin to look at nutritional labels on packaged foods, you may be surprised to learn just how much sugar we ingest each day. The most familiar name for white sugar is Sucrose (table sugar), but you'll also find it listed on labels as Dextrose, Malto-dextrose, High-fructose Corn Syrup, Corn Syrup, Fructose and Evaporated Cane Syrup. The ingredients listed on the contents label are placed in order from the greatest amount to the least amount, so if you must select packaged foods containing simple/refined carbohydrates, make sure that they appear toward the bottom of the ingredient list.

Refined white flour acts in a manner very similar to refined sugar, dumping glucose into the bloodstream too quickly. In addition, foods containing sugar and refined flour usually contain a lot of fat. The calorie totals of these foods can add up quickly and any excess will likely end up in the fat "storage warehouse" you wear on your hips and tummy.

In contrast to the surge of glucose entering the bloodstream after eating refined sugars and flour, foods containing complex carbohydrates, when eaten in their whole-foods form, release glucose into the bloodstream in more of a slow-drip fashion. When this happens, blood sugar levels remain fairly constant so both excessive hunger and fat storage are avoided. Look for the first item on the ingredient list of any packaged foods to be "whole" grain or "bran." If it is, you'll be in good shape. Fresh or frozen vegetables and fruits are also sources of complex carbohydrates that are very good for you. On the other hand, processed fruits, like juices and purees will not be as good at keeping you full, because their fiber content has been removed.

Eating grains, vegetables, fruits, and legumes in their whole-foods form, with as little processing and refining as possible, will fuel your body with quality nutrition and long-lasting energy, as well as help to prevent disease, and keep you feeling full. The Tortoise Diet recommends that approximately 55 percent of your daily calorie total should come from healthy, complex carbohydrate foods, eaten primarily in their whole-foods form. Except for rare treats, refined carbohydrates such as sugars and white flour should be avoided.

THE GLYCEMIC INDEX NUMBER

The Glycemic Index Number is simply one indicator of how quickly a carbohydrate food will be digested and broken down into glucose. The highest glycemic level on the scale is 100, which is the number assigned to pure glucose, since it requires no time at all for digestion and absorption into the bloodstream. Other foods are given index numbers based on how quickly they are absorbed, when compared to pure glucose. Remember, the more rapidly glucose enters the bloodstream, the more blood sugar spikes and then falls, leading to fat storage and hunger.

If this one indicator were the only thing taken into consideration, then the higher the glycemic number, the faster the rise in blood sugar, and the worse the food would be for you. There is much more to be considered however, than simply the glycemic number of any given food. My favorite example is the comparison of carrots and salami. Carrots are a perfectly healthy food that contain a whole host of essential vitamins, minerals, phytonutrients and fiber. Carrots contribute wonderfully to weight loss efforts at a mere 30 calories each, but rank a fairly poor "48" on the glycemic scale. On the other hand, salami, a food that provides very little in the way of vitamins, minerals, phytonutrients or fiber, but does contain plenty of artery-clogging saturated fat, ranks at zero!

My advice is to not worry about the glycemic rating of complex carbohydrate foods, when eaten in their whole-foods form. The way to counteract the effects of any healthy food that ranks high on the glycemic scale is to simply slow down their absorption. This is easily accomplished by making it a habit to always consume carbohydrate foods along with foods containing protein. My advice is to eat lots of carrots ... but eat them with a few almonds, or with a part-skim mozzarella stick!

"My advice is to not worry about the glycemic rating of complex carbohydrate foods, when eaten in their whole-foods form."

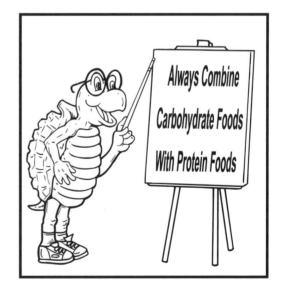

FAT ... WHAT IS IT GOOD FOR?

Fat is the most calorie-dense nutrient, yielding nine calories per gram. Obviously, one good reason to limit fat intake is simply because a high-fat diet will most likely also be a high-calorie diet. In defense of fat, a certain amount is necessary in a healthy diet just as are protein and carbohydrates. Fats circulating in the bloodstream act to transport fat-soluble vitamins (like A, E, and D) and allow the cells to absorb those vitamins. They are also necessary to help form and maintain cellular walls, and they provide the building blocks for various hormones and other necessary compounds. In the stomach, dietary fats allow the contents to empty more slowly so we can feel full for a longer time. Like it or not, a small amount of stored body fat is also necessary for our survival. This stored fat tissue protects organs, and insulates the body to maintain a constant temperature.

It's important to note that there are different types of dietary fat. While similar in terms of calories and potential fat storage, their impact on our health may be vastly different and some types are definitely better for maintaining good health than others.

Saturated fats are found in all animal-origin protein foods, like meats, eggs, butter, milk, cheese, and cream. They can also be found in a few plant foods, such as coconut and palm oil. This type of fat, in excessive quantities, is not good for your health because it raises the sticky LDL cholesterol (the bad one) and increases your risk for heart disease, cancer and stroke. Eating foods containing saturated fats should be kept to a minimum in a healthy diet. Red meat is higher in saturated fat than white meats, such as chicken, turkey and pork. For this reason, the Tortoise Diet recommends limiting red meat to a maximum of two servings per week. Regular milk products are also high in saturated fat, so a healthier and also a lower calorie alternative is to replace these with low-fat or non-fat dairy products.

Hydrogenated or Partially Hydrogenated fats (known as "Trans-Fats") are the Frankensteins of the fat world. They are liquid fats (oils), which have been chemically altered in order to become solid or semi-solid. Margarine and shortening are two obvious examples. These fats are also lurking in many packaged foods because they help to flavor and preserve foods, and extend shelf life. They pack a double bad-health whammy by increasing bad (LDL) cholesterol while at the same time decreasing the levels of good (HDL) cholesterol. After 2006, new laws will require food manufacturers to specifically list the trans-fat content of foods on the nutrient label. Until that time, read the ingredient lists and try to select foods that either do not contain hydrogenated or partially-hydrogenated oils, or foods in which these fats appear very low on the list of ingredients.

Mono-unsaturated fats are the healthy fats found in nuts, and also vegetables that produce oils, like avocados and olives. Olive oil and canola oil are good examples of mono-unsaturated oils. They are considered beneficial because they help lower cholesterol levels and protect the heart against disease. Another type of mono-unsaturated fat is the Omega 3 fat, found in oily fish such as salmon, and also in flaxseed. These have been shown to decrease the risk of cardiac problems and may also fight cancer cell growth. Polyunsaturated fats, like safflower, sunflower and corn oil, also help to lower blood cholesterol, and may be considered to be good fats, as well. All of these types of heart-healthy fats are recommended for good health. Like mono-unsaturated fats, plant sterol esters, found in the new no-trans fat "buttery" spreads are "good" fats. A good example of this is Smart Balance spread. The compounds in

Smart Balance have been found to help reduce LDL cholesterol by blocking the absorption of cholesterol from the digestive tract. They are made with naturally occurring substances found in plants, which are then combined with canola oil. * *Check with your doctor if you are on medications or are being treated for cholesterol management.* *

The American Heart Association recommends that the total fat intake in our diets should be limited to less than 30 percent of the daily calorie total. They further state that 20-25 percent total fat, (including a maximum of 10 percent in the form of saturated fats) is an even healthier goal. For good health, and for weight loss, the Tortoise Diet recommends limiting fat intake to 20 percent of the total daily calorie intake. The emphasis should be on consuming primarily mono-unsaturated fats. Trans-fats should be eliminated.

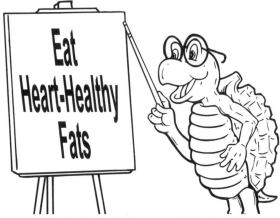

PROTEIN POWER

Protein is part of the structure of every cell in the body. It is essential for building new tissue as well as for making repairs in those tissues. It transports essential substances throughout the blood, contributes to the building blocks of blood, hormones, and bodily fluids, and ensures a strong immune system.

When protein-rich foods are digested, they are broken down into compounds called amino acids. There are twenty-two types of amino acids, eight of which can only be obtained from the foods we eat. Animal-origin protein foods like eggs, meat, milk products, and fish contain all eight of these essential amino acids, and are known as complete proteins. Plant based foods, such as grains, legumes, and vegetables provide some of these essential amino acids, but not all eight of them. Because they provide incomplete proteins, taking in a wide variety of these foods is important in order to get all of the essential amino acids our bodies need. There is one significant exception. Soybeans are not animal in origin, but they do contain all eight of the essential amino acids. Drinking soymilk or eating other soy products, such as tofu, tempeh, or edamame will substitute nicely for meat, egg, or dairy products.

Protein is also a source of energy, providing four calories per gram just as carbohydrates do. The Tortoise Diet emphasizes lean, skinless white meats, fish, legumes, soy and non-fat dairy as main sources of protein. Also, many complex carbohydrate foods contain small amounts of protein, so eating a wide variety of foods will ensure your protein needs are met.

Protein foods can be broken down into glucose for energy if there is a shortage of carbohydrates. This is problematic, however, because if protein is used for energy it cannot accomplish its other essential duties. Since the body prefers carbohydrates for energy, there is really no need to consume excessive amounts of protein unless the body is in a growth phase (i.e. growing children, during pregnancy, people recovering from severe illness or malnourishment, or for individuals who are purposely trying to build additional muscle tissue).

The Tortoise Diet recommends that approximately 25 percent of your total daily calorie intake be comprised of protein. While not being excessive, this is a fairly high protein amount, but this amount is necessary to help prevent excessive loss of muscle tissue during weight loss. If a very high-protein diet (intake of more than 30 percent of the daily diet) is followed, but calories are limited as is common in low-carb diets, the body will compensate for the lack of carbohydrate energy by performing all kinds of complicated physiologic maneuvers to make the glucose that it requires for fuel. By utilizing these alternate pathways to make energy, the body can continue with its various functions. The problem is, the extra work required to make fuel out of alternate energy sources is taxing to the body and may eventually lead to long-term health consequences. A diet containing high quantities of protein foods will probably also fall short in providing the essential vitamins, minerals, phytonutrients and fiber that carbohydrate foods provide, possibly leading to even further health problems.

VITAMINS AND MINERALS

Small quantities of a wide variety of vitamins, minerals, and other nutrients are required each day to keep our bodies functioning properly. These substances assist with many processes in the body. Many people believe that the vitamin and mineral content even in a healthy, whole-foods diet may be lower than it should be, related to changes in the way food is grown, harvested, and stored in our modern world. For this reason, the recommended daily allowance (RDA), which is the amount of vitamins and minerals required for good health, may actually be difficult to obtain from our food alone. The Tortoise Diet recommends that adults should supplement a healthy diet by taking one complete good quality multivitamin/mineral pill or capsule each day. Also recommended is daily supplementation of up to 1000 mg of Vitamin C and 400 mg of Vitamin E for their powerful anti-oxidant effect. To protect against osteoporosis (especially for women), additional supplementation of 1,000 to 1,200 mg of Calcium is beneficial.
** Please check with your doctor regarding their recommendations, especially if you are on medication or are being treated for any medical condition. **

In addition to eating a healthy, whole-foods diet, these supplements are an easy and fairly inexpensive way to help ensure an adequate intake of the many small compounds your body needs to continue at top efficiency. There are, of course, literally hundreds of additional compounds found in health food stores that may, or may not, improve your health. My advice is to not get caught up in spending a whole bunch of money on herbs, powders, pills and potions. Many of the dietary aids that get a lot of press have not been studied long enough for you to entrust your health to them. Just because they're for sale on the supermarket shelf doesn't mean they are good for you. Some of them may be helpful, but in many cases we just don't know yet.

Taking the recommended supplements and improving the nutritional value of the foods you eat will do wonders for your health. Eating a wide variety of nutrient-dense foods is the most important step. Vitamin supplementation, alone, will never ensure that you reach your goals.

YOUR MOTHER WAS RIGHT

There is a revolution occurring in the science of nutrition. Scientists are discovering thousands of compounds found in plant-origin foods, called phytonutrients, which play very important roles in keeping us healthy and preventing major disease. These compounds seem to be able to boost immunity to cancer and other serious diseases, and they can be found only in plant-origin foods. Your mother had no idea how right she was by insisting that you eat your vegetables! If you load up your plate with meat and skimp on vegetables, fruits, legumes, nuts and soy in your diet, you're increasing your chances for developing health problems. Eating a wide variety of phytonutrient-rich foods is a very good insurance policy! Scientists don't yet fully understand all the functions of phytonutrients. What they do know is there are more of these compounds that have not yet been identified, and their role in preventing disease could turn out to be extremely important.

The cost of buying fresh vegetables and fruits on a regular basis may seem to be a little higher than some other foods, but they are a bargain compared to the high costs of treating disease. In my own life, when I heard that I had some pre-cancerous cells, I began to pay a lot of attention to the research I was reading about phytonutrients and cancer prevention. Sure enough, after losing a significant amount of weight and eating lots of fruits and vegetables, when I returned for a follow-up visit to my doctor, there was no longer any evidence of the pre-cancerous cells in my system. That was enough to convince me to keep going with my new healthy eating plan.

Antioxidants and biofavinoids/isoflavones are two of the better known and understood phytonutrients. Antioxidants fight oxidation that causes the cellular damage believed to be the most probable cause of accelerated aging in our bodies. Powerful antioxidants, like Vitamin C and Vitamin E, as well as Magnesium, Copper and Zinc, are contained in brightly colored fruits and vegetables. Bioflavinoids and Isoflavones are compounds found in the highest amounts in SOY products. They are beneficial for lowering the risk of heart disease and may also play an important role in decreasing the risk of estrogen-sensitive cancers of the breast, uterus and prostate by binding with estrogen receptors, with the added plus of lessening pre-menstrual and menopausal discomforts. There is also evidence that eating soy-based foods may also help to lower the levels of LDL cholesterol.
* * Check with your doctor about eating soy products if you have a personal or a family history of breast or prostate cancer. * *

Scientists are discovering more and more amazing phytonutrients every day. There is no pill to take, not even a super multivitamin can begin to cover them all. The best way to protect yourself against aging, cancer and a multitude of other health problems is to "eat" these phytonutrients, especially in their whole-foods form, without overcooking them. Nutrients are always best preserved when foods are eaten either raw or only lightly cooked. It seems that the most brightly colored vegetables and fruits are the richest sources of phytonutrients, so it's also important to eat as many different colored foods as you possibly can. The following is a color-coded list of vegetables and fruits, and the phytonutrients that they are known to provide.

COLOR   FOODS TO EAT   PHYTONUTRIENTS

COLOR	FOODS TO EAT	PHYTONUTRIENTS
RED	Tomatoes Pink Grapefruit Watermelon	**Lycopene** May protect against lung and prostate cancers.
ORANGE	Carrots Cantaloupe Squash	**Alpha and Beta Carotenes** May play a role in preventing cancers of the lung, stomach and esophagus. Important for eye health.
YELLOW / ORANGE	Citrus fruits	**Flavanoids** Play an important role in cancer prevention.
GREEN	All varieties of leafy greens Cabbage Avocado Broccoli Brussels Sprouts	**Lutein** Protects against cardiovascular disease, stroke, macular degeneration and cancer.
WHITE / GREEN	Garlic Onions	**Sulfides** May help prevent cancer in the stomach and gastro-intestinal tract.
BLUE / PURPLE	Grapes and Red Wine Blueberries Strawberries Blackberries	**Anthocyanins** May prevent formation of blood clots. May help to prevent Alzheimer's.

You may have heard that it's important to eat seven to ten servings of fruits and vegetables a day. For maximum nutrition, good health and weight loss, you should also make it a practice to eat as many different "colors" of foods as possible each day. It's easy, really, to develop this habit. In fact, if you did absolutely nothing else except to get into the habit of eating the following foods each day, not only would you take in a minimum of seven servings of colorful fruits and vegetables, you would also meet your goal for including healthy fiber in your diet, and you would certainly lose some weight!

THE DAILY SEVEN FOR SUCCESS

1. Eat an apple and an orange every day.

2. Eat one serving of whole oats every day, such as a bowl of oatmeal or a healthy muffin.

3. Eat a bowl of healthy broth-based (not cream-based) soup, filled with vegetables and legumes every weekday: Minestrone, Split Pea, Lentil, Turkey vegetable, White Bean, Vegetable beef, Chicken noodle, and Turkey Chili are good choices.

4. Each day at dinner, begin the meal by eating a big green salad, dressed either with balsamic vinegar, or a small amount of extra virgin olive oil and vinegar or lemon, or a small amount of low-fat salad dressing. Top the salad with cut up tomatoes, cucumbers, onion, carrots, or other low-calorie vegetables.

5. Eat at least one serving of vegetables at dinner.

6. Eat two servings of whole-grain breads, whole-grain pastas, or brown rice daily.

7. Include a serving of fruit as your after-dinner snack.

"In fact, if you did absolutely nothing else except to get into the habit of eating the following foods each day, not only would you take in a minimum of seven servings of colorful fruits and vegetables, you would also meet your goal for including healthy fiber in your diet, and you would certainly lose some weight!"

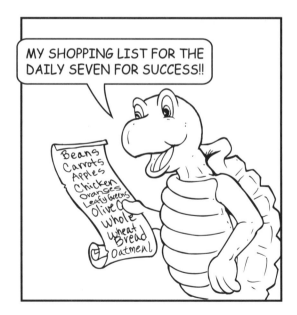

SPY BEFORE YOU BUY

We have learned that it's desirable for both health and weight loss to eat nutrient-dense foods in their whole-foods form with as little refining and processing as possible. Realistically, though, packaged foods will most likely continue to be a part of life. In order to make good decisions about which foods to eat and how large a portion to eat, it's important to know how to read the nutritional labels located on the packaging of prepared foods. These food labels provide information about the size of each serving, the number of servings the package contains, the calories and grams of fat per serving, as well as other important nutritional information.

Keep in mind that the nutritional breakdown given is for EACH SERVING contained in the package. Some labels are quite misleading. A package that looks pretty small may seem, at first glance, to be a reasonable 200 calories. Upon closer inspection, however, you learn the package actually contains four tiny little servings! If you were to eat the entire amount, you would actually be taking in 800 calories, and the associated grams of fat and sugar listed on the label would also be multiplied by four. Yikes! A big percentage of your day's calorie allotment would be blown!

As an example, you might consider the choice of a healthy, high-fiber bowl of cereal with some non-fat milk to be a quick and nutritious breakfast. By reading the nutritional label on the side of the cereal box, you may find that one serving contains only 110 calories, two grams of fat, and a reasonable five grams of sugar. So far so good, right? Then you read further and find that the 110 calorie serving size of the cereal is only half a cup! How many half-cup servings will your cereal bowl hold? My husband, Charlie, who loves cereal, used to pour it into a mixing bowl and eat it with a big soup spoon before I finally got him to realize he wasn't going to lose any weight if he continued to eat his "little breakfast" of 700 calories! After the initial shock, he decided maybe he should cut down on his portion size. Now, instead of a big bowl full, he eats a more reasonable portion by sprinkling a small serving of the cereal he loves on top of a bowl of fresh fruit topped with non-fat yogurt and drizzled with sugar-free maple syrup. Mmm ... an enjoyable treat that is now filling and much more nutrient-dense.

To make the best use of the information provided on nutritional labels, you must know what your own needs are for both total calories and fat grams each day. For weight loss and general good health, you should be aiming for a maximum of 20 percent of your daily calories to come from fat. Multiplying your total daily calorie allotment by 0.20 will give you the total number of calories per day that should come from fat. Now take that number and divide it by nine, since there are nine calories in each gram of dietary fat. This result will give you the number of fat grams you should be eating each day, to stay within your fat allotment. As an example, let's say you are allowed 1,800 calories per day. Multiplying 1,800 by 0.20 results in 360, which would be your daily fat calorie allotment. Dividing 360 by nine means you should be striving to eat a maximum of 40 grams of fat per day.

Dietary labels also break down fat grams into saturated and unsaturated fat. Certainly, limiting intake of saturated fats and hydrogenated (e.g. trans-fats) to the barest minimum is critical to good health, so always think twice about eating any packaged foods containing a high percentage of those unhealthy fats. A good rule of thumb to follow when evaluating labels is to choose products with unsaturated fat, and limit that fat to a maximum of five grams per serving.

Other important information contained on the nutritional label is the number of grams of fiber and the number of grams of sugar. You will note that fiber may be identified on the label as being either "soluble" or "insoluble." Both kinds are good! Sugar, on the other hand, is a refined carbohydrate that will quickly be stored as fat if eaten in excess. You will see sugar listed in many of its various forms as you "spy before you buy."

Remember when looking at nutritional labels to keep in mind that the higher something appears on the ingredient list, the more of that ingredient the food contains. I recommend that you avoid buying products with high-fructose corn syrup appearing near the top of the list. Some experts believe this form of sugar, added to many foods, may be one of the biggest culprits behind the widespread increase in obesity. Also remember, all sugary foods are very calorie dense and should be limited. But I don't advise you to go "cold turkey" and cut sugar out of your life all at once. A good start might be to make an effort to cut down on your sugar intake by simply becoming aware of where it's hidden in the foods you typically eat. If the foods you purchase do contain sugar, aim for a maximum of 15 grams per serving and try to make sure that it appears toward the end of the ingredient list on the label.

Packaged foods have typically been notoriously high in many of the things we should try to avoid, like sugar, saturated fat, trans-fats, processed white flour, preservatives and salt. Fortunately, more companies are now making genuinely healthy packaged foods, but studying nutritional labels carefully is essential to distinguish the healthy products from the pretenders. The pretenders will make their products sound really healthy, but a closer examination of the nutritional contents may reveal something quite to the contrary. It's easy to be fooled, for example, by labels that say "98 percent fat free." That sounds good, but if the total number of fat grams per serving is still high, and if high-fructose corn syrup and/or excess salt has been added to bump up the flavor because fat has been removed, that food won't be the healthiest choice. As I have said, and will say many more times throughout this book, whole, colorful, fresh foods are always the best choice for health and weight loss. Start slow and make small changes that work for you. Change one habit at a time ... like maybe using a smaller cereal bowl!

"I recommend that you avoid buying products with high-fructose corn syrup appearing near the top of the list. Some experts believe this form of sugar, added to many foods, may be one of the biggest culprits behind the widespread increase in obesity."

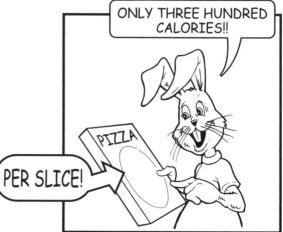

ONLY THREE HUNDRED CALORIES!!

PIZZA

PER SLICE!

A LITTLE DAB WILL DO YA

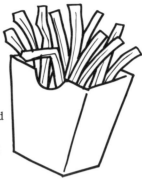

We love salt because it brings out the flavor in food. Unfortunately, we've acquired quite a taste for excessive amounts of it. Many of us shake it liberally onto our food each day. Chips, fries, and most restaurant meals contain very high amounts of it. Salt, just like sugar, is also a major hidden ingredient in almost every packaged food. With this onslaught, it's no wonder most of us go way over the recommended maximum salt intake of about 1,500 mg per day for an adult. Try reading some nutritional labels to see what the salt content per serving is in many common packaged foods, and prepare to be shocked.

So what's the problem? Why is excessive salt intake something to be concerned about? The answer is that it's not good for losing weight and it's not good for your health! The health problem stems from the fact that our bodies require a pretty exact concentration of salt, known by its chemical name of sodium. There are sensitive regulating mechanisms that will work hard to keep the concentration of sodium in the bloodstream just right. Whenever too much sodium enters the bloodstream, the body's first response is to hold on to as much water as possible so the concentration of sodium in the blood can be diluted to the proper level. Unfortunately, when the volume of fluid in the bloodstream is increased, blood pressure is raised, so chronic intake of excess sodium and the fluid retention that accompanies it places excess demands on the heart and kidneys. In fact, many doctors treat patients with heart and kidney problems by prescribing a low sodium diet, along with blood pressure medications that function by releasing excess water from the body.

Some of you may think that it's not possible to enjoy food without added salt. However. as you become more accustomed to eating fresh and healthy foods contained in the Healthy Foods List (Appendix B) in their whole-foods form, and you practice cooking them at home using herbs, fruit juices, salsas, peppers and spices to jazz up the foods, you'll soon come to enjoy the taste of foods without so much salt. Fresh fish, for example, right off the barbecue, topped with some yummy Mango Salsa (Recipe in Appendix C) will be bursting with flavor and color.

There can also be problems if too little sodium is taken in, but that's a pretty rare occurrence for most healthy individuals. Ingesting supplemental sodium and other electrolytes in the form of specially formulated drinks and other products is usually not necessary. Unless you are involved in competitive sports or you sweat buckets during your two to four hour workouts, you're probably safe simply drinking water before, during, and after your workout to replace the lost fluid.

In any discussion of sodium we must also talk about water. After a salty meal or snack, it's natural to feel thirsty. By drinking fluid, the concentration of sodium in the bloodstream can be diluted to the proper level. In the meantime, however, the body will hold onto as much water as possible. Why is this important if you're trying to lose weight? The reason is that one gallon of water equals 128 ounces, which is exactly eight pounds! If just 16 ounces of excess water is retained after eating too much salt, which is entirely possible, the scale is likely to register a gain of one pound, no matter how well you followed your eating and exercise plan the previous day! That could be quite discouraging, if you didn't understand the cause of this weight gain. If you are an essentially healthy individual, with no blood pressure or kidney problems, there is a simple tactic to get rid of this excess water weight following a salty meal. It sounds weird, but the answer is to drink an extra large amount of water. Your healthy kidneys can then flush out the excess sodium, making this temporary weight gain short-lived. It doesn't sound like it should make sense to drink more water to lose excess water weight, but it works!

How much water should a healthy person drink on a daily basis? Typically, at least eight glasses of water per day (64 ounces) is recommended. Actually, fluid requirements are a very individual matter, based on body size, activity level, health, age, the weather outside, and other factors. You might think that getting the right amount of water is as simple as drinking water when you feel thirsty, but it doesn't always work that way. Sometimes people don't experience thirst until they are actually quite dehydrated. Other times people may think that they are feeling "hungry" when their bodies may actually be trying to signal "thirst." Both of these problems stem from the fact that most people simply don't drink enough water.

Concerning the actual amount of water each person should drink, I recommend that you determine whether your fluid needs have been met by simply looking at your own urine (sorry, it's the nurse in me). If it is clear and light yellow in color, and if you empty your bladder several times each day, you're probably adequately hydrated. If your urine turns to a dark yellow color ... drink more water! Keep in mind that drinks containing caffeine, sugar, or alcohol do not meet your body's fluid needs as well as plain water.

ALCOHOL ... THE TRIPLE WHAMMY

Alcohol provides very little nutrition, but at approximately seven calories per gram and over 100 calories per drink, the one thing alcohol does provide is calories! From a health standpoint, it is true that small amounts of alcohol, especially red wine, are actually believed to be beneficial for cardiovascular health. Excess alcohol, however, causes a number of problems. For starters, it can raise triglyceride levels and blood pressure, which may contribute to an increased risk of coronary problems. Additionally, the way our bodies break down the alcohol we drink can also cause liver disease and malnutrition.

For those of us who want to lose weight, the way alcohol is metabolized in the body also presents a big problem. Alcohol is absorbed into the bloodstream almost immediately after it is ingested, especially if taken on an empty stomach. It is the liver's job to break down the alcohol and to detoxify the body of this foreign substance. Because it takes approximately one hour per drink to break down the alcohol, and because the liver becomes totally occupied with this task, it is not available to perform its usual digestive functions. This results in many of the calories from the foods you have eaten being transported directly to the fat storage warehouse to be stocked away for future energy needs. Excess calories from the alcohol, itself, are readily stored as fat, as well. As if that wasn't enough, there is some thought that alcohol also causes the metabolic rate to slow down. We'll be discussing this all-important metabolic rate in great detail later but, in short, it is the rate at which your body burns calories. The effect of this is to further compound the problem of fat storage.

The result of this fat storage will be evident to you for days afterward as you step on the scale, but it will also, unfortunately, be evident during your dinner with drinks. It's well known that alcohol is an appetite stimulant and a willpower destroyer. After having a drink or two before dinner, I guarantee it won't be long before you'll begin to feel pretty hungry. You'll stay feeling hungry too, because the nutrients from the food you eat can't get processed because the liver is too busy breaking down the alcohol. Throw in the fact that after drinking alcohol your self-control usually gets thrown out the window, and with the arrival of the first loaf of fresh, hot bread, you've got the makings of a problem!

Alcohol is a triple whammy for dieters because:

> **1.** It contains a lot of calories, but very little nutrition.
> **2.** It may slow down the metabolic rate and promote fat storage.
> **3.** It stimulates appetite and decreases willpower.

To make a long story short, drinking a lot of alcohol will make it very difficult to lose weight. Because the Tortoise Diet must be viewed as a sustainable way of life, if you do enjoy an alcoholic beverage once in awhile, I'm not going to tell you to give it up. I will tell you, however, that alcohol must be treated as a very high-calorie food.

COFFEE

Centuries ago, when sheepherder's somewhere in the Middle East noticed that their sheep would kick up their heels and frolic with great energy after nibbling on some hard, bright red berries, they knew they were on to something. Merchant trade routes first brought coffee to the Far East and then to the West, and the rest is history. In terms of tonnage, coffee is the most traded commodity in the world today. Millions of people around the world not only wake to a cup of coffee, but also drink it throughout the day. There is no question that we love coffee, the question is whether it should be included in a weight loss plan.

For all you coffee drinkers out there, the news is not so bad! From a health standpoint, coffee has been one of the most studied compounds there is, and in literally hundreds of tests it has been shown to be harmless, when enjoyed in moderation. Pregnant women and people with high blood pressure or other cardiovascular problems should drink decaffeinated coffee, but most other people can enjoy a few cups a day with very little chance of negative health consequences. From a weight loss standpoint, the news is mixed, depending on how you drink your coffee. Some popular diets tell you to stop drinking coffee, period. What we really need to do, however, is change our habits regarding what we regularly add to our coffee.

Although black coffee has very little nutritional value, it also contains no fat, calories or sugar. This cannot be said, though, for many of the coffee concoctions so popular today. Absolutely the worst way for you to begin your day is with a major jolt of sugar, whether you put it in your regular coffee, your latte, or your mocha. Sugar, when coupled with caffeine, will send your blood sugar skyrocketing only to come crashing down a couple hours later. This is guaranteed to leave you starving and looking for more food. Fat, on the other hand, does have a lot of calories. If you order a mocha or latte made with whole milk, or worse yet, a typical sweet blended drink, you're going to be loading up with calories from fat.

So are we all doomed to drink only plain black coffee? Of course not! If you like sweetened coffee drinks, I recommend that you experiment with adding Splenda sugar substitute to your coffee. Splenda, derived from real sugar but containing zero calories, is used to sweeten many of the sugar free flavors available at coffee shops and for home use. Sugar substitutes are not absorbed by the body, so they don't cause blood sugar to skyrocket like regular sugar does. Cutting down on fat is as simple as drinking non-fat milk instead of two-percent, whole milk or worse yet, cream. Learning to like non-fat milk is a lot easier than you'd think. If you drink whole milk now, switch to two-percent for a while before taking the step down to non-fat. If you're a two-percent drinker now, making the change to non-fat shouldn't be too tough.

Taking it one step at a time is the way to change habits. No, you may not enjoy your coffee quite as much at first, but give your new healthy habits a month. If I don't miss my guess, I think that soon you'll be drinking your non-fat, sugar free vanilla latte or sugar free mocha, and it will taste pretty good! And guess what? This is actually a healthy way to begin your day with some necessary fuel, provided by the protein and carbohydrate contained in the milk. Just don't add a six hundred calorie muffin or doughnut loaded with fat and sugar. Those have got to go! My recommendation is to be nutritionally smart, slowly develop some better habits, and enjoy your coffee.

> "What we really need to do, however, is change our habits regarding what we regularly add to our coffee."

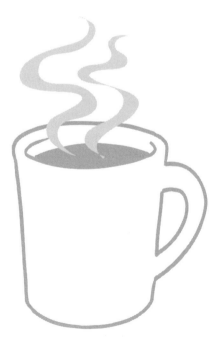

CHAPTER THREE
GETTING GOOD FOODS INTO YOUR LIFE

THE "TOP 40" LIST

To translate the knowledge of good nutrition into successful weight loss and continued healthy eating for a lifetime, it is essential to learn some techniques to fit those healthy foods into your daily life. Although the best diet is one that includes a wide variety of healthy foods, in reality we each have our favorites. Most hare-brained, quick weight loss diets demand that you eat from a limited list of acceptable foods, which may not always coincide with your own preferences. What good does it do if you are only a temporary slave following their rules? You'll drive yourself crazy and you will ultimately fail. Instead of trying to fit into somebody else's plan, the key to success is devising a personalized plan for healthy eating you can live with and enjoy for the rest of your life. Long-term improvement to your health and successful weight loss depends on your decision to eat in a way that nourishes your body with the proper amount of calories from all of the nutrient groups.

One of my secrets is something I call the "Top 40" list. I use my own "Top 40" list to create my breakfast, lunch, and snack food selections. The list helps me to create meals that are quick and easy to prepare, easy to take to work, provide good nutrition and are things I really like. I end up shopping for and preparing a lot of these same foods over and over again, and because I enjoy them, I never feel deprived. I also don't have to spend too much time standing in front of the refrigerator thinking: "What should I eat today?"

Study the menu plans in Appendix A and the Healthy Foods List in Appendix B and begin to identify your own "Top 40" list. Find foods that you like! Not feeling deprived, doomed to a life of eating only salads and plain chicken breasts, is very important to enjoying the Tortoise Diet approach to weight loss. Your "Top 40" list and your routine weekly shopping list should include:

1. Foods that you enjoy and will eat on a regular basis.
2. Foods that provide good nutrition, containing low-fat protein, complex carbohydrates and heart-healthy fats.
3. Foods that are quick and easy to prepare, and don't cost a fortune.
4. Foods that are portable and convenient for you to take along for your busy day.
5. Foods that everyone in your family will enjoy.

Appendix A provides many examples of meals containing my own "Top 40" foods. Each meal or snack contains protein as well as complex carbohydrates, and maybe a little bit of heart-healthy fat. These foods keep me feeling full and satisfied, and I really like to eat them! The more you can select foods and plan meals based on those foods found in Appendix A and Appendix B, the easier it will be to make healthy eating a lifetime habit.

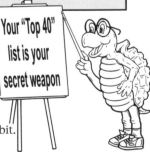

Your "Top 40" list is your secret weapon

THE FIT KITCHEN

The healthy foods you have been learning about won't just chop themselves up and jump onto your dinner plate! To live a healthy new lifestyle, you're going to have to learn some cooking skills, and spend some time in the kitchen. It can be fun to buy a bunch of exotic ingredients, spread out all over the kitchen, and whip up an elegant and complicated meal. In the real world, however, few of us have the time or inclination to exert this much energy to prepare dinner every night. Let's begin by getting the kitchen ready to begin eating in a new way.

Your goals in the kitchen should be to prepare foods that are:

> **1.** Healthy, colorful, flavorful, and as low in fat, sugar and calories as possible.
> **2.** Filling and satisfying, as nutrient-dense as possible.
> **3.** QUICK AND EASY to prepare ... 15 minutes is an achievable goal.

Since the goal is to reduce your intake of calorie-dense foods containing fat, sugar and processed white flour, any of these foods that may be hanging around your kitchen could cause problems! My suggestion is that you just bite the bullet and give away the ice cream, the chips, and anything else that will be a temptation to you. If these junky items are not in your kitchen, it will definitely be easier to avoid eating them. This may be tough for some of you, but remind yourself of those commitments you made! If you have plenty of delicious, healthy foods around, my prediction is you won't have to go hungry, and you're not going to miss the chips ... unless they're staring at you every time you open the cupboard. Once you've cleared out the junky food, you'll have room for a few of these essential kitchen tools:

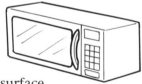

1. a microwave
2. a food processor
3. a blender
4. space in the freezer
5. a really high quality frying pan with a non-stick surface
6. a set of measuring cups and measuring spoons
7. two knives, one large and one small, both high quality and very sharp
8. a large, sturdy cutting board
9. a large selection of various sized air-tight plastic food storage containers
10. a garlic press
11. an inexpensive kitchen scale
12. a notebook or recipe cards
13. a pasta portion-measuring device
14. a really sharp (plane-style) grater
15. a book with calorie counts for various foods
16. a salad spinner
17. a can opener that doesn't leave sharp edges
18. a baking sheet with a non-stick surface
19. a hand mixer
20. non-stick muffin tins, loaf pans and silicone bake-ware
21. a no-oil popcorn popper

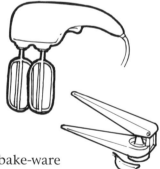

SHOPPING AND FOOD PREPARATION MADE EASY

Now that you have room in the cupboards and all of the equipment you need, it's time to fill the kitchen with delicious, healthy foods. Healthy recipes are readily available in magazines, on the Internet, in cookbooks, on television, in the newspaper, from family and friends, and also here in this book! I've heard it said that the average family pretty much eats the same seven dinners over and over. Some of those seven dinners served at your house may be the ones that have been contributing to your weight problem! To remedy that, your goal is to master a repertoire of new family favorites for dinner that are easy, quick, and healthy. Learning to prepare five to ten new healthy dinners should be an achievable goal, even for a beginner. The recipes I've included in Appendix C and those found at the Tortoise Diet Web site - www.wintheracetolose.com - are ones that have worked well in my own life. I'm a busy person and I'm definitely NOT a pro in the kitchen so believe me, if I can do it, you can too! As with anything new, becoming comfortable with shopping for and preparing healthy meals will take planning and some practice. You may want to start off by making a few core meals enough times until they become second nature and you can make them without having to think much about it. Once you've done that, you can add variety and gradually incorporate new recipes into your weekly meal plans. To streamline your time in the kitchen and make it easier, I recommend you use the following organized approach to shopping for and preparing healthy foods.

1. Evaluate your family's likes and dislikes, and search for recipes that include some of your favorite ingredients and flavors, but are lower in fat and calories.

2. Plan a weekly menu of "Top 40" breakfasts, lunches and snacks that can be eaten on the run. Write down your routine foods and their calorie counts. Put a list on the refrigerator door or in your kitchen notebook so you don't have to think too much about what to eat and how much to eat. Get familiar with the calorie counts and appropriate portion sizes of the foods you enjoy most often so you can make them without much effort or thought.

3. Plan a weekly menu of healthy recipes to prepare for dinner. Pick five to ten of these dinners that you and your family love, and get really good at putting them together quickly.

4. Read each recipe in its entirety and write down ALL of the required ingredients.

5. Take stock of your pantry and refrigerator, and make a shopping list for all necessary items that you do not already have on hand.

6. Shop once a week from your grocery list for staples and all ingredients required for the planned menus. Buy enough of the items to make several batches of the recipes you enjoy most and make most often. This way you'll always have the ingredients on hand when you need them. The other reason to use your shopping list is to prevent "unauthorized purchases." I'm referring, of course, to the not-so-good food choices that the store places prominently at eye level to tempt you. If you have a problem with potato chips, don't buy them! Just walk on by! If you have a problem with ice cream, don't buy it! Eat a healthy snack before you get to the store, arrive armed with a complete shopping list and head for the produce area first! The goal is to get home with easy to make, enjoyable healthy foods.

7. Trim and clean all produce when you bring it home from the store, and re-package it into plastic wrap or plastic containers, to be stored in the refrigerator or freezer for easy use. I call myself the Sunday Chef because my routine is to prepare food for the upcoming week every Sunday after I get home from the store. On one burner of the stove I simmer a big pot of minestrone or some other type of soup. The entire prep time for the soup is about fifteen minutes and that big batch makes plenty to last the entire week. I usually put the soup into small plastic containers and then into the freezer, so they can be placed into an insulated lunch bag in the morning to keep the rest of the food cold while thawing. All I need is a microwave sometime during the day to have a nice hot serving of healthy and delicious soup! On burner #2, I cook a week's worth of oatmeal. Once this has been cooked and cooled, I portion it into individual serving containers, sprinkle each serving with a little cinnamon, a few chopped walnuts, and some no-sugar maple syrup, and place the containers in the refrigerator. Again, all week long they are ready to grab, microwave, add milk and eat. On burner #3, I cook some brown rice and wild rice which I again portion out and place in containers into the fridge. While everything is cooking on the stove, I chop tomatoes, carrots, celery, and whatever else sounds good. I'll wrap these to be kept ready in the refrigerator for lunches and dinner salads during the week. Once a month or so I make homemade healthy muffins or bread while I have my Sunday Chef hat on. These are then individually wrapped and placed in the freezer. This time I spend in the kitchen on a Sunday saves me a lot of time during the week, and prevents me from running out of healthy food to grab for breakfasts and lunches.

8. When making family favorites, cook extra portions or double the recipe. Place individual or family-sized portions in the freezer, ready to pop into the microwave for dinner or to take along for lunch if time is short.

9. Negotiate with family members to find an enjoyable "un-dinner" that can be whipped up at a moment's notice, when you're especially tired or there is no time to cook. By this, I simply mean that dinner doesn't actually have to be "dinner" every night. One favorite of mine for these occasions is to heat up some soup and place open-faced tuna melts made with non-fat mayo and low-fat cheese under the broiler. It's nothing fancy but it's healthy, filling, and the total time spent cooking, eating and cleaning up is about fifteen minutes!

DINNER WILL BE READY IN TEN MINUTES

Organizational skills must be learned to help you accomplish the new goals you've set for yourself and the commitments you've made. It will take some practice for these skills to become habits, but if you begin by identifying the foods you like, making a weekly shopping list, and allowing time when you get home from the store to prepare food for the upcoming week, you'll be off to a great start. The daily life changes you make to regularly put healthy lunches in the bag and dinners on the table are not as difficult as you might think. For one thing, effective organization and planning will definitely save you time. You'll also save money, because you won't be tempted to go out for dinner every night because there's nothing good to eat in the refrigerator or freezer. It may sound like a lot of work at first, but trust me when I say that it will get easier with practice.

HOW LOW CAN YOU GO?

A primary tenet of nutritious eating is that foods are best when eaten closest to their natural state. Most nutritionists would recommend that we eat an apple as, simply, an apple. That's great. Apples in their natural state, unadorned, are a nutrient-dense food full of good things for the body. There will be times in life, however, when merely crunching on an apple will simply not be enough. This is why things like apple pie and apple fritters have been developed to tempt us! A steady diet of apples will contribute to a healthy and svelte existence, but a steady diet of those other more calorie-dense apple products will bring entirely different results. The happy answer to this dilemma is finding new ways to prepare our favorite foods in ways that are lower in fat and calories, but are still tasty and satisfying.

Eating good foods prepared in interesting, enjoyable, and lower-calorie ways will definitely be a part of life for anyone who desires to lose weight and live a healthy life. For this reason, it's important to spend some time experimenting with making the foods you and your family enjoy as healthy, nutritious, low calorie, low sugar, low fat, and satisfying as possible. If you can learn to do this, and still really enjoy these foods, you'll be well on your way to success. If not, it will feel too much like a "diet" for you to persevere. Remember, this is a long-term process. We're looking for a creative and happy compromise.

An important skill to develop is the ability to evaluate recipes for their calorie-dense components and come up with lower-calorie, lower-fat, lower-sugar, and higher fiber ingredients. The following are some substitutions I recommend you try when experimenting with your favorite recipes. Have fun figuring out "How Low Can You Go" with your calorie count when making your recipes.

Recipe component	Substitution
White Flour	Use half white flour and half whole-wheat flour - try to work up to 100% whole-wheat flour, but experiment, as the texture and taste will be altered.
Granulated Sugar or Brown Sugar	Try using half of the specified amount of sugar the recipe calls for, as your "taste" for sweet will be lessened as you eat a more healthy, whole-foods diet. Experiment with no-calorie sweeteners such as Splenda or Stevia (herbal). Use sugar- free maple syrup, molasses, no-sugar applesauce, fruit juices, mashed banana or other fruit.
Eggs Egg whites	Pasteurized real-egg product (like Egg Beaters, ¼ cup = 1 whole egg). Pasteurized egg whites, may use liquid or powdered.
Butter or oil	Try replacing half of specified amount of oil or butter with no-sugar applesauce or non-fat sour cream. Use Canola or Olive oil, or a no trans-fat spread (like Smart Balance) instead of butter or shortening. To add moisture to recipes, in place of using fats experiment by substituting: non-fat or low-fat buttermilk or non-fat sour cream, plain yogurt or no-sugar applesauce.

Cream Cheese	Substitute with non-fat cream cheese or Neufchatel cheese.
Sour Cream	Use non-fat sour cream or yogurt cheese, made from plain, non-fat yogurt. (Place yogurt in cheesecloth, refrigerate and allow the liquid to drain overnight. The firm yogurt that remains is called yogurt cheese).
For dips	Use non-fat dairy products, including non-fat cottage cheese or non-fat ricotta cheese, which has been smoothed in the food processor. Use non-fat yogurt, non-fat cream cheese, non-fat sour cream.
For thickening	Use evaporated non-fat milk combined with a little flour or cornstarch. Reduce pan juices to thicken gravies and sauces. Briefly pulse whole oats in a food processor into a "flour" to thicken fruit-based recipes.
Cream Sauce	Blend non-fat cottage cheese with a little non-fat cream cheese in a food processor, until smooth. Warm gently and add seasonings, and herbs, as desired. Or, thicken non-fat evaporated milk with a little cornstarch. Add grated parmesan cheese and a little trans-fat-free spread (like Smart Balance) to flavor.
Dairy Products	Use non-fat versions of: cream cheese, ricotta, or cottage cheese. Use low-fat or non-fat hard cheeses. Grating cheeses very fine, using either a plane-style grater or the food processor, will allow you to use far less cheese than the recipe calls for.
To add sweetness and moisture	Try grated apples, chopped nuts, fruits, oats, wheat germ, no-sugar applesauce, grated carrots or zucchini, raisins or other dried fruits.

You'll find that many of your favorite foods can be modified to be lower in calories and still taste great. Apples combined with a lot of sugar and a crust made with white flour and lard may taste good, but will cost you dearly in fat and calories. A baked dessert made with apples, cinnamon, raisins, chopped walnuts, sweetened with no-sugar maple syrup and topped with some toasted oats is a very tasty and healthy nutrient-dense alternative. It may take a little time for your taste buds to appreciate treats with less sugar and fat, but as you eat more healthfully this style of eating will become more natural and they'll taste good too! The recipes in Appendix C are some of my own "How Low Can You Go?" creations. I hope you enjoy them! Learn to experiment in the kitchen, and HAVE FUN!

MAKE IT A FAMILY AFFAIR

Just as the rate of adult obesity has skyrocketed, experts are now reporting that the rates of childhood obesity and associated childhood Type-2 Diabetes are rising alarmingly. This condition was previously unheard of in young people, and is yet another indication that there are too many overweight FAMILIES out there. There are pressures on each of us to eat, eat, and eat some more! The entire family is barraged at every turn by ads for convenience and packaged foods. We see them everywhere; on TV, in magazines, on billboards, in vending machines, in school cafeterias, and even on movie theater screens. It's easy to get lured into the habit of eating these fattening convenience foods, and as a society we've fallen for it. It's big business ... and it's making us all big! Unfortunately, we just can't eat the way the marketing wizards tell us to and still be healthy.

Even with all of your best intentions, it will be difficult to establish healthy eating habits for the whole family if it is not made into a team event. Involving your family will not only help you lose weight, but will benefit them as well. You know your family and whether they are struggling with their weight. You know whether they eat too much junky food. You know their likes and dislikes.

Whether members of your family need to lose weight or not, convincing them to deviate from the typical Western fat-producing lifestyle and encouraging them to move toward a new healthier way of eating is important for their health and happiness. As you begin to institute change, your family may expect for everything to return to normal when you give up, just like it has so many times before. Your challenge will be to help them understand that this is not just another temporary period of deprivation and torture. You must convince them that you're ready to start a plan to change your habits forever, and you'd like them to join you.

The best way to enlist your family's help and support is to convince them that this will benefit them as well. Perhaps your spouse would feel better, stop snoring, and have more energy by losing a few pounds. Your teenager may get excited by the prospect of having a clearer complexion, and becoming a better soccer player by eating healthier foods. You have a chance to prevent your toddler from ever having to battle weight difficulties, if you teach him/her early on how to eat properly. For some families, making these adjustments can be traumatic. As with most major life changes, an all or nothing approach is not necessarily the best course. Making small changes and developing new healthy habits may be easier if you tackle them together.

Don't forget to include the family when developing your "Top 40" list, so everyone will be able to find things in the cupboards that they enjoy. When I speak of family, think of your friends also. They will certainly influence you and your ability to continue your lifestyle changes. Let them in on your plans and ask for their help. Along with healthier eating, plan some fun new activities together, preferably ones that don't revolve around eating. Maybe you could initiate a game of volleyball, suggest an after-dinner walk, or challenge someone to a mean game of badminton. Everyone will benefit by following your lead and may even end up having more fun!

> I'd like to add a cautionary note here to remind you that young, growing children require adequate intake of dietary fats and total calories to ensure proper growth and development. Do not limit children under the age of five years old to non-fat or strictly low fat foods. Providing them with adequate amounts of heart-healthy fats as part of a general healthy diet is essential. The same situation is true for pregnant women - don't severely restrict calories and/or healthy fats during this essential period of growth for your baby!

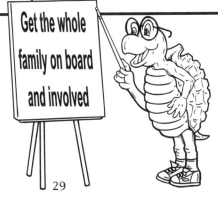

Get the whole family on board and involved

BREAKFAST DOESN'T SCARE ME ANYMORE

I used to be afraid of breakfast. Breakfast was just too early in the day. I was afraid that once I ate breakfast, there would be no stopping me. I knew that once I got started, I would continue to eat all day and by the time I went to bed that night I would have eaten an enormous number of calories. The problem with starting the day with only coffee and willpower, though, was my body was physiologically in need of some fuel. Every night, while sleeping, our bodies continue to work, repairing and restoring the damage from the day. By morning the energy tank is empty and unless fuel is taken in, there will be problems. You know the symptoms ... irritability, mood swings, feeling shaky and an inability to focus. These symptoms are your body's way of shouting "I need food!"

Unfortunately, when all your willpower to avoid eating for as long as possible is placed head to head with the power of real physiologic hunger, hunger will win every time. This sets up a cycle consisting of periods of deprivation, ultimately causing you to become so hungry later in the day that you end up inhaling mass quantities of happy-hour chips and dip, plus an entire dinner, followed by half a package of cookies before bed. This is a sure way to keep you fat!

My new way of eating has been centered on changing my relationship with food. Instead of treating it as the enemy to be battled, I now realize food should be considered as nourishment and strength. Eating nutrient-dense foods throughout the day keeps me feeling satisfied and NOT HUNGRY. All of my energy and willpower, both emotional and physical, can then be directed at living my life instead of thinking about food. This is very different from any other time I've attempted to lose weight. Breakfast doesn't scare me anymore!

Everyone in the family will be more inclined to eat breakfast if it is something they really like and can enjoy every day. Maybe each person will develop their own "special" breakfast and get it ready on their own schedule on busy weekdays, planning more elaborate meals for weekend mornings. Breakfast can be simple and quick, like peanut butter on whole-wheat toast or a glass of milk and a banana. As long as it includes both protein, complex carbohydrates, and possibly a little bit of heart-healthy fat, it will do the job. It will make things easier in the morning if the foods are laid out or prepared the evening before.

One of my own dietary mainstays for breakfast is plain, non-fat yogurt. Yogurt is a good source of complete protein. It also contains live cultures, which are beneficial for your digestive tract, and it's full of Calcium, which is good for your bones and may even help your body to burn more fat. If you choose non-fat yogurt, it is very low in calories and has no saturated fat. For all these reasons, yogurt ranks high on my "Top 40" list. Some people don't like the taste of plain unsweetened yogurt, but I have a witness in my house that will tell you it's possible to learn to enjoy it. My husband Charlie didn't like plain yogurt until he discovered his special waffle breakfast. In Appendix C you'll find the recipe for whole-wheat waffles. On Sundays, I put my Sunday Chef hat on and make a quadruple batch of these healthy waffles. After they've cooled, I wrap each one in plastic, and place them in the freezer. Each morning during the week, Charlie puts a frozen waffle in the toaster and a bowl of frozen berries in the microwave. While they are heating, he gets out some plain, non-fat yogurt and no-sugar maple syrup. When the waffle pops out, he places it in the bowl of heated berries and covers them with the yogurt and a little syrup. This is a delicious, healthy breakfast that he has learned to love, and it fits his calorie requirements. He's able to prepare and eat a delicious, nutritious, fiber-filled, no saturated fat, complex carbohydrate and protein meal in little more than five minutes. After that, he just has to grab a cup of coffee and he's off to work. What a great way to start the day.

YOUR LUNCH WON'T MAKE ITSELF

Even if you eat a good breakfast, by lunchtime your "tank" will be empty again. Hunger is a very powerful thing! If you get too hungry, that hunger will be hard to resist, and the likelihood is pretty high that you'll grab the first food that becomes available. These are situations when you'll hear people say "I blew my diet. I couldn't help it. I was starving." Believe me, if you leave the house for a busy day with only an apple and a yogurt, I can guarantee that hunger, temptation, and plain old physiology will ultimately defeat your good intentions. The good news is you do have a secret weapon to help avoid those diet-blowing predicaments. That secret weapon is called PLANNING and PREPARATION!

The successful Tortoise will make planning and preparing foods for the following day a nightly ritual. Every evening you should ask yourself: "What do I have scheduled for tomorrow?" Evaluating your schedule for the upcoming day will give you a pretty good idea of what you'll need to get ready, so your food is all set to grab the next morning as you're heading out the door. Will you be rushing from morning until night, away from your home or office? If so, you should probably pack an entire day's supply of food and put it into a little insulated bag with a frozen ice pack or a frozen container of soup that you'll be heating up for lunch. If you have a breakfast meeting, will they have healthy foods there that you can enjoy? If not, maybe it would be best to bring along a slice of homemade, whole-grain, banana bread and a piece of fruit, so you could eat a healthy meal rather than having a donut. Do you have an exercise class after work? It's important to eat something within an hour or so before exercise, so maybe you'll need to pack an extra portion of almonds and carrots, or half of a turkey sandwich on whole-grain bread, so you'll have the fuel your body will need. Maybe you typically work at home. If you chop up some vegetables, mix some tuna with non-fat mayo or wrap up a leftover chicken breast from last night's dinner, your chances for a successful day of healthy eating are much improved. Whether at work or at home, if you wait until you're really hungry and find yourself unprepared and facing a full refrigerator or a pastry cart ... well, let's just say there's going to be trouble!

Developing good habits of planning and preparing the foods you'll need for the next day is just that ... developing the habit. Start small if you need to. Make one small change at a time, but just get started. Getting everyone involved and developing family rituals will help. It may be beneficial to review your upcoming schedule together as a family every night at dinnertime. For example, a family "menu" could be developed, so each person in the household will know what to take along for lunch and for snacks. Make sure everyone plans to take enough food to last for the entire time they're planning to be away from home that day.

In the evening when you're preparing your own meals for the following day, pack everyone else a healthy lunch at the same time. Encourage participation by having the kids and/or your spouse help you pack their lunches, and they'll be more likely to actually eat them! Make sure the foods you are preparing contain protein, complex carbohydrates and a little bit of heart-healthy fats. Also include single servings of healthy treats, such as healthy homemade muffins or cookies, pretzels, fruit, vegetables with low fat dips, and nuts. You may find that it's easier to get up thirty minutes earlier in the morning to make lunches and snacks, or perhaps late in the evening when things are quiet after the kids have gone to bed. Find what works for you, and make it happen.

Even with the best planning, it's inevitable that there will be times when you find yourself away from the house for longer than you thought you would be, or unforeseen circumstances arise, leaving you stranded and hungry. If you're not prepared, you could end up blowing all of your hard work on a drive-thru calorie fest that you would regret. Keep a supply of non-perishable, nutritious snacks handy in your briefcase, purse, glove compartment or desk for these occasions. Remember, also, that sports activities or exercise will increase energy (and fluid) needs, so plan accordingly.

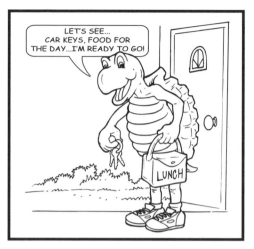

THERE'S SOMETHING ABOUT SOUP

Anytime of the day is really a great time for soup. A good bowl of broth-based vegetable and bean soup has got to be one of the healthiest and most satisfying low calorie foods you can eat. I have certainly made it a routine part of my eating plan. At least two or three times each week I have a bowl of soup for lunch, and quite regularly soup or chili is our main course at dinner. Most people don't think of soup as a choice for their evening meal, but any one of the hearty, healthy, and filling soups found in Appendix C can make a satisfying dinner. If you make your soup ahead of time and freeze it into little containers, you can just pop one into the microwave and dinner will be ready in five minutes. Even if you don't have freshly made or frozen soup handy, a number of healthy, low-sodium, low-fat canned or packaged soups are on the market that taste great and take just a few minutes to prepare. Soup is a great way to eat a bunch of healthy vegetables combined with fiber and protein packed beans, all in one filling and low calorie bowl.

DINNERS YOU MAKE IN YOUR SLEEP

One afternoon Charlie and I were out for a walk in our neighborhood, and it happened to be trash collection day. In addition to large trash containers, our community also provides each household with a small paper goods recycling bin, which is basically an open box that leaves the contents visible. As we were walking down the sidewalk I happened to notice an empty pizza delivery box at one house. The next house had one too. I commented that the typical habit of just calling the pizza delivery service and chowing down on an incredibly fat laden dinner was not a great way for people to be eating. We began to look for pizza boxes as we kept walking. We were shocked! In one block nine out of twelve houses had empty pizza delivery boxes. In another block, eight out of twelve houses had pizza boxes! One block didn't have very many pizza boxes but they had all sorts of big empty soda and beer containers. We decided this block should really get together with the other blocks more often! After awhile we stopped counting, but these observations left an indelible impression.

All those pizza boxes have something to do with why so many of us struggle with our weight. They are an indicator that people have given up on making dinner at home. Those people were all probably tired, stressed, and rewarding themselves with something good to eat after a busy day. I'll admit, it is sometimes difficult to find time to cook, and it's really convenient to just pick something up for dinner when you're tired and hungry. But restaurant and take-out meals are almost always higher in fat and calories than foods made at home. It also costs quite a bit of money to have someone else make all your meals. The result of being stressed out and indulging in too many of these meals is, unfortunately, weight gain ... and even more stress. It is, therefore, absolutely essential to commit a small amount of time in your day to cook some quick and healthy dinners. Some examples of quick and easy dinners are provided in Appendix A and Appendix C.

Once you get to the point where you know what you're going to make for dinner, you've planned it earlier in the week, you've already shopped for it, and it takes you maybe 15 minutes to cook, you'll be on your way to better habits that don't include empty pizza boxes. You'll be able to make healthy dinners in your sleep! After you have served these new healthy meals for awhile and everybody's happy, you'll be able to add variety by branching out a little. You may eventually find that you and your family like more good things than you thought. With any luck, you might be able to sneak a lot of vegetables and other healthy foods into those dinners without them even knowing it!

Getting everyone involved in this "healthy-eating thing" will be easier if you can make it fun by developing some enjoyable and healthy family dinner rituals. Feel free to get creative and come up with fun stuff your family enjoys. Healthy eating doesn't have to be boring! I'll give you some examples of some family dinner rituals that might work in your life.

Monday could be Turkey Chili night (Recipe in Appendix C), and after a really quick dinner like that, there might be time for a walk.

Friday night might be healthy Pita Pizza night (Recipe in Appendix C). Put down that phone ... you can easily make it yourself! Each person could develop their own specialty topping.

On Saturday morning, when you don't have to rush off to work, Greek Omelets or whole-wheat waffles (Recipes in Appendix C) could be on the menu.

While watching the game on Saturday afternoon, even Nachos (Recipe in Appendix C) can be a healthy snack, when made with whole-wheat tortillas, low-fat cheese, non-fat sour cream, and plenty of healthy beans.

On Saturday night, maybe Dad barbeques his famous steak while everyone else pitches in to make a big salad with low-calorie dressing, and some delicious homemade, non-fat, "Baked Fries." (Recipe in Appendix C)

Maybe on Sunday the family will enjoy a big picnic with Healthy Potato Salad, Baked Beans (Recipes in Appendix C), and barbequed chicken ... after taking a long hike.

Creating fun family rituals can do more than make healthy eating easier. With so many activities and commitments that pull everyone in so many different directions, family dinners are an important way for families to bond together ... and get healthy at the same time.

PREPARING FOR WHEN THE MONSTER STRIKES

The "monster" is that overwhelming craving for something crunchy, creamy, salty, chewy or sweet to eat and is something quite different from a little between-meal stomach rumble. In fact, these urges may not have a thing to do with actual hunger. They often have some kind of emotional or hormonal trigger attached, and because of this, they can feel pretty overpowering.

The first thing to do when the monster strikes is try to take a moment and figure out why you are experiencing this craving. If you've skipped a meal or have engaged in a lot of activity, your body may truly be signaling that it needs some fuel. If this is the case, it may be wise to eat your next regularly scheduled meal a little bit early. Another thing that may be happening when you feel hungry is that you are actually a little bit dehydrated. An all-around good habit is to respond to those first twinges of hunger by drinking a big glass of water. In fact, the Tortoise Diet recommends making it a habit to routinely drink 16 ounces of water about one hour prior to each scheduled meal. This is not only a good insurance policy to get you to your next meal without becoming too hungry, it helps you to know that you're getting enough water every day. Give it a try … and make it a habit!

If it's not true hunger and it's not dehydration, most likely this incredible urge you are experiencing to eat some calorie-dense treat may be attached to some other factor. The "trigger" for a craving can be either something happy in life or something sad and stressful. A craving can be caused by an overwhelming day at work, fatigue from lack of sleep because the baby was up teething all night, feeling lonely or frustrated, feeling anxious because you have a date for the upcoming weekend, feeling pre-menstrual and weepy, feeling worried about being able to pay your bills, feeling excited about an upcoming party, or any number of other causes.

If you can identify your feelings, you'll have an opportunity to develop skills to deal with them in ways other than eating. One suggestion is to review your journal to see if there are any recurring patterns related to events in your life that seem to invariably lead to these overwhelming cravings for calorie-dense foods. You may find that every time you have a stressful day at work, the carton of ice cream calls your name. Maybe on the days you are exhausted, a sugary donut with coffee seems to be the only thing that will perk you up. Maybe whenever you're just plain bored you suddenly find an empty bag of chips next to you on the couch. The more you can discover about yourself and how you manage your feelings with food, the better you will become at developing methods to deal with those feelings in more productive ways. Using food to meet needs other than hunger is a very poor health habit. Food is designed to nourish your body and to enjoy, but it is not designed to meet every emotional need you have. You need to honestly ask yourself what is making you so hungry for something you know you shouldn't eat. What is it that is defeating you as you pursue your commitments toward good health and permanent weight loss? Honest answers will lead to solutions.

The last thing you want to do is to give in to these cravings and eat way too many calories or worse yet, go on a binge of uncontrollable eating. The following are some suggestions to keep the "monster" at bay.

1. Again, because sometimes thirst may be mistaken for hunger, try to stave off the urge to eat by first quickly drinking 16 ounces or more of water, flavored seltzer or herbal tea.

2. Stop and take ten minutes to perform a self-care activity to make yourself feel good. Some examples might be:

- Take a long, hot shower, using the luxurious shower gel you usually save for special occasions.
- Call someone who cares and talk.
- Take a short nap.
- Close your eyes and stretch your arms and legs.
- If you're at work, get up from your desk and take a walk down the hall.

3. Try some exercise. Channeling the energy of your feelings and emotions into physical activity will be helpful in stress reduction. Some examples might be:

- Put on some music and dance around and feel your mood begin to lift.
- Try getting up and heading outside for a walk.

It's especially nice to get outdoors and take a fast walk in the fresh air. Once you get moving, your mind may be freed up and you may be able to re-focus on things other than food.

IDENTIFYING YOUR MONSTER

If the craving persists despite all of your delay tactics, you may decide to eat a little something that will "hit the spot" for your specific craving. It will be better to deliberately decide to eat a little something that will really satisfy, so you don't eat a LOT of something else. When it's time to "feed the monster", follow this procedure:

1. First, drink a 16 ounces glass of water before eating anything.

2. Practice portion control. Measure out a single serving of whatever you plan to eat onto a plate or into a glass and then get the heck out of the kitchen.

3. Eat slowly and deliberately, pay attention to the sensation and mindfully enjoy and savor every bite. Remember to include protein and a little fat with carbohydrate snacks, so they will actually fill you up.

4. Drink another 16 ounces glass of water after eating.

5. Picture yourself as strong, healthy, and in control, having resisted the urge to stuff yourself with food that cannot ever truly satisfy all your needs.

Cravings are sometimes very definite for foods that are salty, sweet, creamy, or crunchy. When the "monster" strikes, try to pinpoint just which type of "monster" it is. The weapons required to ward off the "salt monster" are quite different than those needed for the "sweet monster." The following are my suggested healthy foods to combat the various types of cravings.

CRUNCHY

Cut up vegetables and a few nuts
An apple smeared with 1 TBS peanut butter
1 cup crunchy bran cereal with ½ cup non-fat or soy milk
Wasa, RyKrisp, or Ak-Mak crackers spread with 1 TBS peanut butter, reduced fat Laughing
Cow cheese, or non-fat cream cheese
13 almonds or 5 walnuts
A handful of pretzels, with a part-skim mozzarella cheese stick
Toasted whole-grain English muffin with 1 ounce low-fat cheese
No-oil, air-popped popcorn (only 20 calories per cup)

SALTY

Reduced-fat Triscuit crackers, with 1 ounce low-fat cheese
Baked tortilla chips: 1 whole-wheat tortilla cut into wedges, sprayed with non-fat cooking
spray and baked in a 400 degree oven for 3-5 minutes until crisp and served with salsa

SWEET

Non-fat, no-sugar pudding
1 cup no-sugar fruit gelatin, with chopped fruit
A piece of fresh fruit or a serving of frozen fruit
1 small piece of dark chocolate. Let it melt on your tongue and savor it
Fruit smoothie, made with non-fat milk, soy milk or soft tofu
Homemade low-fat and low-sugar baked goods
An oatmeal "cookie": A bowl of hot cooked oatmeal, topped with 1 TBS mini-chocolate chips
and 1 TBS chopped walnuts
Non-fat hot chocolate
1 slice healthy, homemade, Banana Bread or some other healthy muffin. (Recipes in Appendix C)

CREAMY

Non-fat, no-sugar pudding
Non-fat, plain yogurt topped with fruit
Non-fat ice cream bar

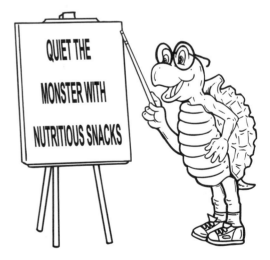

"It will be better to deliberately
decide to eat a little something
that will really satisfy..."

QUIET THE
MONSTER WITH
NUTRITIOUS SNACKS

KID SNACK ATTACKS

If you have children or teenagers at home, you know you've got to have snacks available. For your sake as well as theirs, review the food in the healthy foods list and recipe section with your family to select which types of snacks everyone could substitute for the junky foods they may now be eating. Some examples to put on that "Top 40" list might be: Homemade no-sugar/non-fat whole-grain muffins or cookies, (make extra batches and freeze so they are always available with just a quick zap in the microwave), nonfat milk or soy milk to blend with chunks of fruit and ice for smoothies, whole-grain crackers and low-fat cheese, apples with peanut butter, whole-grain cereal with milk, whole-grain toast with peanut butter, all types of fresh fruit, and no-sugar/non-fat yogurt topped with chopped nuts and fruit.

If you must have packaged snack foods in the house, buy single serving portions instead of the big package, or re-portion the large package into single-serving containers as soon as you bring it home. Write down what the calorie "cost" of that snack portion is. Then put all of these kid snacks on one shelf, and make that the shelf you do not reach for! Designate limited times the kids can eat these calorie-dense snacks, such as one snack food at 4 p.m. after school or a snack cake only on Friday evenings.

Don't underestimate your kid's ability to learn to enjoy healthy snacks. Allow them to experiment with healthy foods and to learn to enjoy them in a fun way. Encourage your smaller children to create (with your help, if necessary) healthy, fun, kid-friendly snack foods like some of the following:

Ants on a Log: Smear celery sticks with peanut butter and dot with raisins.

Colorful "Critters": Cut up fruits and/or vegetables placed onto toothpicks and made into funny shapes on a paper plate, then eaten off the toothpicks.

Fruit smoothies: Allow kids to select the ingredients (fruits, peanut butter, chocolate, etc.) to go into their soy or milk-based smoothie made in the blender. Use some squiggly straws to make it even more fun.

"Smile-y face" on a plate: Smear a plate with bean dip. Use olives, corn, and non-fat sour cream to fashion eyes, ears and noses on the plate. Dive into the dip with baked whole-wheat tortilla chips, whole-wheat pita chips or vegetable sticks.

Mini-Pizzas: On whole-grain pitas (split each pita to make two circles) or whole-grain English muffins, place some tomato sauce, shredded cheese, vegetables, etc. and melt under the broiler.

Fruit swirl: Swirl 1 teaspoon all-fruit jam into non-fat or low-fat yogurt. Drizzle a little chocolate sauce on top and sprinkle with chopped nuts or some whole-grain cereal.

Make these kinds of nutrient-dense foods a regular part of each day. Calorie-dense snack foods should be treated as an exception, rather than the rule. Don't keep ice cream in your freezer. Instead, treat eating ice cream as a special event, something you buy outside of the house. Make baking a cake to celebrate an occasion a special family ritual to be enjoyed once in awhile. Limit trips to fast-food restaurants to the status of a rare treat. Instead, plan and prepare healthy and enjoyable lunches and snacks and learn to develop other rewards to celebrate those special events of life. Develop the new habit of enjoying food as simply part of the activity, and look forward to continuing the fun by playing a game of volleyball or baseball together, or go for a family walk.

IMPRESS YOUR FRIENDS

Socializing and having fun with friends and family almost always involves the enjoyment of food. I don't have to tell you that these occasions can turn into food fests that can certainly present caloric challenges. If you're the one doing the entertaining however, you do have some control over things. Creating healthy, low-calorie, low fat foods for entertaining will definitely require some creativity, but it's actually kind of fun. Keep in mind that your guests may already be very curious about how you have successfully lost weight. They'll start to learn the secret to your success as you dazzle them with your ability to serve tasty and healthy alternatives to the usual fattening party fare. The following guidelines should ensure your confidence and success in the realm of healthy entertaining:

1. Select a style of entertaining that is appropriate for the event, and at the level of formality that best fits your personal style. It's your day, so you should feel comfortable and relaxed. Make it FUN! Use some cute napkins, candles, place cards or pretty flowers to cheer things up and place the emphasis on the entire event, rather than just the food. Organize your serving dishes, plates, glassware, etc. in advance so you are sure to have everything you need.

2. Develop three or four tasty and healthy hors d'oeuvres recipes that you enjoy. Also develop a repertoire of a few low fat, low calorie, low-sugar FABULOUS desserts. Experiment with your favorite high fat and high calorie recipes, using "How Low Can You Go?" techniques to make them lower in fat and sugar, but still a treat. Simply offering choices beyond those tired old greasy chips and dips and sugary cake will make you a standout host or hostess.

3. Shop for the PERFECT vegetables, fruits, meats, and breads for your menu. With minimal fuss and preparation, these delicious foods will make the meal superior to what most people eat every day, and you'll look like a fabulous chef!

4. Practice your entertaining menu in advance. Write down details about the food preparation, including prep-time, ingredients needed, and helpful hints to coordinate the timing of your preparation and cooking. The more comfortable you are with preparing the foods, the less stressful your entertaining will be.

5. Make a detailed shopping list for your menu, and give yourself plenty of time to shop so you are not rushed.

Your guests will be impressed with the low calorie appetizers, meals, and desserts and you will enjoy the self-confidence that comes from successfully losing weight. Invite your friends to join you in your new way of life!

CHAPTER FOUR
THE QUEST TO ACHIEVE YOUR TARGET WEIGHT

APPLES TO APPLES

Scientists have been laboring for many years to understand exactly how
weight loss works, and why the losing part is so darn hard for some of us! By looking around,
it's obvious that we humans come in many different shapes and sizes. Less obvious is the fact
that all individuals have their own unique energy requirements. For this reason, the cruel fact
is that some people may gain weight by eating small amounts of food while their sisters, best
friends, or husbands can go back for second helpings and not gain an ounce. One individual
may also find that despite "dieting" by taking in a measly 1,300 calories a day and exercising
their fool head off they can't seem to lose weight, while their neighbor goes on the same diet,
and loses five pounds. Why? It's not fair! Let's begin to unravel this mystery by discussing
some basic information about weight loss.

WEIGHT LOSS 101

The body is a complex piece of machinery that requires a steady stream of energy to perform
its many intricate functions. As a matter of survival, all bodily systems tirelessly work
together to make sure there is always enough energy available for these functions to continue.
Metabolism is the process of breaking down the foods we eat into their component parts and
releasing the energy they contain. This energy from food is known as calories. The faster a
person's metabolic rate, the higher their calorie-burning rate will be.

Whenever more calories are taken in than the body requires for energy, the excess energy is
stored as fat. Whenever fewer calories are taken in than the body requires for energy, a
calorie deficit is incurred. When there is a calorie deficit, and not enough energy is supplied
from the foods we eat, other sources of energy will be metabolized to provide the necessary
fuel for the body to continue its many functions. Body fat is one of those other sources. Since
one pound of body fat is equal to 3,500 calories of stored energy, many of us carry around
thousands of calories that are just waiting to make up the deficit!

The other major source of stored energy in the body available for use when there is a calorie
deficit is found in muscle tissue. Muscle tissue, however, is the calorie-burning machinery of
the body, so breaking it down to provide energy is not desirable! **The less muscle you have,
the slower your rate of metabolism will be, and the fewer number of calories you will
burn. Always remember that losing too much muscle tissue will defeat any attempts at
permanent weight loss.**

Weight loss can only occur when there is a calorie deficit. The goal of any effective weight loss
plan must be to find a way to tap into the body's fat-storage warehouse of energy, so fat (not
muscle!) is slowly but surely used to make up the deficit.

You might think by just eating 3,500 fewer calories over a period of time it would be possible
to lose one pound of fat. If it were only that easy, losing weight would be a snap.

Unfortunately, the physiology of weight loss is far more complicated, requiring more than merely restricting calorie intake. For successful, long-term weight loss, that flow of the energy being taken in and the energy being burned off must be constantly "managed." The goal is to keep the calorie deficit "just right" so stored fat is utilized to make up the difference, muscle tissue is preserved, and the metabolic rate is kept going strong.

Of course, in the short term, severely limiting calorie intake does indeed cause some weight loss. That's what all the quick weight loss diets count on! Because those diets are based on some form of enforced starvation, muscle tissue will be destroyed and the metabolic rate is slowed. Remember, whenever muscle tissue is lost, fewer calories are required each day. When the dieter can't stand the hunger any longer and returns to eating normally again, it's almost guaranteed that all the pounds they have lost will pile back on, plus a few more for good measure.

Because the metabolic rate has been slowed, that person now won't be able to eat the amount of food they could before the diet began, without actually gaining weight. Overweight people who have tried and failed to lose weight their entire lives may very well have subjected their bodies to periods of "starvation" many times. At this point, their metabolisms may have been slowed to the point that they are telling the truth when they complain of gaining weight while "eating like a bird." This is the way our bodies are designed, and there's just no way to fool physiology. Thus, severely limiting calories as a way of dieting will ultimately defeat any weight loss attempts.

I learned firsthand this principle of eating the correct amount of calories to maintain a "just right" calorie deficit. When I first began my weight loss efforts at 248 pounds, I decided to try to limit my calorie intake to 1,200 calories per day, which I was able to do on most days. During the first eight months of this pretty typical "diet" routine, I lost 70 pounds. But then my weight loss came crashing to a halt and I still had another fifty pounds yet to lose! For a long while, every time I stepped on the scale I could be heard to mutter the phrase "I'm depressed as a dog!" I was stuck in a long, frustrating period that could very easily have caused me to just give up, like I had always done before. What I didn't realize at that time was I had been starving myself into a metabolic slowdown. I wish I had known then how important maintaining a "just right" calorie deficit was. By eating only 1200 calories per day at 248 pounds, I had created a gigantic calorie deficit. This caused my metabolic rate to slow because muscle tissue was being broken down and utilized for energy. It was such a weird concept for me when I finally learned I was eating TOO LITTLE FOOD each day to be able to lose weight!

What is the "just right" calorie deficit that will preserve muscle and promote fat loss? There are many things to be considered when calculating this number because each individual is unique. There is no one-size-fits-all calorie plan. The actual number of calories required each day must be personalized. The process of calculating this number requires several steps, starting with figuring out your "target body weight."

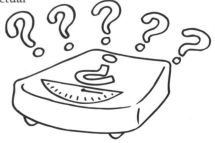

HOW MUCH SHOULD I WEIGH, ANYWAY?

We probably all have a number in our minds of what we'd like to weigh, in a perfect world. We may also have a weight we'd "settle" for. But there is actually a commonly used medical/scientific calculation that can be used to determine what our target body weight should be. When you have finished the following calculations, you will learn that your target weight, according to scientists, may be quite different than the one you had in mind. Calculating that target weight is very important, however, because it helps determine the number of calories you require each day.

I urge you, though, to not be intimidated by a number. Achieving success is all about becoming a healthier person. When you decide that you look great and you feel healthy, even if it's a few pounds over your calculated target body weight, you may decide that the weight you're at is your best weight, and be satisfied. In actuality, the number on the scale is not even the most important target. Rather, it is the percentage of your total weight that is comprised of body fat that tells the real story. We'll be dealing with this in more detail later on, but for now let's start by calculating your target body weight, beginning by determining your frame size.

Don't worry! If math is not your strong suit, there is help for you. By logging onto www.wintheracetolose.com and becoming a Tortoise Diet member, all of the required calculations will be done for you! Many other benefits of membership will be explained later, including having your own personalized and private Web page to track your weight loss progress!

DETERMINING BODY FRAME SIZE

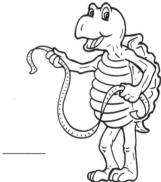

A. MY HEIGHT _____ Feet   plus _____ Inches
    Multiply height in feet by 12   _____
    Add additional height in inches _____
    My total height in inches is   _____
    Multiply total height in inches by 2.54 to convert to centimeters _____
    My height in centimeters is   _____

B. MY FRAME SIZE

Use a tape measure to measure the circumference of the wrist of your dominant hand. Enlist a friend to help hold the tape securely (make sure it is not pulled too tightly). Place the tape just next to the wrist bone, on the side closest to your hand. For accuracy, take the wrist measurement 2-3 times to the nearest 1/8 inch and average together. Convert fractions to decimals as shown below:

    1/8 inch = .125 inch
    1/4 inch = .25 inch
    3/8 inch = .375 inch
    1/2 inch = .5 inch
    5/8 inch = .625 inch
    3/4 inch = .75 inch
    7/8 inch = .875 inch

Example: If your wrist is six inches plus 3/8 of an inch; this would be converted to 6.375 inches.

My wrist circumference in inches is   _____

Multiply that number by 2.54 to convert to centimeters   _____

My wrist circumference in centimeters is   _____

From the earlier calculation, my height in centimeters is   _____

Divide height in centimeters by wrist circumference in centimeters _____

Compare the result of this calculation to the numbers on the following chart:

Frame Size	Men	Women
Small	(>) 10.40	(>) 11.00
Medium	9.60 - 10.40	10.10 - 11.00
Large	(<) 9.60	(<) 10.10

My Body Frame Size is _____

Example: A 5' 4 ½" woman with a wrist measurement averaging 6 3/8 inches:

Wrist measurement of 6.375 inches x 2.54 cm = 16.19 cm

Height of 5' 4 ½ = 64.5 inches x 2.54 cm   = 163.83 cm

Therefore, 163.83 cm divided by 16.19 cm   = 10.11 cm

As you can see, this woman has a MEDIUM FRAME, because 10.11 is less than (<) 11.00, but larger than (>) 10.10.

DETERMINING TARGET BODY WEIGHT

A commonly used general rule is the following:

For women, 100 pounds should be allowed for the first 5 feet in height,
Plus 5 more pounds for each additional inch in height.

For men, 110 pounds should be allowed for the first 5 feet,
Plus 5 more pounds for each additional inch in height.

Based on my sex and height, my target body weight is _____ pounds

ADJUSTMENT TO TARGET BODY WEIGHT BASED ON FRAME SIZE

If you have a Large Frame, add 10% to your target body weight
(target body weight) x (1.1) _____ pounds

If you have a Medium Frame, add 0 / subtract 0 _____ pounds

If you have a Small Frame, subtract 10% from your target body weight
(target body weight) x (0.9) _____ pounds

After adjusting for frame size,

My Target Body Weight is _____ pounds

MORE "APPLE" INFORMATION

Calculating your target body weight, based on your basic body type, was the first step toward determining your unique calorie requirements. There are other mathematical formulas, though, that reduce every person, no matter how different, to the proverbial "apple" for comparison with other "apples." These formulas further refine the process of determining individualized calorie needs by taking into consideration other factors that impact each person's highly individual basic energy needs; such as age, muscularity, activity level, and genetics. By incorporating this personalized information into the calculation, the specific number of calories required each day to meet each person's metabolic needs can be determined.

FREE CALORIES FOR LYING AROUND

The next step toward developing an individualized calorie plan for effective weight loss is to calculate your minimum daily calorie requirement. The basal metabolic rate (BMR) represents the bare minimum number of calories you would require to sustain your bodily functions if all you did was just lie around all day on the couch. The charts located in Appendix D are based on the Harris-Benedict Formula, which is considered the "gold standard" for calculating BMR because it takes sex, age, height and weight into consideration to determine calorie requirements.

Use the charts in Appendix D to determine your own personal BMR, based on your target body weight. Please notice that there are separate charts for men and women. On Chart #1 read across the top from left to right until you locate the number that represents your current age. Next read the column on the left side of the page from top to bottom to find your height. Follow that line from left to right until you locate the number where your height and age intersect. Write this number down, as the Chart #1 number. Next, on Chart #2, locate the number that represents your target body weight in pounds. Write down the number located next to that weight as the Chart #2 number. Add the Chart #1 and the Chart #2 numbers together to determine your BMR at your target body weight.

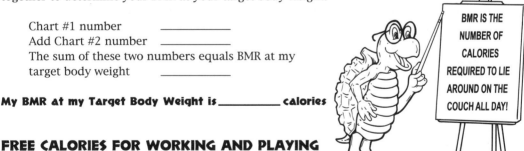

Chart #1 number   _____
Add Chart #2 number   _____
The sum of these two numbers equals BMR at my
target body weight   _____

My BMR at my Target Body Weight is _____ **calories**

BMR IS THE NUMBER OF CALORIES REQUIRED TO LIE AROUND ON THE COUCH ALL DAY!

FREE CALORIES FOR WORKING AND PLAYING

In addition to BMR, further energy is required to fuel the process of digestion as well as the typical amount of activity you engage in each day. Just how much additional energy is required will be influenced mostly by your usual level of activity, as determined primarily by your occupation. The more your muscles work as you engage in your occupational activities, the higher the rate of calorie burn will be throughout the majority of the day. A person whose workday consists mostly of driving or sitting at the computer, for example, will require fewer calories than someone who is lifting boxes all day, or someone who actively chases after a busy toddler. By applying the appropriate Activity Factor, the amount of energy required for fuel during a typical day can be predicted.

Multiplying your BMR at your target body weight by your Activity Factor, and then adding 10 percent to account for the energy required for digestion, will result in the total number of daily calories required to maintain your body at that target body weight. I've made the calculation a little easier by including the calories you burn by digesting food with the Activity Factor. The appropriate Activity Factor, then, includes your total additional energy expenditure, above and beyond your BMR, for your normal daily activities excluding purposeful exercise. We will talk about the effect of exercise on calorie needs later.

ACTIVITY FACTORS

Men and Women: Sedentary - 1.3
Use this Activity Factor if you spend most of your day sitting or driving, with minimal movement.

Some examples of this level of activity are: office work, lab work, phone work, computer work, playing cards, sewing, light housework, and watching television.

Men and Women: Light Activity - 1.4
Use this Activity Factor if you spend most of your day performing activities that require you to be somewhat mobile and to use your upper body as well.

Some examples of this level of activity are: working as a janitor or maid, gardening, auto repair, electrician, welder, restaurant worker, hospital worker, caring for children, light carpentry work, cashiering or stocking in a store or warehouse, and standing assembly line work.

Women: Moderate Activity - 1.5
Men: Moderate Activity - 1.6
Use this Activity Factor if you spend most of your day being moderately active, in an occupation that requires significant walking and/or physical labor.

Some examples of this level of activity are: walking a postal route, package delivery person, and moderately active landscaping or construction activities.

Women: Heavy Activity - 1.7
Men: Heavy Activity - 1.8
Use this Activity Factor if you spend most of your day being very active, in an occupation that requires significant amounts of heavy manual labor.

Some examples of this level of activity are: furniture movers, lumberjacks, working with a pick and shovel, hard digging, anything where throughout the day you are hauling around heavy things, like bricks, tile, wood, heavy boxes or bags of soil.

Based on my usual level of activity, as determined by my daily occupation, my Activity Factor is _____

MY LIFETIME CALORIE PLAN

The Activity Factor that best describes your usual level of daily activity, as determined primarily by your occupation, is now used to determine your own personal calorie requirements at your target body weight. **By calculating this number you will learn the number of calories you will be able to eat, once you arrive at your target body weight and target body fat percentage!** And that doesn't take into consideration that when you exercise, you'll be able to eat even more! You may be pleasantly surprised to learn you won't have to live forever at the starvation level, because your body truly does need plenty of calories for energy.

BMR at my target body weight   _____

Multiplied by my Activity Factor   _____

Equals my Lifetime Calorie Plan   _____

MY WEIGHT LOSS CALORIE PLAN

Your Lifetime Calorie Plan is the number of calories you will be able to eat to maintain your target body weight and target body fat percentage, once you get there, if you engage in your usual amount of activity. Maintaining your current, heavier weight, however, requires a larger number of calories. As previously discussed, a calorie deficit is required for weight loss. Our challenge is to ensure that the gap between the calorie requirements at your current weight and the number of calories to be eaten during weight loss is that "just right" deficit. If it is too large, muscle tissue may be lost and metabolism may be slowed. If it is too small, no fat loss will occur.

> Adjusting your Lifetime Calorie Plan to create the proper calorie deficit will result in your Weight Loss Calorie Plan. This is the amount of calories that should be eaten during weight loss, to provide that "just right" calorie deficit.

Since men and women at the same amount of pounds over their target body weight have different calorie needs, there is a scale for men that is different than the one for women.

If you are 176-200 pounds over your target body weight: After calculating your Lifetime Calorie Plan, round that number down to the nearest 100.
    MEN ADD 800 CALORIES, WOMEN ADD 400 CALORIES

This is my Weight Loss Calorie Plan _____

If you are 151-175 pounds over your target body weight: After calculating your Lifetime Calorie Plan, round that number down to the nearest 100.
    MEN ADD 700 CALORIES, WOMEN ADD 300 CALORIES

This is my Weight Loss Calorie Plan _____

If you are 126-150 pounds over your target body weight: After calculating your Lifetime Calorie Plan, round that number down to the nearest 100.

MEN ADD 500 CALORIES, WOMEN ADD 200 CALORIES

This is my Weight Loss Calorie Plan _____

If you are 101-125 pounds over your target body weight: After calculating your Lifetime Calorie Plan, round that number down to the nearest 100.

MEN ADD 400 CALORIES, WOMEN ADD 100 CALORIES.

This is my Weight Loss Calorie Plan _____

If you are 76-100 pounds over your target body weight: After calculating your Lifetime Calorie Plan, round that number down to the nearest 100.

MEN ADD 200 CALORIES, WOMEN ADD ZERO CALORIES.

This is my Weight Loss Calorie Plan _____

If you are 51-75 pounds over your target body weight: After calculating your Lifetime Calorie Plan, round that number down to the nearest 100.

MEN ADD ZERO CALORIES, WOMEN SUBTRACT 200 CALORIES.

This is my Weight Loss Calorie Plan _____

If you are 26-50 pounds over your target body weight: After calculating your Lifetime Calorie Plan, round that number down to the nearest 100.

MEN SUBTRACT 200 CALORIES, WOMEN SUBTRACT 300 CALORIES.

This is my Weight Loss Calorie Plan _____

If you are 25 pounds or less over your target body weight: After calculating your Lifetime Calorie Plan, round that number down to the nearest 100.

MEN SUBTRACT 300 CALORIES, WOMEN SUBTRACT 400 CALORIES.

This is my Weight Loss Calorie Plan _____

Yes, you've probably figured out that you will be asked to count calories when following the Tortoise Diet. You may think counting calories sounds like a pain. Believe me, so do I! Don't worry ... I promise I'll show you a little later on how to make keeping track of your daily calorie intake an easy task.

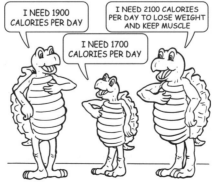

TALL TALES OF THE SCALE

While the ordinary bathroom scale is certainly a useful tool, it doesn't begin to tell the whole story. **An essential component of the Tortoise Diet is understanding that the total number of pounds the scale registers is made up of both fat weight and lean weight.** Lean weight is everything in the body that isn't fat, but for our purposes, when we refer to lean weight we'll be talking about muscle.

> The problem with the scale is that when it is indicating weight loss (or gain), it can't differentiate whether the loss came from fat weight or lean weight.

During weight loss, monitoring the number of pounds of lean weight you are preserving, and the number of pounds of fat you are losing is essential to ensure that the weight being lost is truly fat, rather than calorie-burning muscle tissue. Why is preserving muscle so important? The reason is that each pound of muscle, at rest, burns about 15 calories a day for fuel, and even more with increased activity. Conversely, each pound of happy fat sitting there enjoying the ride around town the muscles are giving it, is burning only two calories a day for fuel! The importance of preserving muscle as you lose weight is illustrated by the following example: If Mary loses twenty pounds (according to the scale), with ten pounds of that weight being muscle, she will have lost the calorie burning potential of approximately 10 lbs. x 15 calories = 150 calories per day! In other words, she can eat 150 fewer calories each day, just to remain at her present weight! You can easily see how every precious pound of muscle lost will make it harder to reach your target body weight, and then be successful at staying there.

Aging also works against us. Because the typical person at age forty has already lost ten pounds of muscle, that person is using at least 150 calories less energy each and every day than when they were younger. Now you know why you could eat so much more when you were twenty without gaining weight!

I hope I've made my point that muscle preservation is essential! It is the biggest mistake the average person makes when losing weight. Unfortunately, rapid weight loss always causes the loss of muscle!

With quick weight loss, the scale tells a "tall tale" of temporary success that isn't really the whole story. Slow weight loss, on the other hand, tends to preserve muscle, which allows you to eat more calories, maintain your metabolic rate, and prevent weight loss plateaus!

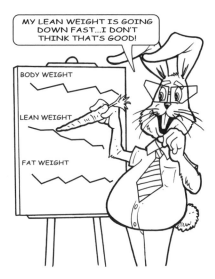

47

TARGET BODY FAT PERCENTAGE

Because it is so important to preserve lean weight while you lose fat, you must now determine how many pounds of your target body weight should be made up of body fat and how many pounds should be lean weight. To learn this, you first need to determine your target body fat percentage.

There are many different opinions regarding what percentage of your total body weight should be comprised of fat. Many researchers simply offer a range of numbers for acceptable body fat percentages, while others offer ranges for athlete, lean, normal, over-fat, and obese. For our purposes, I'm going to give you a single number for your target body fat percentage that I believe realistically corresponds with your target body weight. However, as with your target body weight number, you may decide when you get close to your target body fat percentage that you're happy with the way you look. That's fine! As I have said before, the Tortoise Diet is about being healthy and happy. I think it's important, however, to have a single number to aim for.

Table 4-1 shows my recommendations for target body fat percentages. These goals should be considered even more important than your target body weight! You'll notice that the percentages for women are higher than those for men. You can blame it on hormones, ladies. Women's bodies require a little more body fat to function effectively. You'll also notice the numbers for people over age forty are higher than for people under forty. This is because of that natural process of aging, causing muscle tissue to be replaced by fat tissue over time. Strength training exercises, performed on a regular basis, can minimize this process to a large degree. Unfortunately, muscle tissue is lost for both men and women simply due to hormonal changes, so it becomes increasingly more difficult with age to preserve muscle.

Table 4-1

MEN	Under 40 years old	12%	Fat Weight
	Over 40 years old	15%	Fat Weight
WOMEN	Under 40 years old	18%	Fat Weight
	Over 40 years old	21%	Fat Weight

My Target Body Fat Percentage _____

TARGET LEAN AND TARGET FAT

Now that you know your target body fat percentage, it's possible to determine the target number of pounds of fat weight and the target number of pounds of lean weight that should comprise your target body weight. Of course there are more calculations for you to do! In these calculations, you must express your target body fat percentage as a decimal. Example: 21% is converted to 0.21 and 15% to 0.15.

My target body weight _____
Multiplied by my target body fat percentage expressed as a decimal _____
Equals my Target Fat Weight _____

_____

My target body weight   _____
Minus my target fat weight
Equals my Target Lean Weight _____

Let's use 35-year-old Paula as an example. Paula's target body weight is 125.0 lbs, based on her height of 5' 5" and her medium frame size. Because she is under 40 years old, her target body fat percentage is 18. Plugging in Paula's target numbers shows:

Paula's target body weight   <u>125.0 lbs</u>
Multiplied by Paula's target body fat percentage expressed as a decimal (0.18)
Equals Paula's target fat weight   <u>22.5 lbs</u>

Paula's target body weight   <u>125.0 lbs</u>
Minus Paula's target fat weight   <u>22.5 lbs</u>
Equals Paula's target lean weight   <u>102.5 lbs</u>

Therefore, when Paula reaches her target body weight of 125 pounds, her weight should be comprised of 22.5 pounds of fat, and 102.5 pounds of lean weight.

CALCULATING YOUR CURRENT BODY FAT PERCENTAGE

So far, you've calculated some important target numbers:

1. Your Target Body Weight
2. Your Target Body Fat Percentage
3. Your Target Fat Weight
4. Your Target Lean Weight

These are the target numbers you must pay close attention to throughout your weight loss. These numbers represent your goals, and clearly defined goals are important in any endeavor. However, now that you know where you are heading, to be able to measure progress you need to determine where you are starting from. You need to determine your current numbers. To calculate your current fat weight and current lean weight, you'll start by figuring out your current body fat percentage.

There are many ways to determine your current body fat percentage. One easy way is to purchase a digital weight/body fat scale. A digital body fat scale doubles as a good quality digital weight scale, which you should have anyway. A digital weight/body fat scale is accurate and consistent each time you step on it. There's no little needle to manipulate by stepping a little to the left or right, so there's no cheating! Make sure to tap a digital scale before stepping onto it, so the read-out is zeroed before you begin. This type of scale utilizes electrical impedance in your body (don't worry, it doesn't hurt!) as a way to determine the percentage of fat in your body, relative to your body weight. It's important to know that if you are dehydrated, over-hydrated, or having hormonally related water retention, the reading will be affected, so a single reading may or may not be significant. Jot the numbers down in your journal each week and keep track over the long term to realistically see true changes and trends.

I usually get on the scale first thing in the morning, after using the bathroom and before eating or drinking anything. If you choose to take body fat readings at this time of day, be aware that the reading will probably be about 1-2 percent higher than your actual body fat percentage. This is because you're usually a little dehydrated first thing in the morning, and being dehydrated causes the body fat percentage reading to be artificially raised. But unless you're very near your target body fat percentage, you don't need to worry about this ... it's consistency we're after.

Some people like to weigh and take body fat readings just once a week. That's fine, just pick a day and time that is the same each week. In the interest of research, I record my own numbers every day. It's been fascinating for me to watch what my body is doing, and how amazing it is that eating a salty meal, for instance, can put two pounds on the scale the next morning. When this happens, I don't despair, though, because I realize that it's just excess water weight, and not a gain in fat. If you do take readings every day, average your daily readings to determine your average weight and body fat percentage for the week. Record these numbers in your journal.

** Anyone who has an electronic, implanted medical devise, such as a pacemaker, should not use a fat monitor scale utilizing electrical impedance. **

CALCULATING CURRENT LEAN WEIGHT AND CURRENT FAT WEIGHT USING THE BODY FAT SCALE

After you have determined your body fat percentage by stepping on the body fat scale, you can now easily determine your current lean weight and current fat weight. Remember to convert the body fat percentage to a decimal. If your reading is 29.2 percent, for example, 0.292 is the number to use for your calculation.

My current body weight _____
Multiplied by my current body fat percentage expressed as a decimal _____
Equals my current fat weight _____

My current body weight _____
Minus my current fat weight _____
Equals my current lean weight _____

CALCULATING CURRENT BODY FAT PERCENTAGE, CURRENT LEAN WEIGHT AND CURRENT FAT WEIGHT USING THE TAPE MEASURE

If you don't have a body fat monitor scale, there is another fairly easy way to measure body fat percentage. You can calculate your important numbers with this method, requiring only a cloth tape measure and a few calculations. Use the tape to measure your abdomen at the level of your belly button. When doing the measurement, hold the tape against the skin without being pulled too tightly, and make sure the tape is held parallel to the floor. The result of this measurement is then inserted into the following YMCA formula to determine current body fat percentage.

MEN	WOMEN
Multiply waist measurement by 4.15	Multiply waist measurement by 4.15
Equals _____	Equals _____
Minus (98.42)	Minus (76.76)
Equals _____	Equals _____
Minus (.082 x current body weight in pounds)	Minus (.082 x current body weight in pounds)
Equals _____	Equals _____
Divided by current body weight in pounds	Divided by current body weight in pounds
Equals my Current Body Fat Percentage _____	**Equals my Current Body Fat Percentage** _____

Again, we'll use Paula as an example:

Paula's current body weight is 162.0 pounds. Her waist measurement at the navel is 33.0 inches. Convert fractions of an inch to a decimal using the chart on page 41.

(4.15 x 33.0)	
Equals	136.95
Minus	(76.76)
Equals	60.19
Minus	(0.082 x 162.0)
Equals	46.906
Divided by	(162.0)
Equals	0.2895

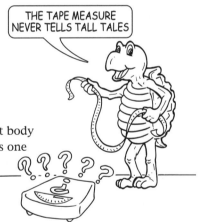

THE TAPE MEASURE NEVER TELLS TALL TALES

The results of this calculation indicate that Paula's current body fat percentage is 28.95 percent. This easy measurement is one that anyone can use to monitor trends in their changing body fat percentage.

CURRENT VERSUS TARGET

It's finally time to compare where you are now (your current numbers) with where you want to be (your target numbers).

Let's again use Paula as an example:

Paula's current body fat percentage	0.295
Multiplied by Paula's current body weight	162.0 lbs
Equals Paula's current fat weight	47.8 lbs
Paula's current body weight	162.0 lbs
Minus Paula's current fat weight	47.8 lbs
Equals Paula's current lean weight	114.2 lbs

| Paula's earlier calculated target fat weight | 22.5 lbs |
| Paula's earlier calculated target lean weight | 102.5 lbs |

By subtracting Paula's target fat weight from her current fat weight, you can see that she has 25.3 pounds of body fat to lose. Paula's situation is a good one, however, because her current lean weight of 114.2 lbs is greater than her target lean weight of 102.5 lbs.   During the time she is losing fat weight, she can afford to lose some muscle, but only a maximum of 11.7 pounds. As she loses weight it will be important for her to pay close attention, to make sure she does not lose too much muscle too quickly. The best way for her to stay on track is to regularly monitor her current lean weight and fat weight measurements and to record those readings.

To figure out where you stand, simply compare your fat weight and lean weight at your current body weight to your target numbers.

The difference between your current numbers and your target numbers will reveal the amount of fat you need to lose and the maximum amount of muscle that you can afford to lose.

My current fat weight   _____
Minus my target fat weight _____
Equals fat weight to lose   _____

My current lean weight   _____
Minus my target lean weight   _____
Equals maximum lean weight to lose _____

Almost certainly you're now carrying around a few more pounds of fat than your target fat weight number indicates you should have. It's also likely that at your current heavier weight you have more lean weight than you will need to have when your reach your target body weight. Often this is simply because you have been lifting and moving a larger body. Your calculation shows how much lean weight you can afford to lose as you are losing body fat. Keep in mind that this is the maximum amount of lean weight you should lose. Losing less muscle is always better. Some of you might find that you have a negative number for the maximum lean weight you can lose. You're not in a good situation because you have less than zero pounds of muscle you can afford to lose! In other words, your negative number indicates the amount of lean weight you need to BUILD while losing fat weight. Not to worry, we'll address that problem a little bit later to help you know what to do.

WEIGHT LOSS EXPECTATIONS

The hare-brained quick weight loss diets are notorious for making outlandish claims, promising miraculous things like: "Lose a pound a day with our miracle diet." These diets make weight loss sound fast and easy, but they ultimately fail. They fail because you'll always end up quitting the diet, either because you can't stand starving any longer, or because your metabolic rate slows down to a crawl and your weight loss hits a long and frustrating plateau.

Let's talk about weight loss expectations. What really happened the last time you went on that quick weight loss diet? For every five pounds lost, according to the scale, probably three pounds was just water weight, destined to come right back on, and one and a half pounds was precious calorie burning muscle, destined to not come right back on. Of the entire five-pound weight loss, then, only half a pound came from that store of body fat that you want to get rid of. A measly half pound, after all of that struggle and starvation! Not only is that pretty discouraging, but also, because of the muscle tissue lost, you must now eat fewer calories each day.

The promise of the Tortoise Diet is that weight loss will happen, but to be successful at preserving muscle, it must be a slow and steady process.

WEIGHT LOSS HAS TO BE SLOW TO BE PERMANENT!

About now you've got to be wondering just how fast you can realistically expect to lose weight while following the Tortoise Diet. Before I answer that question, I want to ask you something. What do you think is the main reason most people fail on a diet? The answer is because they have unrealistic expectations regarding how quickly body fat can be lost. Losing body fat is far more difficult that simply losing "weight."

PREDICTED WEIGHT LOSS

Predicting weight loss is difficult because two people starting at exactly the same weight, eating the same amount of calories, and exercising the same amount, may each lose entirely different amounts of weight. This is perfectly normal and there's no need to become discouraged. Each individual should monitor his or her own progress by monitoring loss of fat weight versus lean weight over a period of weeks. If you and your friend are following the Tortoise Diet, you WILL both lose body fat. If your friend seems to be losing weight more quickly than you are, don't get sidetracked, just keep on running your own race. The Tortoise Diet is about real life, and losing weight while actually continuing to enjoy your life!

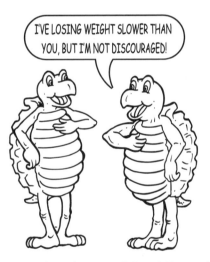

I'VE LOSING WEIGHT SLOWER THAN YOU, BUT I'M NOT DISCOURAGED!

Having said all of that, however, it can be expected that somewhere between 0.5 to 1.5 pounds of body fat can be lost per week by following the Tortoise Diet. If you are less than twenty-five pounds over your target body weight, you'll almost certainly be at the half pound of fat range, maybe even less. If you're 100 pounds or more over your target body weight, you might be closer to the one and a half pound of fat per week range. Again, talking about total weight loss is meaningless, as losing fat weight is the important thing. However, because fat weight does come off so slowly, I'm presenting these guidelines so you can have realistic expectations about the typical rate of fat loss.

One critical point in the weight loss experience where having correct expectations is especially necessary is when a person is just beginning their "race." Whenever people begin to restrict calorie intake, especially if salt intake is also reduced, a huge amount of water weight will be lost in the first couple of weeks. It is quite natural for a person to get pretty excited when they lose five pounds in the first week. Excitement stays high when another three or four pounds are lost in week two. Usually, however, by the start of week three most of the water weight is already gone, and by the end of the week, the average person loses only a relatively small amount of weight. Many people who start a diet with great enthusiasm become discouraged and quit at this point. Others may continue on for one more week, hoping to again see the kind of weight loss they had during week one. But by the end of week four, the hard reality of true fat loss has set in. This is when the average person who is only interested in quick weight loss, discouraged by the lack of progress, simply gives up.

Again, because you need realistic expectations, I am going to give a general approximation of how fast you will lose water weight in the first three weeks of the Tortoise Diet. Table 4-2 indicates the predicted amount of water weight the average person closely following the Tortoise Diet might expect to lose during the first three weeks.

Table 4-2 ESTIMATED WATER LOSS
(All figures are in pounds)

Pounds over Target Body Weight	125+	100+	75+	50+	25+	< 25
First week water loss	6.0	5.0	4.0	3.0	2.0	1.0
Second week water loss	3.0	2.5	2.0	1.5	1.0	0.5
Third week water loss	1.0	0.75	0.75	0.25	0.25	0.25
Total water loss, first three weeks	10.0	8.25	6.75	4.75	3.25	1.75

As with fat loss, you can see that heavier people will lose initial water weight faster than lighter people. Let me reiterate, these numbers are all general guidelines, and your water weight loss may be quite different from the numbers shown in Table 4-2. The real value of this table is to show that the initial rate of weight loss can be expected to slow dramatically by the end of the second week. After that time, the slower, more realistic rate of fat loss begins. You can see how easy it would be to become discouraged at the end of week three, if you thought that large initial rate of weight loss was going to continue. You need to know this, understand this, and please, don't quit the Tortoise Diet after week three!

YOUR PERSONAL WEIGHT LOSS RATIO (PWLR)

Previously, you calculated the number of pounds of fat you have to lose to achieve your target body weight and target body fat percentage. You also determined the target number of pounds of lean weight you must have when you arrive at that point. To make sure to hit those targets, close attention must be paid to not only how much "weight" is lost, but what that weight is comprised of. Because we know the scale can sometime tell tall tales, additional tools must be utilized to gauge the amount of muscle being lost, compared to the amount of fat being lost.

For most of you, the number of pounds of fat you have to lose is greater than the maximum number of pounds of lean weight you can afford to lose. Those two numbers comprise the total number of pounds of "weight" you have to lose to reach your target numbers.

A comparison of those two critical numbers can be expressed as a ratio. I call this ratio Your Personal Weight Loss Ratio (PWLR). If, for example, you have 25 pounds of fat to lose and can lose a maximum of only 8 pounds of muscle, the ratio of the two numbers would be expressed as 0.32 (8 pounds divided by 25 pounds = 0.32). A PWLR of 0.32 means that for each pound of fat lost, a maximum of 0.32 pounds of lean weight can be lost, to ensure that target numbers will be met.

Because lean weight includes not only muscle, but also water, your initial PWLR ratio should not be calculated until after the end of your first three weeks on the Tortoise Diet. As we just discussed, this is due to the large amount of water weight lost during those initial weeks. When you do calculate your initial PWLR, it will be an invaluable tool to gauge how well you are progressing toward your goals of preserving muscle while losing fat. In general, the larger the PWLR number, the more muscle you can afford to lose while you are losing fat, so the bigger the number ... the better!

To calculate your initial PWLR at the end of week three, use the following procedure.

---

1. Calculate the number of pounds of fat weight and the number of pounds of lean weight that make up your current body weight.

2. Subtract your target fat weight from your current fat weight to determine the total number of pounds of fat you still have to lose.

3. Next, subtract your target lean weight from your current lean weight to reveal the maximum number of pounds of lean weight you can afford to lose.

4. Using these two numbers, divide the maximum number pounds of lean weight you can afford to lose by the number of pounds of fat you still have to lose. The resulting number is your initial PWLR.

Repeat the same procedure each week to determine your current PWLR ratio. You'll know your weight loss is staying on track if your current PWLR remains equal to or greater than your initial PWLR number. Your aim is to keep your PWLR number as high as possible. These calculations can be done for you each week if you choose to log on to www.wintheracetolose.com and become a Tortoise Diet member.

To illustrate how to determine your PWLR, let's look again at the numbers we calculated for Paula. Paula's numbers at the end of week three on the Tortoise Diet (after initial water loss has occurred) were the following:

Paula's current body weight   162.0 lbs

Paula's current fat weight	47.8 lbs
Minus Paula's target fat weight	22.5 lbs
Equals fat weight to lose	25.3 lbs

Paula's current lean weight	114.2 lbs
Minus Paula's target lean weight	102.5 lbs
Equals maximum lean weight to lose	11.7 lbs

Paula can lose a maximum of 11.7 pounds of lean weight while she works to lose 25.3 pounds of fat weight. Dividing 11.7 by 25.3 results in 0.46, which is her initial PWLR. This ratio is unique to Paula, and it means that, for right now anyway, she should lose a maximum of only 0.46 pounds of lean weight for every 1.0 pounds of fat weight.

The following are Paula's numbers after four more weeks (after the end of week seven).

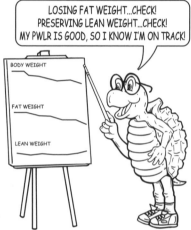

Paula's current body weight	158.0 lbs
Paula's current fat weight	44.6 lbs
Minus Paula's target fat weight	22.5 lbs
Equals her fat weight to lose	22.1 lbs
Paula's current lean weight	113.4 lbs
Minus Paula's target lean weight	102.5 lbs
Equals maximum lean weight to lose	10.9 lbs

According to the scale, Paula has lost a total of four pounds in four weeks. If Paula wasn't keeping track of her numbers, she might be discouraged by such a small weight loss. Let's delve a little deeper and see how she's really doing. Paula first subtracts her target lean weight(102.5 lbs) from her current lean weight (113.4 lbs) to learn that the difference between those two numbers is 10.9 pounds. This NOW is the maximum number of pounds of lean weight she can afford to lose while she continues to lose weight. She would next subtract her target fat weight (22.5 lbs) from her current fat weight (44.6 lbs) to learn she has 22.1 pounds of fat remaining to lose. Therefore, of the four pounds she lost, 3.2 lbs was fat weight and 0.8 lbs was lean weight.

Using her new numbers, she can calculate her current PWLR. By dividing 10.9 (the maximum number of pounds of lean weight to lose) by 22.1 (the number of pounds of fat weight to lose), she determines her current PWLR to be 0.49. Since 0.49 is a number larger than her initial PWLR of 0.46, she can happily know that her weight loss is going great! Rather than being discouraged at the loss of only four pounds in four weeks, she can be really excited that she has successfully been able to preserve most of her calorie-burning muscle tissue, while losing body fat. Her body composition is changing, and it's changing in a good way.

"You'll know your weight loss is staying on track if your current PWLR remains equal to or greater than your initial PWLR number."

CHAPTER FIVE
EXERCISE - WALKING & WEIGHTS

A WALK IN THE PARK

I'm sure you've been patiently waiting for me to eventually get around to the subject of exercise. I can almost hear the groaning. You may have never exercised before in your life, or maybe you've tried it a few times, but gave up because it was too hard. You may not feel like exercising because you're too heavy, too embarrassed, too out of condition, too busy, too hot, or too "whatever" to begin. I'll be honest with you though, right up there with healthy eating, daily exercise is an essential component of a healthy lifestyle, and successful fat loss depends on making the commitment to spend some time moving your body every day. I know that putting on those gym shorts is just about the last thing you want to do, but before you gather up your arsenal of excuses and immediately skip ahead to the next chapter, just give me a minute to tell you what I've learned about effective exercise. Effective exercise for fat loss is easy. Yes, I promise! Please read on.

The Tortoise Diet exercise program will be easy because, once again, it's based on the way our bodies actually work. During exercise, energy to fuel your muscles may come from glucose (foods you have recently eaten), from a limited supply of glycogen (glucose energy stored in the muscles), from your stored body fat, or from a combination of all three. If your goal is to lose weight, your primary concern is to exercise in such a way that stored body fat is used for energy. Here's the great news. In conjunction with eating the appropriate number of calories, Low Intensity Fat Burning aerobic exercise (LIFB) is a great tool to use to help achieve this goal, and it can truly be as simple as taking a walk in the park! That's right, an enjoyable walk in the park, a walk around your neighborhood, or a lunchtime walk at work is one of the best things you can do to lose body fat.

IF YOU CAN'T BREATHE ... SLOW DOWN!

What is the LIFB aerobic zone, and how do we know when we are in it? The word aerobic simply means "uses oxygen," and the word anaerobic means "works without oxygen." When you move your large muscles with continuous, regular movement while keeping your heart rate elevated to 60-85 percent of its maximum range, your muscles use vast quantities of oxygen as they work. You can tell by your breathing how hard you are exercising and how much oxygen is being used. In general, the harder you exercise the deeper and harder you'll have to breathe, and the more energy your muscles are using. As long as there is plenty of oxygen and fuel for the muscles, this type of activity can continue.

When your heart rate climbs above 85 percent of maximum, the activity becomes anaerobic. At this level, no matter how hard you try you can't provide the muscles with enough oxygen. In addition, during this all-out effort, a byproduct called lactic acid will build up in the muscles. Lactic acid build up will lead to muscle cramping and the feeling like they're on fire! Anaerobic exercise can only be tolerated for very short bursts of time, **so if you feel like your lungs are burning, your legs are cramping up, and you can't breathe ... slow down!**

The Tortoise Diet recommends that aerobic exercise be done mostly in the LIFB aerobic zone, with the heart rate kept between 60 percent and 70 percent of maximum range. This is your low intensity zone, the walk in the park aerobic level. To know what the appropriate zone is for you, personally, you must first determine your maximum heart rate. Maximum heart rate is the maximum number of times your heart can beat each minute, which decreases as we age. The following is a simple formula to help you determine your maximum heart rate, as well as the proper heart rate for each of the exercise zones.

220 Minus my age
Equals _____ (100% of my Maximum Heart Rate (MHR)
My low-intensity aerobic zone is   MHR x (.60) _____ to MHR x (.70) _____
My high-intensity aerobic zone is   MHR x (.70) _____ to MHR x (.85) _____
My anaerobic zone is   MHR x (.85) _____ or higher

After you have performed this calculation you will know what your heart rate should be as you exercise to stay in the correct zone. There are several ways to determine whether or not you're safely and effectively exercising in this proper zone.

1. Heart rate monitor

The optimal way to keep track of whether or not you are in the correct aerobic zone is to wear a heart rate monitor that continuously reads your heartbeat, so you can adjust your activity level immediately if you see that your heart rate is either too high or too low. These monitors range from basic models that record the time and heart rate, to more advanced models with features that record the number of calories burned and what percentage of those calories came from body fat. The basic models are fairly inexpensive, and I highly recommend that you get one.

2. Check your pulse

If you don't have a heart monitor, you'll need to periodically check your pulse. To check your pulse while you exercise, slow down your pace a little bit and place the pads of your index and middle fingers under the side of your jaw. Run the fingers down the groove in the side of the neck, next to your windpipe, until you feel the rhythmic pounding of your pulse. Make sure that you don't press too hard. Continue to move the entire time, but slow down enough so you're not bouncing around too much to be able to feel the pulse. When you're sure you have the right spot, use a watch with a second hand and count the number of heart beats in a six second period. Multiply that number by ten to determine your heartbeats per minute. Now compare that number against the heart rates you figured out for each of your aerobic zones. Either step up your effort if it's below the range you desire to be working in, or slow down and take it a little easier if it's too high.

3. Level of perceived exertion (LPE)

How hard are you working? Are you strolling along, smelling the flowers along the way, feeling like you could go on for hours, breathing with about as much effort as you do while sitting on the couch? Or are the flowers blurry as you speed on by with arms pumping, sweat pouring, and your breathing sounding like an out of shape rhinoceros? By rating your level of exertion on a scale of 1 to 10, you'll be able to determine your level of aerobic effort, and make adjustments in your activity to match your current goals for the exercise session.

LPE 1 The amount of effort required for surfing the net, watching TV, and other similar activities.

LPE 2 Warm-up activities requiring easy effort. You could sustain this level of activity for several hours. Your breathing is not labored, and you could recite the entire pledge of allegiance without difficulty.

LPE 3 Easy to moderate activity. You could sustain this level of activity for an hour, or even longer. Your breathing is a little deeper than when at rest, but you can still speak in full sentences.

LPE 4-5 Moderate activity. You could sustain this amount of effort for 30 minutes or longer. Your breathing is deep with effort, but not gasping or labored. You can speak in short sentences, which are then followed by a deep breath.

LPE 6-7 Vigorous activity. You could sustain this amount of effort for only 15-30 minutes at a time. Your breathing is very deep with effort. You are probably able to speak just a few words before taking your next deep breath. This level of activity requires some concentration.

LPE 8-9 Very intense activity. You could sustain this amount of effort for just a minute or so. You are very focused, and there's no time or energy for talking! After the activity has ended, you will continue to breathe deeply for a few minutes, as your heart rate returns to normal.

LPE 10 All-out effort. You could sustain this amount of effort for just a few seconds. You feel like your lungs may burst, your heart is beating wildly and your muscles are burning. No talking!! Pure focus!! After the activity has ended, you will continue to breathe deeply for several minutes, as your heart rate returns to   normal.

The LIFB aerobic zone is LPE 3-5. Most of us could go for a walk lasting an hour or more without becoming aerobically winded. If you are really out of shape, your muscles might get too tired to walk for an hour, but from the standpoint of lung capacity, unless you have health limitations, you probably wouldn't have to quit because of a lack of oxygen.

4. The "talk test"

As you exercise, try saying something encouraging out loud like, "I'm moving and taking good care of myself so I can be a happier and healthier person." Or, how about, "I'm getting stronger and healthier so I can hike the Grand Canyon, participate in a charity walk-a-thon, play a game of basketball with my kids, or just walk up the stairs without wheezing." Your breathing and your ability to talk or not talk is a quick and easy gauge of how intensely you are exercising. Before I got a heart monitor, I could easily gauge my own exercise intensity by calling my friends while I was exercising. They sometimes laughed and called me their obscene phone caller because of my heavy breathing, but I knew if I could talk to them easily in short sentences, followed by a big breath, I was safely working in the 60-70 percent aerobic zone. The talk test works, but I don't recommend you make business calls this way, unless you tell the person you're speaking with why you're such a heavy breather!

It is important to note that your perceived level of exertion may change from day to day, even as you perform the very same activities. How hard you feel you are exercising may be affected by many things. These could include your level of hydration, the weather, the amount of sleep you've been getting, the amount of stress you've felt that day, when you last had a snack, whether you have done a particularly heavy workout the day before, your hormonal cycle, or other factors. Jot down your perceived level of exertion each day in your journal, along with what type of activity you did and for how long. Evaluating this information over a period of time will help you to identify your own individual patterns. When do your exercise sessions feel effortless and enjoyable? When do your feet feel like lead? When do you quit after ten minutes and when are you able to continue for an hour or longer? Based on this data, you may be able to better plan your exercise activities, not only for the best weight-loss results, but also for the most enjoyment possible.

WHY LOW INTENSITY AEROBICS IS BEST

My critics are bound to say if you exercise in a higher aerobic zone you burn calories faster, so why waste time walking. Wouldn't a heart-pounding workout provide more bang for your workout buck? My answer is to review one more time the commitments you've made. Your goal is to improve your health and achieve permanent weight loss. Everything about the Tortoise Diet revolves around these commitments, and therefore, any activity or habit involving health or weight loss has to be fully supportive of these two goals. There are four reasons why I recommend LIFB aerobic exercise over higher intensity aerobics, not only for overweight beginners, but for everyone else as well.

1. To achieve permanent weight loss, exercise is a daily habit you have to develop, and you must make the commitment to do it for the rest of your life. Working out at a breakneck pace to burn as many calories as possible for an hour, five days a week is not something that most people can keep up forever. I believe it's more likely that a person can actually find twenty minutes or longer to walk sometime during the day, and will be able to continue to do this enjoyable activity for the rest of their lives. Whether you walk, swim, cycle, or do some other kind of aerobic exercise in the LIFB zone, it's most important that you find something you love to do! Exercise has to be something you look forward to, not something you dread.

2. Exercise performed in the LIFB zone burns a higher percentage of body fat than exercise done at a higher intensity. At this modest level of exercise, the total number of calories burned may not be huge, but after the first twenty minutes approximately 50-60 percent of what is burned will be taken directly from the fat storage warehouse. Because LIFB aerobic exercise burns primarily stored body fat, circulating blood glucose as well as glycogen stores remain available to supply the

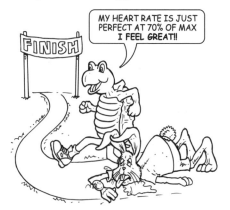

MY HEART RATE IS JUST PERFECT AT 70% OF MAX I FEEL GREAT!!

FINISH

60

body's ongoing energy needs. This means that blood sugar levels remain fairly stable, so excess hunger does not occur. Also, since the energy supply from fat is virtually endless and muscle fatigue does not set in, as it does with higher intensity exercise, this type of activity can be sustained for long periods of time. When you are eating at your "just right" calorie deficit by following your Weight Loss Calorie Plan, the goal is NOT to burn off a lot of calories and make the calorie deficit even larger. Instead, your goal is to have your working muscles burn body fat. Thus, LIFB is a great way to burn body fat, and the longer it is done - the better. If you eat according to your Weight Loss Calorie Plan and walk on a treadmill at a moderate pace with your heart rate in the LIFB zone, you're achieving your goal of burning fat from the storage warehouse as well as the person next to you who is gasping for breath!

3. Injury is a definite concern whenever anyone starts an exercise program, but especially if you're not a kid anymore. As we age our muscles weaken, our tendons and ligaments become less flexible, and injury occurs much more frequently than when we were young. And unfortunately, when middle-aged people injure themselves it can take a long time to heal. Therefore, diving into a vigorous exercise (or sports) program without first working up to a better level of fitness is risky, not only for injury but also for a heart attack. This is definitely not supportive of our goal to improve our health. You are much more likely to enjoy safe exercise without hurting yourself with LIFB exercise.

4. The final reason I recommend LIFB exercise over higher intensity aerobics is preservation of lean weight, which is muscle tissue. You know how important it is to preserve muscle tissue during weight loss. For the purpose of our discussion, however, it's important to remember that if you're eating at a calorie deficit, which you will be if you're trying to lose weight, LIFB exercise will preserve muscle tissue while high intensity aerobics tend to cause the breakdown of muscle tissue. Because muscle burns so many more calories than body fat, this is counterproductive to our weight loss efforts.

"AVOID THE PLOP"

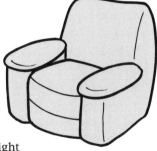

For many people who are overweight, exercise is not a big part of life. In fact, for many of us, moving from the car to the desk to the couch and searching for the remote may be the most activity we do in a day. Believe me, I know, because I certainly was once at that point. But when I learned that a large percentage of the fat calories I burn when I exercise in this easy fat-burning zone come right off my body, I got motivated to go for a walk! I suggest walking because it's something that is enjoyable, it doesn't cost a thing, and the only equipment required is a good pair of shoes. There are many other choices for LIFB activities, of course, and whatever activity you choose is really up to you.

Actually, the type of activity you choose has a lot to do with your general fitness level. For some of you who are quite overweight and have not been exercising, merely standing in front of the television and marching in place while rhythmically moving your arms up and down may raise your pulse to the LIFB aerobic zone. If this is the case, try doing this effective LIFB exercise for at least 20 minutes, even longer if you can. As your health and fitness progress and as your weight decreases, it will take more effort to achieve the same aerobic heart rate, so you'll have to step up the pace and increase the intensity a bit. An easy walk around the neighborhood that used to cause you to breathe deeply and get your heart rate to the correct level might now need to be a brisk walk. When you get in really good shape, you may have to include some hills to keep your heart rate in the LIFB zone. When you do find that you need to push a little harder to remain in the proper aerobic zone, congratulate yourself ... you've made progress.

If it sounds like I'm an advocate of walking, you're right. My husband and I love to walk after dinner to "avoid the plop." Afterward we look forward to coming home and enjoying our evening snack. It's our ritual on most nights. It has become a good health habit! But please let me restate that it's really important to find something YOU love doing. Activities such as step aerobics or riding a stationary bicycle while watching the news, exercising to a video while your kids do their homework after dinner, dancing around the living room to your favorite music, or swimming laps in the pool might work for you. Be creative. Just find something you love to do, and start doing it!

HOW LONG EACH DAY SHOULD I DO LOW-INTENSITY AEROBICS?

When you are overweight, your heart, lungs, and every joint in your body are already working under a heavier load than they were designed to bear. You may know what I'm talking about ... the aching knees and back, or feeling winded when taking the stairs. When I was really heavy, I wasn't able to walk much because of a sore foot. I actually had something called a Morton's Neuroma in my right foot. Every time I walked for any length of time the ball of my foot would get numb and I would start to limp painfully. I went to a podiatrist who, instead of saying "Ma'am, you need to lose some weight," injected the foot with cortisone. That wasn't the cure I needed though, and it wasn't until I lost weight that I noticed it was getting better. Now, 120 pounds lighter, my foot doesn't bother me anymore!

When I was just beginning my weight loss, I wasn't up to doing a lot of aerobics. Also, I never would have been caught dead wearing shorts to exercise at a gym. I was ready, however, to make the commitment to myself to simply get moving a little bit every day. I just had to put my shoes on and get started. I decided to begin by exercising for 20 minutes, at least four days a week. Because of my sore foot I decided not to walk, but every day when I got home I put my tennis shoes on and headed to the garage. I had an exercise bike and a stair climber out there and, even though for many years they had served only as clothes hangers, now that I was ready, they came in handy. I began slowly, placing the tension on the lowest level, because I was in very poor condition. Early on, just barely moving my legs caused my heart rate to jump up. I purchased an inexpensive heart rate monitor wristwatch, because I wanted to be sure to keep my heart rate in the 60-70 percent range. I'm sure I didn't look graceful or athletic, but because I was in the privacy of my own garage, I didn't care. It was so convenient to just step out the door to begin my exercise that I never had the excuse of not being able to get around to it.

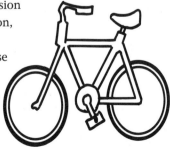

On days when I was feeling kind of tired, I put my shoes on and told myself that if I was still too tired after five minutes, I would quit. What almost always happened was that five minutes became ten, and pretty soon the twenty minutes was over and I felt great! After a few weeks of consistently exercising for twenty minutes a day, I began to increase the duration of my daily exercise by a little bit each week. By the end of the first year, I had worked up to a full hour of daily aerobic exercise. Eventually my foot didn't hurt so much and I was in good enough shape for Charlie and I to start our after dinner walking program. To this day, we try to walk almost every evening. If we have a free weekend, we go on a long hike in the canyons near our home, sometimes walking in the LIFB zone for two or three hours.

With continued exercise, I got stronger and I lost more weight. As I progressed, I became very interested in the effects various types of exercise had on my body and how they impacted the way I felt. I began to experiment with other exercise techniques and combinations of activities, and jotted down how I felt and how they affected my weight loss. I kept track of these results, and learned a lot about what did and what did not work. I read everything I could to try to find out the physiologic reasons why certain things worked better than others. The culmination of my own experience, as well as my research on the subject has evolved into the exercise recommendations of the Tortoise Diet.

Don't think you can't exercise because you're too overweight or out of shape. Exercise is mandatory if you want to lose weight and be healthy! It may help you to visualize me, at 248 pounds, starting out by simply doing what I was able to do. That's the place for you to begin, as well. You may take a smaller step, or move at a slower pace than someone who is more fit, but even that amount of movement will be beneficial. As your fitness level improves, the effort and intensity required to achieve the same effect will have to be cranked up a little bit. It's a constantly evolving process, and you will amaze yourself with what you will eventually be able to achieve with the committed, daily effort to put those shoes on and get going!

Once you are in better shape and have been exercising for awhile, my recommendation is for LIFB exercise to be done for at least forty minutes a day, four to six days each week. If twenty minutes of LIFB exercise is all you can handle, or fit into your busy day, then that's the place to start, increasing your time as you are able. Because of the way your body uses energy during exercise, fat doesn't come out of storage very easily until after you've been doing your LIFB exercise for at least twenty minutes. For this reason, the longer you can exercise the better. Some good news, though, is that it's important to rest one day per week. Give your body some down time. This is when muscle tissue fibers repair themselves and get rested for the next round of workouts. But notice I said rest one day per week ... not four or five!

* * Never perform any kind of exercise that causes pain. As was my case, if walking causes you discomfort, figure out a different way to do your LIFB aerobics. Good alternative choices for LIFB exercise might be swimming or riding a stationary bicycle. Please check with your doctor before beginning this or any other exercise program. It is a good idea to rule out any underlying physical conditions, so you'll be able to exercise safely. * *

YOU GOTTA KEEP THOSE MUSCLES

It's likely that you have more muscle at your current heavier weight than you will have when you reach your target body weight. It's important to take steps early, as opposed to later, to preserve most of that muscle during your weight loss process. As you know, if you lose too much muscle tissue, your weight loss will slow to a crawl. Maintaining your personal "just right" calorie deficit is the first key to lean weight preservation. Performing LIFB aerobic exercise is the second key component for fat loss and muscle preservation. The very important third key to preserve muscle is the other half of the Tortoise Diet "Walking & Weights" program ... the strength-training part.

How important is exercising with weights? YOU WILL NEVER REACH YOUR TARGET BODY WEIGHT AND TARGET BODY FAT PERCENTAGE IF YOU DON'T PRESERVE MUSCLE AS YOU LOSE WEIGHT. Sorry, I need to stop shouting now, but I just wanted to dispel any notion you might have that you can achieve your goals without strength training. Ohhh ... nooo, you just knew it had to get worse! As with LIFB exercise, however, I promise you it's not going to be that tough.

CHANGE YOUR LIFE ... ONE WEIGHT AT A TIME

The Tortoise Diet "Walking & Weights" exercise program involves, as the name implies, working with weights! Strengthening your muscles by using them to push and pull against increasing levels of weight resistance will help preserve, and may even build additional lean weight. It may sound daunting at first, but an effective strength program doesn't have to be long and complicated. In fact, each strength-training session should take only about twenty to thirty minutes. And here's the great news. It's really important to rest your muscles between weight lifting sessions, so strength-training exercise will be limited to two sessions each week. Twenty to thirty minutes, twice each week ... see, I told you it wasn't going to be that tough!

Strength training is beneficial for many important reasons. Not only will these exercises burn body fat and preserve or even build calorie-burning muscle, they will also help to condition the heart, maintain strong bones, and keep joints flexible. In addition, strength-training will just plain make life, in general, easier for you. When your muscles are strengthened you will have better functional fitness and less chance of injury while performing the routine activities of your day. Lifting babies or bags of groceries, running to catch the bus, playing tennis on the weekends, or whatever it is you do in your life will become much easier as you become stronger.

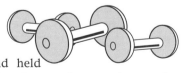

You don't need fancy weight machines to get started with a strength-training program. If you're going to work out at home, the only equipment you'll need are some hand held dumbbells. I don't recommend the type of hand-held weights that you have to change plates on a bar, because they are too cumbersome and time consuming. Buy individual hand weights, two of each weight. If you are brand new to strength training, it's not necessary to go overboard in the beginning and buy super heavy weights. I currently have pairs of

2 lb., 5 lb., 8 lb., 10 lb. and 15 lb. hand-held weights. I didn't add the 10 lb. and 15 lb. weights, however, until I had been exercising for a number of months. Men might want to add a pair of 20 lb. and 25 lb. weights to their collection, as well.

Don't worry, ladies, the Tortoise Diet strength-training program is NOT designed to "bulk you up." You don't have enough testosterone in your system to develop gigantic muscles. Instead, your body will appear smaller, sleeker, and shapelier by developing strong and lean muscles that look absolutely feminine and beautiful.

THE TORTOISE DIET STRENGTH TRAINING PROGRAM

As mentioned, strength-training exercises will be performed twice each week, allowing a minimum of 48 hours of rest between sessions. Always perform a five-minute aerobic activity prior to beginning your routine. This activity will elevate your heart rate and warm up your muscles to make them more pliable and ready to work. The Tortoise Diet strength-training program includes two different exercises for each of the five major muscle groups. For each of the exercises, one complete movement of the weight up and down or back and forth, through the entire range of motion of the joint, is considered one repetition. For maximum effect, it is desirable to lift the weight using a one-two-three-four count, pause at the top of the movement and squeeze the muscle, and then return back to the starting position on a one-two-three-four count. Don't swing the weights around and let momentum do the work. Always keep your movements controlled. Get into the habit of inhaling while lowering the weight and exhaling while lifting the weight. Don't hold your breath! It will be common for the heart rate to rise higher than the 60-70 percent level. It will, in fact, be quite normal for your heart rate to climb into the anaerobic (>85% of maximum) range as you exert yourself. When this occurs, just keep breathing and slow down your pace a little. Keep a record in your journal of the exercises you perform, the number of repetitions and sets of each exercise and how much weight you use for each set. Also note how you felt during and afterward, and what your heart rate and breathing were like during the exercise session.

Completion of the entire number of repetitions for each exercise comprises one set of the exercise. You will be doing two sets for each of the ten different exercises during every strength-training session. Keep moving at a steady pace, from one exercise to the next, only taking as much time as necessary between sets to allow yourself to catch your breath.

The amount of weight you select for the first set of each exercise should be one that allows you to complete a minimum of eight and a maximum of sixteen controlled full repetitions, while maintaining excellent form. In other words, you are to select a weight that is heavy enough that, at somewhere between eight and sixteen repetitions, you just won't be able to lift the weight any more with good form. This is very important. In order to get the full benefit from a strength-training program, muscles must be worked to the point of "failure."

The amount of weight you select for the second set of each exercise will be a heavier weight that allows you to complete a minimum of four repetitions and a maximum of eight controlled full repetitions. As you did for the first set, select a heavy enough weight that allows you to work the muscle until it is totally fatigued. When you have finished the entire strength-training routine, drink some more water and perform some long, easy stretches of your major muscles. When stretching, the key thing to remember is to do easy stretches that don't hurt. If you feel any pain at all during the stretch, you're pushing the muscle too far. Also, try to hold each stretch for about 30 seconds. Slow and easy, that's the key to avoiding injury.

You will find the Tortoise Diet strength-training exercises in Appendix E, along with illustrations and further instructions.

Just a word of caution ... when you begin any strength-training program it's extremely important to take precautions to avoid injury. Warming up before your workout, and using a slow and easy controlled technique when lifting weights is absolutely essential each and every time you perform your routine. If at any time during your workout you experience any joint pain or other sharp pain ... **STOP**. Take as many days off as necessary to be able to start your workouts again without pain.

SHOULD I JOIN A GYM?

A question you may have at this point is whether you need to join a gym to start a strength-training program. My answer is no. You might want to, and it's okay to do so, but it's certainly not necessary. For me, I found that by the time I could get my gym attire rounded up and put on, get in the car and drive to the gym, park, walk in and find the machine I wanted to use, I could have already finished a complete workout at home. If you prefer the social aspect however, or it's convenient for you to go to a gym, by all means do so. If you do work out at a gym, ask a staff member to show you the correct adjustment of any machines you decide to use. A machine adjusted for a person 6' 2" will not fit you if you're 5' 2"! Also, you may find it helpful to enlist the assistance and instruction of a qualified personal trainer. Whether at the gym or at home, especially as you are first learning the exercise routine, a trainer will be able to make sure you are performing the exercises with correct technique.

MY PWLR IS GETTING SMALLER, WHAT DO I DO?

Two situations require your immediate attention during weight loss. The first is if your weekly calculations indicate that your current PWLR has become smaller than your initial PWLR. The second also involves PWLR, but it is when your current lean weight is smaller than your target lean weight, and your PWLR is a negative number. In both cases, your job is to start your PWLR headed back into bigger numbers! What should you do if your Personal Weight Loss Ratio is drifting downward or has "gone negative?" In other words, when the amount of muscle you can afford to lose during weight loss is getting smaller all the time. The prescription is to hit those weights!

BUILDING THE EXERCISE HABIT

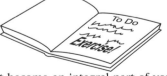

The Tortoise Diet "Walking & Weights" program must become an integral part of your new good health habits if you plan to live up to your commitments of achieving good health and permanent weight loss. Unfortunately, it's one thing to know how important exercise is, but it's quite another to successfully turn it into a daily habit. Your appointment book is probably pretty full! In fact, right now you may be getting your excuses ready. But remember that discussion about dropkicking and prioritizing in Chapter One? The decision to include exercise in your life is just a daily obligation, and like everything else, it must be prioritized and have a time allocated for it or it won't get done. It's not important what time of the day it's done, but simply that it is done. Set the goal and, make it happen! Finding time to exercise is something anyone can do, with a little creativity and with an eye fixed on the goal of good health, increased energy, increased self-esteem, and a firm and fit body. I've already mentioned some of the ways I have found time in my life to exercise. However, based on your own preferences and your schedule, you'll need to identify your own best time to include exercise in your day.

CLIMB A MOUNTAIN ... WHEN YOU'RE 80!

Before leaving our discussion of exercise, I want to go back over some key points I believe are important for you to understand and take to heart. If you're under 40 years old, you may not believe the day is coming when you're going to start feeling old. It seems for many people that age 40 is about the time when your back starts hurting, your joints become a little stiff, you don't sleep as well, little injuries take a lot longer to heal, and that fast metabolism you've always had seems to be slowing down. Maybe some of these things sound familiar, and you definitely know what I'm talking about! Worse yet, maybe you're under 40 years old and you know what I'm talking about! The great news for all age groups is that, with a healthy diet, along with a serious strength training and aerobic program, you don't have to age! You will, of course, grow older, but the physical deterioration and disease that we commonly associate with aging is, to a very large degree, something that doesn't necessarily have to occur. With a healthy eating plan you can dramatically reduce your risk of dying of heart disease, cancer, or diabetes. With a strength training program to retain your muscle mass and to keep your bones strong, there is no physiologic reason you can't be nearly as strong at 60 as you were at 20. Add those two components to a good aerobic exercise program and there is no reason why you can't climb a mountain ... when you're 80!

"The decision to include exercise
in your life is just a daily obligation,
and like everything else, it must be
prioritized and have a time allocated
for it or it won't get done."

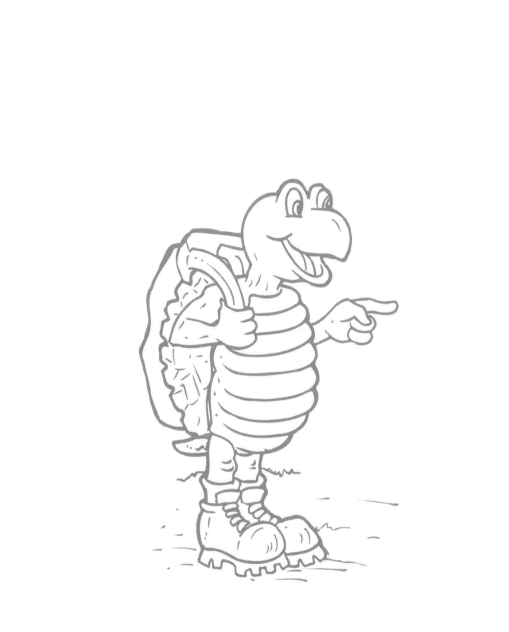

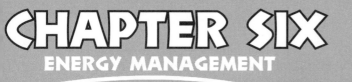

CHAPTER SIX
ENERGY MANAGEMENT

PUT ON YOUR ENERGY MANAGER HAT

To achieve your goals, you need to "put on your energy manager hat." By this I mean you must become adept at being able to tell when your body's energy tanks are empty, need refilling or are already full enough. At anytime during your day if your energy tanks get too full they may be in danger of overflowing into the fat storage warehouse.

You have already learned what kind of food to eat and how to exercise effectively. It is now time for the successful energy manager to learn the important skills of knowing how and when to eat. This require developing an understanding of how to make adjustments to the energy inflow, based on the energy outflow that has occurred. It sounds complicated, but by the end of this chapter you will be a top-notch "energy manager" and a fat-burning machine.

IT'S ALL IN WHEN YOU EAT IT

The very process of digesting food actually increases the metabolic rate, and accounts for about 10 percent of the energy you require each day. Therefore, it is very important to know that eating small quantities of nutrient-dense foods regularly throughout the day will not only prevent you from feeling hungry, it will help to maintain your metabolic rate. This is yet another key to weight loss success!

I've noticed that many people who are overweight eat a big majority of their daily calories from afternoon through bedtime. If you are one of these people, this could be one of the more difficult habits to change ... but change you must! The Tortoise Diet recommends dividing the total number of calories allotted by your Weight Loss Calorie Plan into six meals per day, in the following proportions:

Meal #1   20% (breakfast)
Skipping breakfast is a big mistake! The longer you wait to eat in the morning, the more your body will go into starvation mode, and the more your metabolic rate will slow down. Also, if you wait too long, by the time you do get around to eating you'll be so hungry you'll probably be tempted to eat everything in sight. So when your alarm goes off in the morning, wake up your metabolism by developing the habit of eating within an hour after rising. Breakfast can be something simple and quick, but it absolutely must contain protein as well as complex carbohydrate foods, plus a little heart healthy fat, if desired. Also make sure to drink 16 ounces of water within the first hour of the morning.

Meal #2   10% (mid-morning snack)
You'll be a little hungry by the time three hours has passed. Make sure you have a portable, enjoyable snack, containing protein and complex carbohydrate foods that meet your particular calorie needs. Become very familiar with these "Top 40" list foods. Shop for them, prepare them, have them handy, and eat them regularly.

Meal #3   25% (lunch)

Three more hours have passed and you'll again be a little hungry. Be sure to include protein, complex carbohydrates, and a little bit of heart healthy fat in this meal. Develop two or three lunches that you enjoy and meet your calorie needs, shop for them, prepare them, have them handy, and eat them regularly. I found it particularly helpful to make soup a regular part of my lunch menu.

Meal #4   10% (mid-afternoon snack)

Same information as for Meal #2.

Meal #5   25% (dinner)

Three more hours have passed, and it's time to eat again. Remember to drink a 16 ounce glass of water when you feel the little twinge of hunger, usually about an hour before the next scheduled meal. I strongly encourage you to develop a repertoire of 5-10 healthy dinners that you and your family can enjoy eating every week. If you're not eating a green salad as a main course, try to eat a green salad to begin each dinner. Include at least one, preferably two, additional vegetables along with some lean protein with the meal. I recommend taking a nice walk or performing some other form of LIFB exercise for 20-60 minutes after Meal #5 if you can. There are so many health benefits associated with simply "avoiding the plop" after a larger meal. In addition to burning calories and fat, you'll enjoy better sleep, better digestion, more relaxation, and some fun family time or enjoyable "me" time.

Meal #6   10% (evening snack)

This meal can be eaten from 2-3 hours after Meal #5. Make sure that Meal #6 does not contain any fats, otherwise, just as you usually do, include protein and carbohydrate foods.

Developing this good habit of eating every three hours throughout the day will provide adequate energy to keep you feeling fairly satisfied. It's normal to feel some mild hunger before each meal and before you go to bed at night. However, if you're eating the correct amount of filling, nutrient-dense protein and complex carbohydrate foods, the hunger you experience should never be overwhelming. Experiencing a small amount of hunger is actually a good sign and means you're losing weight correctly, but you should never get to the point of feeling ravenous and uncomfortable.

If you leave the house every day for work, as many of us do, it's obvious that to eat every three hours, you're going to have to take food with you. You may have a concern about having to eat so many meals while at work. My response is that most people get a mid-morning and mid-afternoon break, which is the perfect opportunity to eat a quick meal. And even if you don't get a break, we're not talking about a five-course meal. Meals #2 and #4 don't consist of very many calories, and shouldn't take more than a minute or two to eat.

I CAN EAT SIX MEALS A DAY SO I NEVER FEEL DEPRIVED!

MEAL #1   MEAL #2   MEAL #3   MEAL #4   MEAL #5   MEAL #6

MAINTAINING THE BALANCE

Most people won't have a problem understanding the unfortunate fact that if you eat too much in a given day you will gain weight. A much more subtle problem is how eating a large meal, even in a day when we don't go over our total daily calorie limit, affects weight loss.

Because it takes approximately four to six hours to digest a meal containing complex carbohydrates, proteins and fats, there is about a four-hour window for the body to use up the energy from a meal. Whenever we sit down to a large meal and take in more calories than our bodies require for the next few hours, whatever isn't needed at the time will be stored away for later use. This stored energy is what we know (and hate) as fat, and it's being stored right there on your hips and tummy.

This means eating large amounts of food at one sitting is a bad idea! One way to prevent fat storage after eating an extra large meal is to get out there for a walk, or some other form of LIFB exercise, to burn off the excess calories you've taken in. Obviously, the other way to prevent fat storage is to simply limit the calories taken in at any one sitting to the amount your body is able to use for energy in the next few hours. These are your two choices if you want to prevent fat storage ... you can either choose to not eat too much, or you can plan to get up and move.

I AM CONSTANTLY MONITORING CALORIES TAKEN IN AGAINST CALORIES BURNED!

ENERGY IN

ENERGY OUT

To prevent fat storage, while still providing the calorie deficit required for weight loss, the maximum number of calories you should eat at any one sitting is 35 percent of your total Weight Loss Calorie Plan. Therefore, although not ideal, it is allowable for a 25 percent meal to be combined with a 10 percent meal. This is okay as a way to occasionally enjoy a bigger breakfast, lunch or dinner. Whenever you combine two meals, the 10 percent meal scheduled for either just before or just after that 25 percent meal should be deleted.

You may wonder how to make adjustments if you do eat more than 35 percent at any one meal. The correct response would be to skip the next scheduled 10 percent meal and get right back on your regular Tortoise Diet eating schedule. A mistake so many dieters make is to try to compensate for periods of over-eating by not eating for the rest of the day. The binge/starve cycle of dieting just doesn't work, so get back on track as soon as you can.

Conversely, eating too little throughout the day can also present problems. Spreading the calorie deficit provided by your Weight Loss Calorie Plan throughout the day is ideal. Increasing the calorie deficit by skipping meals and under-eating is not recommended.

Another situation in which the calorie deficit is increased, which must be accounted for, is when energy is expended during exercise. This is good news, because exercise increases energy needs. When you exercise you must replace of the portion of the calories burned to ensure that the calorie deficit is kept "just right."   What you must realize is that your

Weight Loss Calorie Plan provides the minimum number of calories your body must have each day to prevent your metabolic rate from slowing down. Exercising like crazy as a way to hurry up weight loss is just another "hare-brained" approach that doesn't work.

Therefore, when you exercise you must add calories to the meal closest in time to when the exercise is performed, to keep that "just right" calorie deficit. Add calories based on the following:

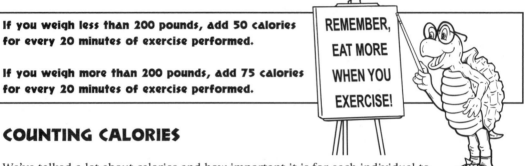

If you weigh less than 200 pounds, add 50 calories for every 20 minutes of exercise performed.

If you weigh more than 200 pounds, add 75 calories for every 20 minutes of exercise performed.

REMEMBER, EAT MORE WHEN YOU EXERCISE!

COUNTING CALORIES

We've talked a lot about calories and how important it is for each individual to follow their own personalized Weight Loss Calorie Plan to keep that "just right" calorie deficit for fat loss. How can you get this important facet of energy management to work in real life? Many people find that counting calories is just too cumbersome and difficult. As I've said earlier, I whole-heartedly agree! Fortunately, there is an easier way to keep track of your all-important daily calorie totals. I find that the more I regularly eat the foods I like, and eat them in the specific quantities I have determined to be correct for my own calorie needs, the easier it is to keep track of how many calories I am taking in.

When I developed my own personal "Top 40" list, I wrote down the calorie counts of the foods I liked and the appropriate portion size for my own calorie needs. These were the foods I used to develop what are now my favorite meals. I kept a list of these foods and their calorie counts up on my refrigerator until eventually I became very familiar with the number of calories they contained. Now it's pretty easy for me to know how many calories I'm eating for breakfast and how many calories I pack into my insulated bag to take to work. This is the point you need to get to, as well.

The calorie counts of many healthy, nutrient-dense foods are listed in Appendix B. Complete meals with specified calorie totals are listed in Appendix A. Appendix C contains recipes in which the calorie total for the entire recipe has been determined, so you can select the serving size that meets your specific calorie needs. If you use these resources to develop your own "Top 40" list of routine foods and meals, you too can get to know the calorie counts of your own favorites without having to look them up each time. At that point, you won't need to count anymore!

HARA HACHI BU

In a part of Okinawa, Japan, there are a large percentage of people who live to be more than 100 years old. These people, as a group, are slim and remain vigorous and active well into old age. There are probably a number of factors contributing to their health and longevity, but an important one may be their practice of Hara Hachi Bu. Hara Hachi Bu simply means making it a practice to stop eating when you feel about 80 percent full.

The dietary habit of Hara Hachi Bu is effective because it is based on sound physiologic principles. When we eat food, many complex hormonal, chemical, and physical interactions occur. There is about a twenty-minute delay between when we have eaten enough food, and the time our brain gets the message. That means that if we wait to stop eating until we become aware that we feel full, we will already have eaten more than we should.

It's all too easy to sit down to eat, only to suddenly find you've consumed an entire plate-full, bowl-full, or bag-full of food. You didn't mean to eat that much, you just weren't paying attention. Hara Hachi Bu is simply developing the ability to pay attention to how your body feels as you eat and to learn to effectively gauge when you have eaten enough and have satisfied your body's need for fuel. It takes effort to stop eating before we feel pleasantly full, but as with all good habits, it becomes easier with repetition and time, especially once you truly believe that when your brain eventually gets its signal, you won't feel hungry.

I encourage you to try it for yourself the next time you sit down to a meal. Consciously enjoy the total experience of relaxation and conversation while you eat. Take in the aroma, the color, the texture, and the taste of your food. Eat slowly and savor each bite. Periodically, take a sip of water and try to rate your hunger. Pay attention to how full you are beginning to feel, and when you think you've reached the 80 percent full level, STOP eating. Take another sip of water and turn your attention to something besides the food. The very process of slowing down the experience of eating will give your brain a chance to receive the full signal from the stomach. After twenty minutes or so, I predict that you'll truly feel 100 percent full!

Mindful eating has benefits for both health and weight loss, and is a good habit to develop. Make an attempt to practice Hara Hachi Bu as often as you can. Learn to experience what the sensation of being about 80 percent full feels like. Learning to put on your energy manager hat will prevent you from mindlessly finishing off a huge amount of food. If you practice Hara Hachi Bu at home, where you know the approximate calorie content of the foods you are eating, you will be better able to gauge your calorie intake in situations where you are not so sure of the number of calories in the food, like at a restaurant or a party. On those occasions, because you have learned to pay attention to how your body feels when you are about 80 percent full, you will be able to keep calorie intake under control and enjoy the experience.

There are, of course, times when I neglect the practice of Hara Hachi Bu and end up feeling too full. I call those times "HARA HACHI BOO BOO!"

TGIW AND "FOOL YOUR BODY" TO REV UP THAT METABOLISM!

I'll be the first to admit that food is not only a physical necessity, but is inextricably and pleasurably woven into the many occasions of our lives. If consistently practiced as a lifestyle, however, the Energy Management techniques and habits you learn will accommodate events such as restaurant meals, birthday parties, business lunches, vacations, and even the seemingly endless holiday season, when most thoughts of healthy eating and weight loss are usually abandoned with the first piece of pumpkin pie.

A secret I learned early on that has really worked for me was dividing the long process of weight loss into small "chunks" of time. I found that if I divided the week into three or four day segments of closely following my Weight Loss Calorie Plan, I could then look forward to a special meal twice each week. Usually on Wednesdays and Saturdays, I enjoy a dinner out at a restaurant or a night with friends. Because Wednesday's are one of the nights I look forward to, I started calling them my "TGIW" meals. This ability to let loose a little bit and enjoy foods I wasn't eating on a daily basis, was a practice that made my new healthy eating plan seem pretty painless. TGIW is a great thing for several reasons. Despite our best efforts to incorporate the habits aimed toward maintaining an optimal metabolic rate and that "just right" calorie deficit, our very smart bodies will still sense we're not providing it all the calories it wants. Because of this, the metabolic rate will gradually slow down a little. Thus, besides the pure livability and enjoyment factor, believe it or not, a couple times a week it actually helps in your long-term weight loss efforts to bump up your calorie intake and eat a little more! The key here, of course, is to "Fool Your Body" just a little. It is not a license to over-stuff it by eating a huge number of calories. **That's why effective energy managers will make it a habit to add back 400 calories to their Weight Loss Calorie Plan twice each week while enjoying a TGIW meal.** This will essentially "fool" the body into revving up the metabolic rate and to not worry because starvation is not going to happen anytime soon.

To calculate how many calories you can eat during a TGIW meal, use the following guidelines. The maximum calories allotted for a TGIW meal should be:

> 25% of daily calorie total allotted by your Weight Loss Calorie Plan (a meal)
> + 10% of daily calorie total allotted by your Weight Loss Calorie Plan (a snack)
> + 400 additional "Fool Your Body" calories
> + Any calories to be added for exercise
> = TGIW meal calorie allotment

Let's use a Weight Loss Calorie Plan of 1,400 calories as an example:

> 25% (meal #5) = 350 calories
> + 10% (meal #6, which would be omitted that evening) = 140 calories
> + 400 "Fool Your Body" calories = 400 calories
> + the calories to be added for 60 minutes of exercise = 150 calories

Total calorie allotment for the TGIW dinner = 1,040 calories.

This may sound like quite a bit, and it's certainly more than you would usually eat for one of your Weight Loss Calorie Plan meals. However, since the calories at a restaurant meal can add up very quickly, 1,040 calories is not enough to go crazy and eat everything in sight.

I must caution you about drinking alcohol while eating a TGIW meal. It's a big challenge to manage energy and prevent fat storage when alcohol is consumed. For this reason, I recommend that the calories for each alcoholic beverage you consume should be counted as DOUBLE their actual caloric value! To illustrate, let's say before arriving at your favorite restaurant, you've calculated your calorie allotment for a TGIW meal to be 1000 calories. A cocktail, a glass of wine or a beer each typically contains about 150 calories. For every glass, then, you should count the total as a whopping 300 calories! A typical dessert might also contain 300 calories ... and that's if you plan to share it with your dining partner. If you go out to this meal with the idea that you're going to have two drinks and share a dessert, that's already 900 calories! That doesn't leave much for the salad and bread, much less the entree.

Here's a suggestion. If you are going to drink, how about limiting your alcohol consumption to one alcoholic beverage at your TGIW meal. Then go home and enjoy a non-fat hot chocolate or a non-fat chocolate pudding for less than 100 calories per serving, instead of ordering dessert? If you do that, you can prevent going over your TGIW calorie allotment while still enjoying the things you like to eat and drink.

The purpose of TGIW/"Fool your Body" is twofold, one being to maintain the metabolic rate and the other being a way to make the Tortoise Diet a plan that can last a lifetime. It's important to note that on these two days each week, there will be no calorie deficit. On those days, then, you will NOT lose body fat. This is why it is so critical to limit TGIW meals to twice weekly, and to limit the meal to the maximum number of calories allowed, based on your calculations. If you follow these TGIW rules, the other five days each week will feel easier to you mentally and emotionally, and on those days you will have the calorie deficit needed for fat loss.

TGIW meals really helped me during my weight loss. Because I could always look forward to an enjoyable meal a couple times each week, I was able to really focus my energies on sticking with my healthy eating program during the other days. It felt pretty easy, because I knew it would only be a few days before I could TGIW again. Also, because I didn't feel perpetually deprived and hungry all the time while following my Weight Loss Calorie Plan each day, I didn't feel the need to indulge in every fattening thing on the menu during a TGIW meal. It's a new and very freeing experience to be able to treat food in this fashion.

Even now, after having lost all the weight I need to lose, I continue to incorporate this newly developed habit into my life. For you, it could be a Sunday breakfast, Tuesday lunch with a friend, a Saturday barbeque or party, or maybe just an opportunity to cook a decadent long-time family favorite at home. Maybe instead of TGIW, you'll say TGIM or TGIT, or whatever days you choose! Eating nutritious foods in the proper portions is a great thing, and is essential to be able to meet your goals for weight loss and health. But, never again enjoying a steak dinner with a baked potato, Caesar salad and a few bites of mud pie for dessert may be just too much to ask!

> "TGIW meals really helped me during my weight loss. I found that because I could always look forward to an enjoyable meal a couple times each week, I was able to really focus my energies on sticking with my healthy eating program during the other days."

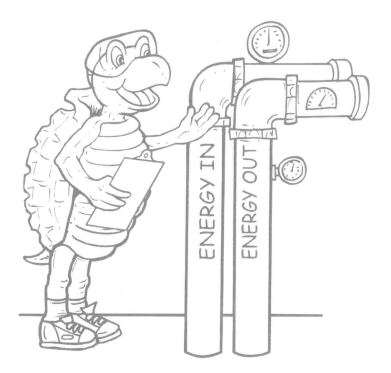

CHAPTER SEVEN
CHARTING YOUR SUCCESS

A MAP FOR YOUR JOURNEY

You've come a long way toward preparing yourself and you are almost ready to begin your "journey of a thousand miles." You've determined your goal numbers that may, as you begin, seem like they are truly about a thousand miles away! The reality is that they're entirely within your reach, so don't be discouraged! However, because the journey may be long, and because the scale will tell "tall tales," it is critical for you to regularly measure your ongoing progress toward achieving your goals. Taking weekly measurements of your body weight, body fat percentage, fat weight, lean weight and current PWLR, recording that information, and comparing those current numbers against both where you started, and where you ultimately are headed, is a practice I highly recommend.

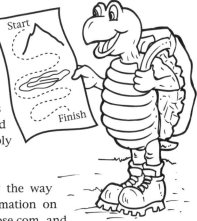

Plotting your weekly numbers on a graph will provide a clear visual record of how well you are doing toward reaching your target numbers. Over time, you will be able to make adjustments to your eating and exercise, if necessary, based on the reality of how your body composition is changing. A graph will plainly show this information and help keep you motivated and encouraged as you continue to work to lose fat ... rather than simply losing "weight."

The following are examples I have constructed to show the way Tortoise Diet members will see their personalized information on their Web page. You can log on to www.wintheracetolose.com and follow the instructions to become a member, and your graphs will be done for you. If you are not a member, and you choose to keep your own records and construct your own graphs, your charts at home should follow this same format.

MARY'S CHART

Let's use Mary as an example. Mary has logged on to www.wintheracetolose.com and become a Tortoise Diet member. She has selected a personal password to use to view her private Web page. She will now type in her sex, age, height, current weight, and wrist measurement. She will then select the appropriate Activity Factor, based on her occupational activities, and type it in. She then provides her body fat percentage from her scale or, if she doesn't have a body fat scale, she provides her waist measurement. All of the appropriate calculations, based on this information, will be instantly done for her, and her personal Web page will be ready.

Mary will see three charts on her Web page as shown in Figure 7-1.

FIGURE 7-1 MARY'S BEGINNING CHARTS

NAME: MARY

LIFETIME CALORIE PLAN: 1900
CURRENT BODY WEIGHT: 171.2 LBS
CURRENT LEAN WEIGHT: 111.3 LBS
CURRENT FAT WEIGHT: 59.9 LBS
CURRENT BODY FAT PERCENTAGE: 35.0
INITIAL PWLR: n/a
CURRENT PWLR: n/a

WEIGHT LOSS CALORIE PLAN: 1600
TARGET BODY WEIGHT: 127.5 LBS
TARGET LEAN WEIGHT: 104.5 LBS
TARGET FAT WEIGHT: 23.0 LBS
TARGET BODY FAT PERCENTAGE: 18.0

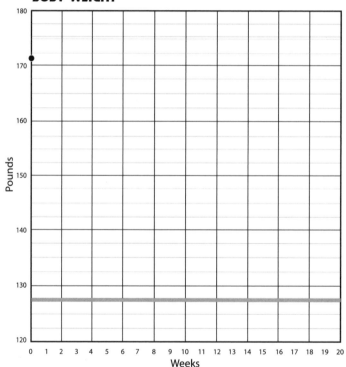

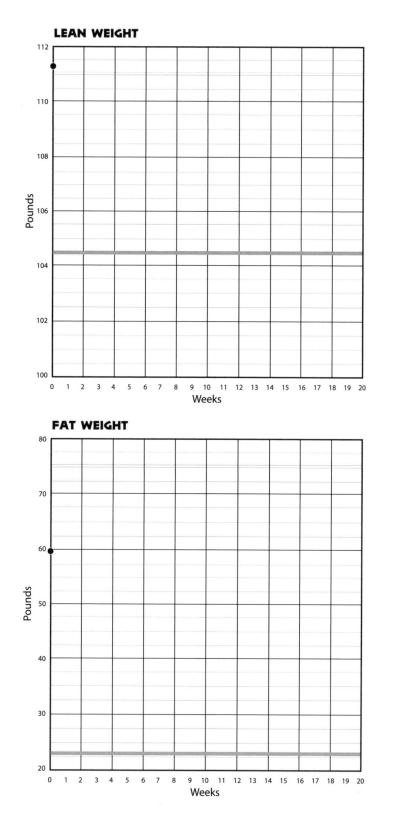

LEAN WEIGHT

FAT WEIGHT

In each of the three charts the solid horizontal lines reflect Mary's target numbers for body weight, lean weight, and fat weight. Mary's beginning current numbers for this same information are indicated, as well, as points on the graph. Because Mary may be losing significant water weight for the first couple weeks, her initial PWLR will not be calculated until the end of week three.

Once each week, Mary should update her information on her Web page. Ideally, information should be updated on the same day each week, as this will provide the best representation of her progress for the week. When Mary enters her current body weight for the week, as well as a new body fat percentage (or waist measurement), her updated information will be instantly plotted. At the time she types in information for week three, her initial PWLR will be calculated. Each week after that, her current PWLR will be recalculated, based on the new information she provides. Mary will be able to clearly see how she is progressing by comparing her target horizontal lines against the corresponding "in progress" graph. She will also be able to compare her current PWLR with her initial PWLR to see if it is higher or lower.

> "Once each week, Mary should update her information on her Web page. Ideally, information should be updated on the same day each week, as this will provide the best representation of her progress for the week."

Figure 7-2 shows Mary's progress after fifteen weeks.

FIGURE 7-2 MARY'S PROGRESS AFTER FIFTEEN WEEKS

NAME: MARY

LIFETIME CALORIE PLAN: 1900	WEIGHT LOSS CALORIE PLAN: 1500
CURRENT BODY WEIGHT: 151.0 LBS	TARGET BODY WEIGHT: 127.5 LBS
CURRENT LEAN WEIGHT: 107.5 LBS	TARGET LEAN WEIGHT: 104.5 LBS
CURRENT FAT WEIGHT: 43.5 LBS	TARGET FAT WEIGHT: 23.0 LBS
CURRENT BODY FAT PERCENTAGE: 28.8	TARGET BODY FAT PERCENTAGE: 18.0
INITIAL PWLR: 0.13	
CURRENT PWLR: 0.15	

BODY WEIGHT

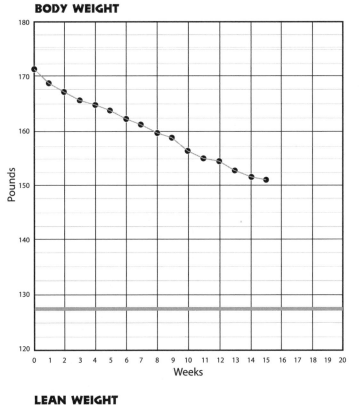

LEAN WEIGHT

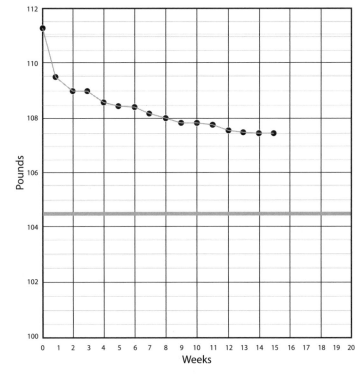

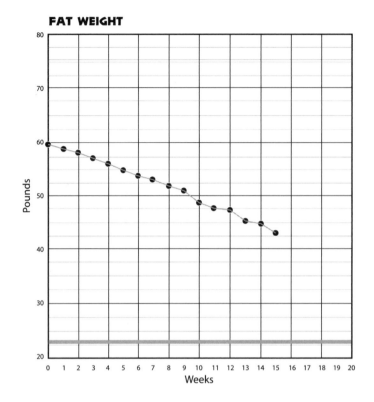

Mary's graphs reveal that after fifteen weeks she's doing great! To reflect the fact that she has gone from being 26-50 pounds over her target body weight to 0-25 pounds over target, her Weight Loss Calorie Plan has been reduced by 100 calories. By looking at Mary's lean weight graph, you will notice that she has lost several pounds of lean weight in the first two weeks. Remember that because water is a part of your body's lean weight, her lean weight graph reflects her (expected) large initial water weight loss! This is why her Personal Weight Loss Ratio was not calculated until week three.

Mary's situation is typical of what many of you may encounter when you start the Tortoise Diet. Her initial PWLR is only 0.13, which means that she can lose only a small fraction of a pound of muscle for every pound of body fat she loses. Basically, a number this small means that nearly all of her existing muscle tissue must be preserved while fat is being lost. Mary's fifteen-week graphs show she has definitely succeeded in this task. She has kept her current PWLR above her initial PWLR. By staying consistently above her initial PWLR, she is on track to lose her fat weight without losing too much lean weight. This chart reflects the progress of someone who is on her way to successfully reaching her target body weight and target body fat percentage!

TOM'S PROBLEM

Let's look at another example. Tom, a 53-year-old 6-foot tall man, with an medium frame size, has just become a Tortoise Diet member. His initial PWLR will not be calculated until week three. Figure 7-3 shows his beginning charts.

FIGURE 7-3 TOM'S BEGINNING CHARTS

NAME: TOM

LIFETIME CALORIE PLAN: 2300
CURRENT BODY WEIGHT: 218.4 LBS
CURRENT LEAN WEIGHT: 151.1 LBS
CURRENT FAT WEIGHT: 67.3 LBS
CURRENT BODY FAT PERCENTAGE: 30.8
INITIAL PWLR: n/a
CURRENT PWLR: n/a

WEIGHT LOSS CALORIE PLAN: 2300
TARGET BODY WEIGHT: 170.0 LBS
TARGET LEAN WEIGHT: 144.5 LBS
TARGET FAT WEIGHT: 25.5 LBS
TARGET BODY FAT PERCENTAGE: 15.0

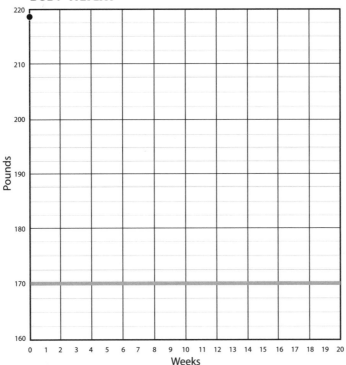

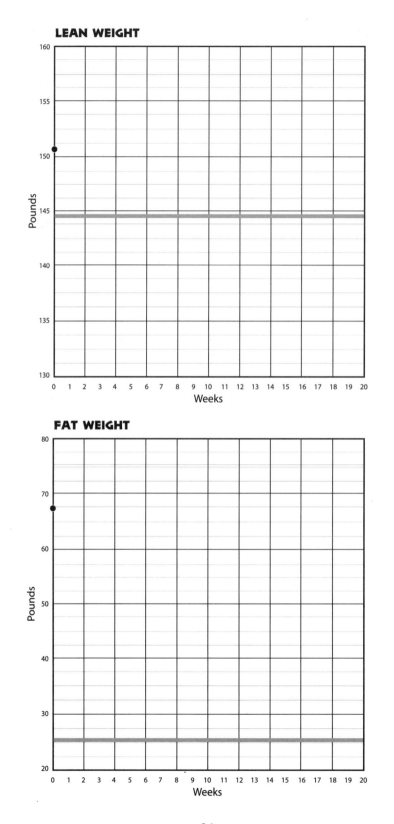

LEAN WEIGHT

FAT WEIGHT

Figure 7-4 shows Tom's progress after fifteen weeks.

FIGURE 7-4 TOM'S PROGRESS AFTER FIFTEEN WEEKS

NAME: TOM

LIFETIME CALORIE PLAN: 2300
CURRENT BODY WEIGHT: 198.4 LBS
CURRENT LEAN WEIGHT: 138.9 LBS
CURRENT FAT WEIGHT: 59.5 LBS
CURRENT BODY FAT PERCENTAGE: 30.0
INITIAL PWLR: 0.08
CURRENT PWLR: -0.16

WEIGHT LOSS CALORIE PLAN: 2100
TARGET BODY WEIGHT: 170.0 LBS
TARGET LEAN WEIGHT: 144.5 LBS
TARGET FAT WEIGHT: 25.5 LBS
TARGET BODY FAT PERCENTAGE: 15.0

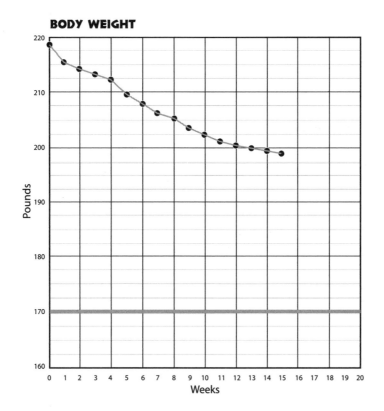

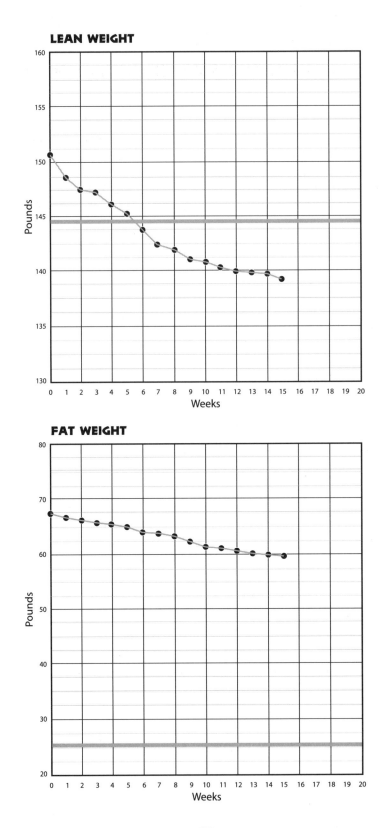

After fifteen weeks, Tom's body weight is down to 198.4 pounds. His Weight Loss Calorie Plan has been reduced by 200 calories because he's gone from 51-75 pounds over his target body weight, to 26-50 pounds over target. Tom has made good progress at losing "weight," but is the 20 pounds he's lost the right kind of weight? Tom's current body fat percentage is 30.0 percent, which is down only 0.5 percent from where he started! That's not good. It means that of the total body weight he's lost, only 7.8 pounds of that weight was actually fat weight. What's even worse is that he's lost 12.2 pounds of lean weight. Some of that can be attributed to water loss during the first couple weeks, but most of it was muscle. In fact, his current lean weight has become lower than his target lean weight. Tom has "gone negative!"

Tom's situation is typical of the way so many people attempt to lose weight. Tom probably thinks he's doing great. He's lost 20 pounds. He's basking in the congratulations from his friends. What he's not hearing from his friends however, is that he looks good. He doesn't look good because that negative PWLR means he's lost way too much muscle. Additionally, because he's lost 12.2 pounds of muscle, and because each pound of muscle lost costs him at least 15 calories per day, he can now eat about 180 fewer calories per day just to stay even. Tom is very likely headed for a major plateau, and he won't understand why the scale just won't budge.

Tom's problem is simple. He hasn't started a strength-training program. He can turn this situation around if he starts seriously hitting those weights! It certainly would have been a lot easier, however, if he had started a strength-training program in the beginning. Tom, like so many people, needs to understand that the goal is to lose fat, not muscle.

ANN'S PROBLEM

Ann has a problem many people who begin the Tortoise Diet with relatively little weight to lose will experience. Ann is 37-years-old, 5 feet 5 inches tall, with a medium frame size. When she first became a member she weighed 147 pounds. After three weeks her current body weight is down to 140 pounds, indicating that she only needs to lose fifteen more pounds to achieve her target body weight of 125 pounds. Unfortunately, as she looks at her charts after three weeks she realizes she is **starting off with a negative PWLR.** Her charts after three weeks are shown in Figure 7-5.

FIGURE 7-5 ANN'S CHARTS AFTER THREE WEEKS

NAME: ANN

LIFETIME CALORIE PLAN: 1800
CURRENT BODY WEIGHT: 140.0 LBS
CURRENT LEAN WEIGHT: 98.3 LBS
CURRENT FAT WEIGHT: 41.7 LBS
CURRENT BODY FAT PERCENTAGE: 29.8
INITIAL PWLR: -0.22
CURRENT PWLR: -0.22

WEIGHT LOSS CALORIE PLAN: 1400
TARGET BODY WEIGHT: 125.0 LBS
TARGET LEAN WEIGHT: 102.5 LBS
TARGET FAT WEIGHT: 22.5 LBS
TARGET BODY FAT PERCENTAGE: 18.0

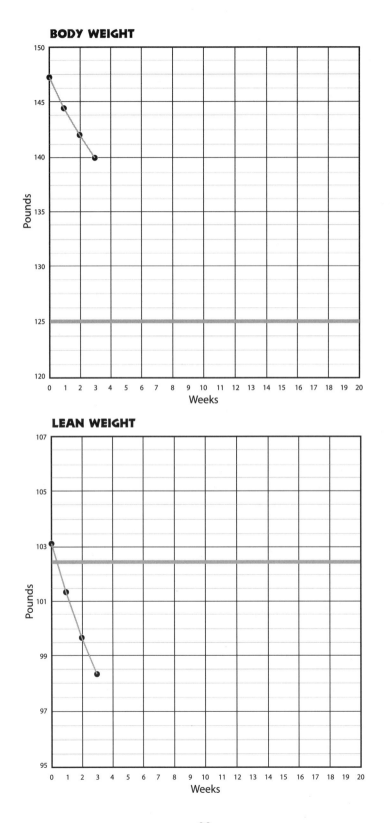

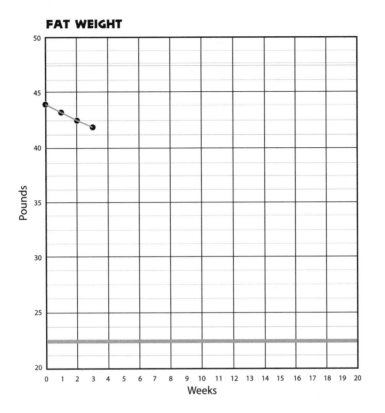

It's tempting for Ann to disregard her negative initial PWLR and only focus on those fifteen more pounds to lose. After all, her goal is within sight, correct? Not true! Her goal is not nearly as close as it seems. Her negative initial PWLR is telling her something is wrong. A quick glance at her numbers indicates that to reach her target body fat percentage, she needs to **gain 4.2 pounds of muscle, while losing 19.2 pounds of fat.** The 19.2 pounds and the 4.2 pounds add up to a 23.4 pound body composition change! Body composition is the term that describes what I've been talking about all along ... how much of your total body weight is fat weight and how much is lean weight? Ann needs to gain lean weight while losing fat weight. The problem is that it takes a very real effort to actually gain muscle while losing fat. Ann needs to start a strength program!

MY OWN VERY GOOD PROBLEM

My own experience with losing the last few pounds necessary to achieve my target body weight illustrates yet another situation that could happen to you. If you will recall, I described earlier my own experience with hitting a long and frustrating weight loss plateau. I now know this situation occurred because my calorie deficit had been too large, and I was not dedicated to performing my strength-training exercises. The result of these two factors was a slowed metabolic rate and the loss of too much muscle, which, of course, caused my plateau.

Fortunately, these important concepts were things I did eventually learn. I was able to successfully reverse course by eating the correct number of calories and initiating a strength-training exercise program, in addition to LIFB aerobics. Because I did start to faithfully do strength training, I actually ended up having a very good problem. I ended up with more lean weight than my target amount. This good problem is one that could also happen to you, if you pay attention early in your weight loss to preserving as much muscle as you possibly can.

Preserving more muscle than I needed to while I continued to lose fat allowed me to actually arrive at my target body fat percentage of 21.0 percent before I reached my target body weight of 118 pounds. I was actually ten pounds heavier on the scale, and I did have 2.1 pounds more fat than my target fat weight, but I also had 7.9 more pounds of muscle than my target lean weight.

I got really excited when it became clear to me that it wasn't necessary to worry about arriving at 118 pounds on the scale. Because those extra ten pounds were comprised of mostly muscle, not fat, it enabled me to get to my target body fat percentage at a body weight of 128 lbs. What?!! Can it be true that I achieved all my weight loss goals at a weight that was ten pounds above my target body weight? The answer is yes because here's a little secret: **The target body weight you have calculated is not your goal. Your real goal is to achieve your target body fat percentage!**

It's true. Reaching your target body fat percentage is your true aim and the goal that will enable you to achieve that fit and firm look you want. If you only look at the scale's "tall tale," you won't ever know if you have ten pounds too little muscle. Again, why is this so important? Because if you have ten pounds too little muscle ... you must have ten pounds too much fat! The scale might indicate you are at the weight you were aiming for, but you certainly won't have achieved the look you were hoping for!

And ladies, trust me when I say that a little extra muscle, over and above what you need to achieve your target body fat percentage, looks great! I'll take those 7.9 pounds of extra muscle I ended up with any day. Another plus for building a little extra muscle is that because of those 7.9 pounds, I can now eat about 120 more calories every day and not gain weight!

www.wintheracetolose.com

I hope these examples have illustrated the value of charting your lean weight and fat weight. Charting my progress was invaluable to me, as there were so many times that the scale showed very little progress. That could have been pretty discouraging, but because I was graphing my fat weight and lean weight, I was able to see that my body was actually changing, and changing in a good way. A glance at your chart can answer many questions and help you understand exactly what is happening as you lose weight. Are you losing weight too quickly? Are you losing too much muscle to be able to sustain your weight loss? Do you need to eat a little more? Will you be able to reach your target body fat percentage? Your chart will help you make the immediate corrections necessary to keep you on track.

This important habit of charting weight loss progress is one that very few people consider. But believe me, whether you become a Tortoise Diet member and allow us to do all the calculations and draw your graph on a weekly basis for you, or you do it yourself with some graph paper and colored pencils, charting is something you really need to do.

By logging on to www.wintheracetolose.com and becoming a Tortoise Diet Member you can get started right away. Becoming a member will cost you less than just one of those restaurant dinners per month that you are giving up to become a healthier and thinner person! In addition to monitoring your progress towards your weight loss goals, you'll also find ongoing information and support that can encourage you and help you succeed. A Tortoise Diet membership will provide you to the following valuable services each week:

1. A personal and private Web page for you to access anytime you like!

2. All the necessary calculations to help you succeed are done for you! Your personalized results instantly appear on the screen.

3. Each week, as you log onto your page, your chart will be instantly updated with the information you enter.

4. Your Lifetime Calorie Plan will be calculated and then adjusted to show your Weight Loss Calorie Plan. You will be alerted when it is time to further adjust your Weight Loss Calorie Plan, as you get closer to your target body weight.

5. Your current body weight, current fat weight, current lean weight, and current PWLR, along with all your target numbers will be graphed on a full color chart!

6. You will also received helpful information, support, recipes and encouragement.

All of this information will serve, over the long haul, to help you stay motivated, encouraged, and empowered. If you see your current numbers drifting in the wrong direction, you'll know to make necessary adjustments to your eating and exercise patterns, and your chart will help you know what those adjustments should be.

"Charting my progress was invaluable to me, as there were so many times that the scale showed very little progress. That could have been pretty discouraging, but because I was graphing my fat weight and lean weight, I was able to see that my body was actually changing, and changing in a good way."

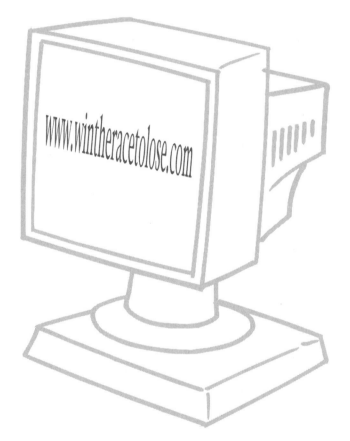

CHAPTER EIGHT
A LOOK AT THOSE "HARE-BRAINED DIETS!"

THOSE "HARE-BRAINED" DIETS!

Changing poor habits into good habits will take some time. You can only begin your successful lifetime race toward improved health and permanent weight loss if you believe deep in your heart that the slow and steady way is truly the only way. You must discard the idea that quick weight loss diets, pills, potions, or surgeries will in any way help you reach your goals.

Before you commit to changing your life by following the Tortoise Diet, I believe you should first review what the other diet alternatives are, and the reasons why I encourage you to reject them. Hopefully, by the time you finish this chapter, you'll have decided once and for all that those diets don't work and you'll be totally convinced that the Tortoise Diet offers the solutions you're looking for. With that in mind, let's review some of the most popular diets and weight loss methods.

LOW-CARBOHYDRATE DIETS

Is bread really bad? Can the lowly potato actually be ... EVIL? The popular low-carbohydrate diets promote the idea that "carbs" are bad for you, and they are to blame for your excess weight. These diets typically consist of very low calorie plans containing vast quantities of protein and unhealthy saturated fats, which may lead to kidney disease, gout, stroke, cancer, blocked arteries ... literally, a "heart attack on a plate!" While encouraging protein consumption, these plans allow very little of the complex carbohydrates our bodies need for energy. I will agree with them that simple refined sugars and processed white flour, like those found in pastries, chips and cake are carbohydrates that don't contribute much to health or weight loss. We all know these sugary and refined carbohydrates are calorie-dense, and can quickly pack on the pounds, but really ... no whole-grain bread? No fruit? No giant green salads? No romantic Italian dinners?

The real truth about the role of carbohydrate foods in a diet for weight loss and health is in stark contrast to the low-carb diets. Good health, vitality, anti-aging, disease prevention and successful long-term weight loss all depend on eating a wide variety of foods containing complex carbohydrates, eaten primarily in their whole-foods form.

What happens, then, when intake of carbohydrates is considered off limits? A shortage of any of the major nutrient groups, whether proteins, fats, or carbohydrates, will cause the body to have to adjust itself as best it can to continue to perform its many complex functions.

We have very smart and resilient bodies, however, so no matter what foods we eat or don't eat, all systems will be working toward providing the brain and other tissues with the energy they need to function.

A small supply of carbohydrate energy, called glycogen, is stored in the liver and muscles. Glycogen serves as a back-up supply for those times when no circulating blood glucose is available. When inadequate amounts of carbohydrates are eaten, that limited supply 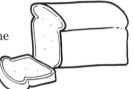 of glycogen gets used as an emergency supply for the glucose energy the body requires. After the glycogen is gone, the body will begin to make glucose by breaking down proteins either from the foods we have eaten, or by breaking down muscle tissue. Lastly, fat will be removed from the storage warehouse in an attempt to meet glucose energy needs. The only problem is, fats cannot be broken down into glucose. The energy contribution from the breakdown of fats is something known as "ketone bodies."

The hare-brained diets that place "carbs" in the "off limits" category rave about the benefits of these ketone bodies, which they claim melt body fat away, and eliminate hunger. In actuality, the ketone bodies are a low-quality fuel that can take the place of glucose in providing some, but not all, of the body's energy needs. The brain using ketones instead of glucose for fuel is somewhat like an old car running on only seven cylinders and belching out black smoke, compared to the smooth purring of an expensive sports car engine running on high-octane fuel. The body would simply prefer to have its higher-quality carbohydrate fuel to provide glucose, rather than being forced to function with lower-quality energy from ketone bodies.

Performing this extra work of breaking down other energy sources to compensate for the lack of its usual preferred fuel is taxing to the body, which can cause several problems. First, the acid-base balance is affected, which causes the kidneys to have to kick it into overdrive to adjust the pH back to normal. Extra water is pulled from the body's tissues to help the kidneys flush out the acid, which causes tissues to become dehydrated, much like a piece of jerky. Secondly, because ketones are unable to provide enough fuel for the brain and other tissues, some of the body's existing muscle tissue will have to be broken down and converted into glucose.

Additionally, when proteins are used to make glucose energy, rather than carbohydrates, the proteins usual function of tissue repair and general body maintenance will be neglected. This means the immune system will be weakened, making the individual more vulnerable to illness. The lack of vitamins and phytonutrients from not eating enough colorful vegetables and fruits may also contribute to illness, and the lack of fiber those foods contain may increase not only the discomfort from constipation and hemorrhoids but also the risk for cancer.

The important concern regarding these types of diets may be their long-term negative impact on health. After all, what good is it to lose weight in this manner if the long-term risks increase for colon cancer, breast cancer, cardiovascular disease, stroke, and kidney failure?

Many people are tempted by these diet plans because losing weight while being encouraged to eat foods full of protein and fat, like steak, bacon, butter, and cream sounds so darn un-diet-like and good! However, let's evaluate what really happens on a low-carb diet plan. Just like these diets promise, there usually is a large initial weight loss. This seems very encouraging and would be great, except the scale is telling a "tall tale" because the weight loss is primarily from water being flushed out (remember how hard those kidneys are working!). Some of the weight being lost does indeed come from the body's fat stores. Body fat broken down to form ketone bodies, however, will also lead to muscle tissue being broken down to provide glucose.

Therefore, as you see the scale dropping, in addition to the large amount of water weight, a significant amount of the weight lost will be precious calorie-burning muscle tissue. Losing too much muscle tissue is a hare-brained idea, doomed to failure. No matter how hard a person keeps trying, weight loss, at some point, will begin to stall.

Meanwhile, all of the steak, bacon, butter, and cream being eaten are getting old. You're feeling constipated, dry-mouthed, and sluggish, and you'd gladly give it all up for a sandwich! Your body craves carbohydrates like crazy, because they provide its most desirable fuel and it's getting pretty tired of running on those seven cylinders and belching out black smoke! It may be possible to resist the urges for awhile but they'll only continue to grow stronger. Eventually most people succumb to temptation, taking a small bite here and a little taste there. Pretty soon every "carb" in sight is being eaten with wild abandon.

The body's response to once again being fed the carbohydrates it craves for energy is YIPPIE! THANK YOU! NOW, THAT'S WHAT I NEED! The truth of the matter is you just can't fight physiology. Once carbohydrates are re-introduced, the body will do everything it can to prevent that state of perceived starvation from ever occurring again. Inevitably, all of the weight that was lost is very likely to be regained, and it will be even easier to gain weight in the future because of muscle tissue loss and a slowed metabolism.

It is true that eating too many "carbs" can make us fat. It is also true that eating too much protein or fat can cause the exact same result! I will agree that it's really easy to consume too many calories by eating calorie-dense foods made with processed flours and sugar. If it were true, however, that all types of carbohydrates make you fat, then how do you explain the fact that two-thirds of the people on the planet eat a diet very high in complex carbohydrates, with very limited quantities of expensive protein foods, and they're not overweight! What they don't do is eat white bread and other processed grains all loaded with sugar, trans-fats, high fructose corn syrup, salt, and whatever else is in the stuff we eat too much of.

As I've said before, it all comes down to exchanging poor health habits for better habits. Once you get used to the taste of whole-grain flour, less sugar, and less salt, you don't miss the bad stuff any more. Many processed foods that you used to enjoy will start to taste too sweet, too salty and too greasy. After eating healthy for a number of months, you may actually eat something really rich that wouldn't have fazed you before, but it now almost makes you feel sick to your stomach. So when indulging in some of those refined, processed foods, my recommendation is to try taking just a few bites instead of polishing it off.

People who follow these low carb diets, or any other fad diet, are "hares" in the race to lose weight. At first, by cutting out carbohydrates these hares may speed on ahead of the Tortoise, and probably will quickly lose some "weight." But, remember that it's most important that the weight lost is body fat, rather than merely water or precious calorie-burning muscle tissue. After these hares run out of steam, they will be left derailed and disappointed by the side of the road. Meanwhile, those following the Tortoise Diet will continue to make slow but steady progress toward achieving their goals by shedding body fat, preserving muscle tissue and maintaining the metabolic rate. They'll be able to do all of this while continuing to eat all kinds of enjoyable foods, and yes ... even enjoying a romantic Italian dinner once in awhile!

WHAT ABOUT A PILL TO MELT FAT?

An effective diet pill seems to be everyone's fantasy. It is entirely possible that sometime soon a drug company will succeed in developing a diet pill that really does help you lose weight without harmful side effects. I'm sure the company that develops this pill will be wildly successful, but I, for one, won't be taking such a pill. Why, you ask? Because I don't believe taking any kind of diet pill will support my commitment to lose weight permanently and improve my health, even if the FDA deems these drugs "safe."

Let's evaluate the two types of drugs that are currently in the works. One is touted as being able to somehow block the absorption of calories. What do you think is going to happen to your health if you take a pill to lose weight, but because of this pill you are able to get away with eating even more of the junky foods that have contributed to your excess weight? If a pill promises to magically "melt fat" with no effort on your part, you will almost surely be incredibly tempted to eat even more junky, salty, sweet, and fattening foods than you do now. There may not be any weight consequences whatsoever for this kind of eating, but it's likely that your health will suffer. You will have very little incentive to work at improving your health by changing your eating habits, and you probably won't make exercise a top priority either! My prediction is by continuing the poor health habits that have caused you to become overweight, you will eventually have a serious health crisis on your hands. Yes, you might lose weight by taking such a pill, but possibly at the expense of a serious disease. Will it be worth it? After a doctor visit or two, I'm sure your answer will be no. Then you will be faced with exactly the same problem you have now ... changing poor nutritional habits into good ones.

A second type of pill may act by reducing the appetite, which will damage your health in yet another way. Most people don't include enough healthy foods in their diets now to prevent disease, let alone after artificially reducing their appetites. Remember when I talked about phytonutrients and how important they are in fighting disease? Phytonutrients are only found in colorful foods like vegetables and fruits, foods that also contain many vitamins and essential minerals. What about fiber and its role in preventing colon cancer and other diseases? As with the pill that "melts fat", if you haven't developed good eating habits before this kind of pill is available, you could be setting yourself up for major health problems.

If all that isn't enough to convince you not to take pills to lose weight, how about the fact that you're still going to have to exercise to prevent losing too much muscle? Quick weight loss, whether it's by starving yourself, or whether it's done with the help of a pill, doesn't work. The old adage of "let the buyer beware" applies. My advice is simple: Don't pop pills or swallow potions to lose weight. Eat healthy food, take a few vitamins, and spend the rest of the money you save on a good pair of walking shoes!

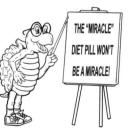

THE "MIRACLE" DIET PILL WON'T BE A MIRACLE!

VERY LOW CALORIE DIETS

Very low calorie diets come in all different forms. I have had patients, for example, who've had their jaws surgically wired together, so they wouldn't be able to eat any solid food at all! I also took care of quite a few people who had to have their gall bladders removed because they had been following an extremely low-calorie, protein-sparing fast. This type of diet was originally designed to be a drastic, medically supervised regimen of severe calorie restriction, intended only for those people who were extremely overweight. By drinking only a little packet of reconstituted protein powder for each meal, the total calories are limited to about 400 per day!

Not only are these diets taxing to the body, sometimes causing electrolyte imbalance and kidney problems, in addition to those gall bladder problems, they are also tough on the person's mind and emotions. I have been personally acquainted with several people who made a stab at losing weight on this type of medical program, and they were miserable all of the time. None of them could stick with the program for long. Most people simply can't go through daily life without any semblance of enjoyment, and it's really hard to think of anything pleasant when your body is starving.

Many other diets have calorie plans that fall in the 700 to 1000 calorie range. This is not enough energy for an adult to prevent the metabolic rate from slowing dramatically. Again, at first weight loss will be dramatic, due to a large amount of water and muscle tissue loss, but after suffering through this regimen a plateau will inevitably occur. When the scale just won't budge and the starvation and suffering get to be too much, the diet will likely be abandoned. When normal eating is resumed, it will be nearly impossible to maintain even the pre-dieting weight, because of the muscle-tissue that has been lost.

WHAT ABOUT GASTRIC BYPASS SURGERY?

There is another drastic quick fix measure that is becoming increasingly popular. I'm referring to the various surgical techniques many people are using to lose weight. These surgeries are all variations of a single concept, which is to make the stomach smaller and prevent the absorption of calories in the gut. The normal stomach has the capacity to hold about one quart in volume. These surgeries decrease that capacity down to only a few ounces, so the stomach will be filled after only a couple bites of food. It's pretty much a no-brainer that if a person can only eat a serving-spoon full of food, they'll lose a lot of weight.

As always, because too few calories are taken in, the body will have to resort to its usual methods for survival and will break down its own muscle tissue for energy. You know by now that the ultimate effect of the state of starvation is a metabolic rate that is slowed to a crawl. In addition to being deprived of adequate calories, the person's diet may end up being deficient in many of the vitamins, phytonutrients and minerals that our foods usually provide, so the immune system may not function well. Also, because the gastro-intestinal tract is usually surgically shortened, the absorption of nutrients and water is compromised, so many people experience something called "dumping syndrome." This is just another term for nausea, cramping, and big-time diarrhea!

These surgeries were originally indicated only for individuals who were severely and dangerously overweight, and were suffering from severe health problems that made the risk of undergoing major surgery a potentially life-saving option. Over time, however, the surgery has become more commonplace, and many people now consider it just another viable weight-loss technique. In addition to the potential health problems already discussed, what gets lost among the glowing celebrity testimonials are the potentially dangerous risks and side effects associated with this major surgery. These surgeries are drastic measures, and should never be considered as a first, second, third, or even fourth resort!

Interestingly, following these radical procedures, the patient is always advised to eat small, frequent meals of high-quality, nutrient-dense foods. If they don't do this, they'll stretch that tiny stomach back out and can potentially gain the weight back. Hmm ... eating small, frequent meals of high-quality, nutrient-dense foods. That's exactly what the Tortoise Diet promotes, and without all the associated risks.

VERY LOW FAT DIETS

Very low fat diets recommend limiting fat intake to 10 to 15 percent of the total daily calories. These diets are very healthy in many respects, but miss the mark in an important way. It is certainly true that eating a very low fat diet makes it easier to eat fewer calories, but the "real life" thing gets in the way. When fat intake dips below 15 percent or so, we start to feel unhappy and deprived. And when we're not happy, we eventually break down and eat a double cheeseburger with fries. This is good for getting happy, but not good for losing weight.

Besides, it is not merely eating fat that can make you fat, because whenever more calories are being taken in than the body requires for energy, whether from fats, carbohydrates, or protein, the excess energy will likely end up being stored as fat. Therefore, my recommendation is to include heart-healthy fats in an amount that helps you achieve satiety. Satiety is a nutritional term that means when you're done eating you're satisfied. In other words, you're happy!

LIQUID DIETS

These hare-brained diets are usually over-the-counter meal replacement drink concoctions that tell you to drink two or three of their liquid meals each day, and to then enjoy a "sensible" dinner. I'm glad they recommend you have at least one sensible meal each day, because liquids cannot begin to provide the same sense of fullness and satiety as crunchy, chewy, real food, not to mention it gets pretty monotonous to drink only a little can of something and call it a meal. If you follow the Tortoise Diet you'll be able to enjoy eating real food all day long. You won't be hungry and your meals don't have to be boring.

WHAT ABOUT THE LITTLE EXPENSIVE CARTONS OF FOOD DIETS?

The "little expensive cartons of food" diet plans are not a cheap way to eat! Another problem with these little cartons of food are, well ... they're little! Because they're so small, they don't usually fill you up, so when you're done, you'll still find yourself foraging through the cupboards for more food. Not having to do that is the whole reason you paid dearly for the little carton of food in the first place! Freshly prepared food almost always means more fiber, more crunching, more chewing, more taste, and more satisfaction. For the same amount of calories, freshly prepared foods fill you up to a much greater degree.

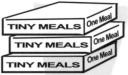

The most important reason I don't recommend these programs is because they short-circuit the good health habits you need to develop. This goes to the heart of what I hope the Tortoise Diet will do for you. You need to get to the point where it's a habit to plan your family's meals each week, make a shopping list, and come home to spend some time in the kitchen. What is your family going to eat if you're eating little cartons of frozen food? What are you going to eat if you get caught without a microwave? What are you going to eat if you get tired of these foods? What I'm saying is they just don't support the "commitment to lose weight permanently" test. I can't see myself eating these little dinners for the rest of my life, and if I stop eating them I haven't developed the habits necessary to prevent myself from going back to eating exactly the way I did when I was overweight.

THE QUICK FIX MENTALITY

I am convinced that taking the slower path is the only way to achieve permanent weight loss and good health. The Tortoise Diet is designed to achieve these goals, and because it is based on sound physiologic principles that result in true FAT LOSS, the truth is this is anything but a "quick" process. I'll admit, believing that you can reach your goals by committing yourself to losing body fat in a slower but correct way can be a challenge. It's tough to get over the "quick fix mentality" because it's always attractive to take the "easy way." Always remember, however, that the body doesn't respond well to starvation and deprivation and it will fight back if it is subjected to such treatment. We've all lost weight temporarily, only to just gain it back again. Remember your commitment to ... this time ... lose weight permanently.

The good news is, it's not necessary to torture and starve yourself, and you don't have to waste your money on surgeries, gadgets or pills. The Tortoise Diet is a very livable nutritional and exercise program that really works. There is power in taking control over your own life, and in becoming stronger and healthier while losing weight. There is also power in taking the slow way ... truly the only way in the long run.

"I am convinced that taking the slower path is the only way to achieve permanent weight loss and good health."

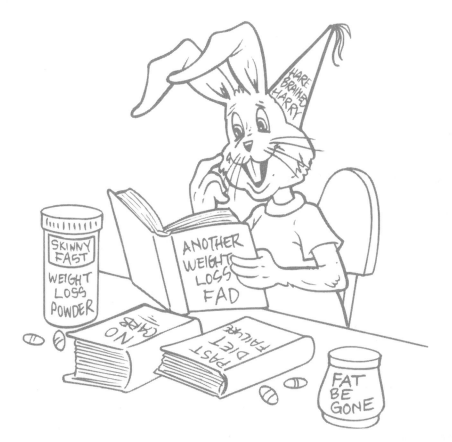

CHAPTER NINE
TWENTY-FIVE HABITS OF THE SUCCESSFUL TORTOISE

NEW HABITS

Many acquaintances of mine during my weight loss process were very curious about what I was doing to lose so much weight. I always felt frustrated because there just wasn't a quick and simple answer that would begin to explain the many things I was learning and practicing. This entire book is quite literally the result of that frustration, but this chapter, in particular, is the answer I always wanted to share with people. You'll note by its length, however, how difficult it would have been for me to tell somebody in twenty-five words or less how I lost weight! I usually ended up saying to people that it was just a lot of little things, and it was ... a lot of little things called habits!

In this chapter you will learn the twenty-five essential health habits that were crucial to my success. If they sound familiar, it is because this entire book to this point has been focused on introducing you to these habits and the reasons why they are so important. They are the "secret" to my success. By making very small bits of progress each day, gradually and over a period of many months, I turned a lifetime of poor habits into new and healthy ones. There's nothing super-human about me, though ... I'm just a person who simply decided to change my health and my weight by doing it one day at a time. These new habits that I gradually acquired not only helped me to succeed in losing weight, they now help me to keep that weight from ever coming back!

These same habits can also help you to achieve your goals without having to endure deprivation and hunger. With time and repetition, they will come to feel as easy and natural as your old habits. Learning to practice all twenty-five of them is essential for you to be able to fulfill the two commitments you made to improve your health and achieve permanent weight loss. Make a copy of the habits and put them on the refrigerator, tape them to your mirror, or place them prominently on your desk so you can be reminded daily how to stay on the path toward success. They are the keys to achieving your weight loss goals.

Self-Awareness and Stress-Management Habits

1. Prioritize yourself as being important and take responsibility for your life and happiness. "Dropkick" the time-wasting activities from your life that are preventing you from achieving your goals.

2. Practice mindfulness. Keep an informal journal and learn to identify your own emotional or stressful "triggers," and develop healthier responses.

3. Develop realistic expectations and personalized goals. Reject the "hare-brained" notion that improved health and permanent fat loss can be achieved quickly.

Nutritional Habits

4. Improve your health and decrease your hunger by including as many fresh, colorful, healthy, nutrient-dense and fiber-filled complex carbohydrate foods as you can each day. An easy way to do this is to eat the "daily seven for success" foods every day: An apple, an orange, a serving of oatmeal, a bowl of broth-based vegetable and legume soup, a green salad, a vegetable at dinner, and some whole-grain bread or pasta. Limit your intake of refined carbohydrates (table sugar, high-fructose corn syrup, white flour, and processed foods).

5. At every meal, eat protein foods together with complex carbohydrate foods. If you eat some carrots, eat some low-fat cheese; if you eat an apple, eat some peanut butter, etc.

6. Decrease saturated fat and include mostly mono-unsaturated heart-healthy fats. Eliminate trans-fats.

7. Drink 16 ounces of water an hour before each meal, more if you're really hungry.

8. Take a good multiple vitamin each day.

9. Make an efffort to get an adequate amount of sleep.

10. Gradually learn to eat foods without added salt.

11. Limit alcohol. Count any calories from alcoholic beverages as DOUBLE their actual caloric value.

Food Planning and Preparation Habits

12. Develop a repertoire of healthy dinners that you and your family really enjoy, and that are easy enough to make every night, even when you're tired. Also develop your own "Top 40" list of healthy foods to use in making your other meals.

13. Plan your meals for the week and put together a shopping list of items you need to purchase. Go to the store and buy everything at once. When you arrive home, rinse, chop, portion-out, freeze, and, if you'd like, make soup, oatmeal, healthy muffins, etc. to refrigerate or freeze for the upcoming week. Get as much food preparation done in advance as you can. Do not ever run out of healthy food, for you or your family.

14. Plan ahead so whenever you leave the house you take enough food with you to last for as long as you'll be away. Always be prepared, so you'll never be caught without enough healthy food available when hunger strikes.

Exercise Habits

15. Do some type of enjoyable LIFB aerobic exercise for a minimum of twenty minutes, a minimum of four days each week. For even greater fat-burning, perform LIFB exercise for a minimum of forty minutes each session, up to six days each week. One day of rest each week is recommended.

16. Dedicate yourself to performing the Tortoise Diet strength-training program twice each week. Use weights heavy enough for each set to fatigue the muscle being worked.

Energy Management Habits

17. Try to eat the total number of calories each day that your Weight Loss Calorie Plan allows. Learn to count calories easily by getting to know the calorie totals of the foods you eat regularly.

18. Eat within an hour of getting up each morning and then continue throughout the day to eat a meal approximately every three hours. Spread your "just right" calorie deficit out throughout the day by dividing your Weight Loss Calorie Plan allotment into the following portions:

Meal #1	20%
Meals #2, #4, and #6	10%
Meals #3 and #5	25%

19. Occasionally, it is acceptable to combine a 25 percent meal with a 10 percent meal, for a total of 35 percent at one meal. When this is done, omit the next regularly scheduled 10 percent meal. Do not eat more than 35 percent of your Weight Loss Calorie Plan total at any one meal, unless it is one of two TGIW meals allowed each week.

20. TGIW/"Fool Your Body" by adding 400 calories to your Weight Loss Calorie Plan during two meals each week. Look forward to these two special meals each week, but don't overdo them and blow all your hard work.

21. Practice Hara Hachi Bu, especially when eating a big meal. Become very familiar with the way your body feels and how much food it usually takes to make you feel 80 percent full.

22. When you exercise, eat more to compensate for the calories burned. Add calories for exercise to the meal either just before or just after the exercise is performed, based on the following:

If you weigh less than 200 pounds, add 50 calories for every 20 minutes exercise performed.
If you weigh more than 200 pounds, add 75 calories for every 20 minutes of exercise performed.

Charting Your Progress Habits

23. Chart your current body weight, fat weight, and lean weight once each week. Compare these numbers to your target numbers. Calculate your current PWLR each week and compare it to your initial PWLR to make sure the current number is equal to or larger than the initial number. Calculate your body fat percentage each week. Evaluate your progress by looking at periods of at least three weeks in length, to see true changes.

Lifetime Success Habits

24. Constantly remind yourself of your commitments to improve your health and achieve permanent weight loss.

25. Continue to practice all of the new and healthy habits you have learned! Congratulate yourself as you progress toward your goals. Don't be discouraged if your weight loss seems slow. Quick weight loss doesn't work.

You may be feeling a little overwhelmed! After all, twenty-five life-changing habits is a lot to learn. But remember my earlier example of "moving the mountain." Big projects must be broken down into smaller tasks. In the next chapter you will find out how to slowly and steadily begin the job of changing your life!

"By making very small bits of progress each day, gradually and over a period of many months, I turned a lifetime of poor habits into new and healthy ones."

CHAPTER TEN
ON YOUR MARK, GET SET, GO!

THE TORTOISE DIET TRAINING ASSIGNMENTS

To make it easier for you to incorporate these new habits into your life and get started toward your goals, the Tortoise Diet offers a series of assignments. These step-by-step training assignments are designed to help you learn to incorporate all twenty-five essential habits into your life. Each week's assignments will build upon those learned during the previous week, until eventually all twenty-five are included in your daily practice. Step by step, slowly but steadily, you will make progress.

The assignments are organized into three phases. The first phase is called "Preparing To Win The Race To Lose." In this phase you will begin the Training Assignments by first taking a few important days to prepare. Once you're prepared to begin, you'll start the second phase, consisting of an initial three-week period of retraining called "The Tortoise Takes Off." Week One will be spent learning the most important healthy habits. During Week Two and Week Three you will continue to practice the habits you've already learned, in addition to some new ones each week. Meal plans containing healthy foods in specific calorie amounts and proper nutrient combinations will be provided for you to choose from based on your own personalized calorie needs. In addition to the eating plan, you'll also begin the "Walking & Weights" exercise plan. Other healthy habits, besides those directly concerning eating and exercise, will also be addressed. The third phase is called "Making Your Own Plan." In this last phase you will learn all the remaining habits needed to make the Tortoise Diet a lifetime plan.

PREPARING TO WIN THE RACE TO LOSE

During these first few days, your goal is simply to prepare to begin your race. This preparatory period will not be wasted time, as you will be working on some important habits. Your goal prior to beginning Week One of the Training Assignments is to successfully complete the following initial eleven assignments.

Assignment #1
Make the commitment to improve your health and to lose weight permanently.

This is the important first step as you begin your "journey of a thousand miles." You must decide once and for all that those other hare-brained diets don't work. You must also realize that it has taken time, perhaps years, to develop the habits that have caused you to become overweight. It is only logical, then, that it will also take time to develop new habits that will help you lose weight and achieve better health.

Assignment #2
Create an environment for success.

Right from the beginning, it's important for you to "go public." Enlist your family and close friends to join you in your efforts. This will go a long way toward keeping you motivated. Also, try to rid your kitchen of all tempting, junky foods that will no longer fit into your eating program. Once you've cleared out space in your refrigerator, freezer, and the cupboards, you'll be able to equip your kitchen with the tools you'll need to prepare and store healthy foods. Lastly, review your daily schedule and "dropkick" the unnecessary or undesirable time-wasters from your life, so you'll have time to incorporate new and healthy activities.

Assignment #3
Buy a notebook and begin to jot down your thoughts.

A big part of learning new habits is simply becoming aware of your current behaviors, and how those behaviors impact your life. Begin the habit of keeping a record of what you eat during the day, when you eat it and why you eat it. Be honest! Review this information to see if you can identify any of your current eating behaviors that may have contributed to where you are today. By starting this practice early on, you'll have a great deal of information to help gauge your progress.

Assignment #4
Figure out some numbers.

If you haven't already done the required measurements and calculations to determine your own personalized information, it's time to do so. I encourage you to do all of your calculations twice to make sure you haven't made a mistake. Also, when taking measurements, do them three times and take the average. Jot all of this baseline information in your journal. Refer again to Chapter Four, as well as Appendix D for the specific calculations to determine the following essential pieces of data. Log on to www.wintheracetolose.com and become a Tortoise Diet member if you would like both the initial and the ongoing weekly calculations done for you.

Current body weight _____ Target body weight _____
Current body fat percentage _____ Target body fat percentage _____
Current fat weight _____ Target fat weight _____
Current lean weight _____ Target lean weight _____

Number of pounds of fat to lose _____
Maximum lean weight to lose _____
BMR at target body weight _____
Appropriate Activity Factor _____
Lifetime Calorie Plan _____
Number of pounds currently above target body weight _____
Weight Loss Calorie Plan _____

Assignment #5
Set up your weight-loss graph to chart your progress.

Tracking the ongoing changes in your fat weight and lean weight is critical to your success. Watching the lines on your graph move in the correct direction is exciting! Seeing the numbers on your graph going in the wrong direction is motivating! As a Tortoise Diet member, your graphs will be done for you. If you choose to do your own graphs, now is the time to get some graph paper and set up some charts similar to those found in Chapter Seven. Write down the number of pounds of fat weight to lose and the maximum pounds of lean weight to lose. Write down your current body weight, current fat weight, and current lean weight, and also your target body weight, target fat weight, and target lean weight. Now plot these numbers on your graph in similar fashion to the graphs in Chapter Seven.

Assignment #6
Purchase an assortment of hand-held dumbbells.

Maybe you already have some lying around. If so, it's time to dust them off! If not, go to the sports store and purchase a few. Don't go overboard and buy really heavy weights. You can always buy those later if you need them.

Assignment #7
Calculate the number of calories needed for each of your six daily meals.

To determine your calorie needs for each meal, multiply your Weight Loss Calorie Plan total by the following:

For Meal #1	Weight Loss Calorie Plan total	x .20	_____
For Meals #2, #4, and #6	Weight Loss Calorie Plan total	x .10	_____
For Meals #3 and #5	Weight Loss Calorie Plan total	x .25	_____

Put these calorie allotments for each meal up on your fridge so you can easily refer to them every day.

Assignment #8
Choose meals from Appendix A that add up to approximately the number of calories you are allotted for each meal, and are foods that sound the best to you.

From the meal plans provided in Appendix A, select two breakfast meals, three or four lunch meals, and three or four snack meals that are appropriate, based on your calorie requirements. Also review the provided dinner meals and pick four or five that you and your family could enjoy. These are meals you will be eating during Weeks One, Two and Three. The only requirement is you must choose meals that will ensure you eat each of the following foods every single day: an apple, an orange, a bowl of vegetable and legume based healthy soup, and a small green dinner salad. On days you eat a large main course salad for dinner, or on TGIW days, you may omit the small green dinner salad requirement. Write down each meal you have selected, along with its calorie count and place it on the refrigerator, so you can easily refer to it as you are preparing your food each day.

Assignment #9
Plan and purchase healthy foods for the entire first week.

Based on the meals you chose in the previous assignment, make a complete shopping list for the entire first week, for you and everyone else in your family. Don't buy any foods that are not on your list. Make sure you have a good supply of plastic storage containers, and consider purchasing an insulated bag or some other container, if necessary, to take food with you when you leave the house each day. Be sure to eat a healthy snack before you go shopping so you're not too hungry!

Assignment # 10
Prepare as much food as possible for the entire first week.

When you get home from the store, wash, rinse, cut, chop, cook, portion-out, store, and freeze the food. Do as much food-prep as possible before your busy work week starts. Use this opportunity to make a batch of soup, oatmeal, brown rice, salad greens, etc. to save yourself some time later.

Assignment #11
Prepare your next day's meals the night before.

On the night before you are ready to begin Week One, plan and prepare what you are going to eat for each of your six meals on the following day. Start day one off right! Place all of the foods you plan to eat for meals #1 through #4 into a single bag, box, or container. Know that this is the total amount of food you should eat during the day, until it's time for dinner. Make sure to tuck away an extra protein bar, some almonds, or a packet of instant soup in your car or at the office, in case you find yourself away from home for longer than you anticipated. Always be prepared! If you're going to eat breakfast before you leave the house, get it ready the night before. You may have to set the alarm a little bit earlier so you have time to prepare and eat your breakfast.

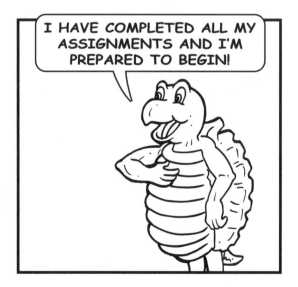

THE TORTOISE TAKES OFF

WEEK ONE

Now that you've completed the first eleven assignments, it's time to begin changing your life! The first phase is called "The Tortoise Takes Off," because not only will you be taking off some weight, you'll also be "taking off" on your quest to win the race to lose. During this three week training period you may be pleasantly surprised by the amount of weight you lose. Some of that initial weight lose is, of course, the loss of some water. A good portion of it, however, will be taken from your fat storage warehouse, never to return!

During "The Tortoise Takes Off," you should closely follow the menu plans and dinners found in Appendix A for every meal. Select any of the meals that are appropriate for your Weight Loss Calorie Plan. The exception to this will be the two TGIW meals allotted for each week. Here are your twelve assignments for Week One.

Assignment #1
Write in your journal every day.

For some people this will be easy and natural. If you are one of those people who have never been inclined to write in a journal before, just make an effort for a few minutes each day to jot down the foods you eat, the exercise you do, and some general observations about how you feel. Take note of how the food you have eaten affected you. Did you feel full? Did it meet that "crunch" craving? Did it look good on the plate? Did it taste good? Did you feel satisfied? Rate your level of hunger between meals and note whether drinking 16 ounces of water helps satisfy you until your next meal. Jot down the number of minutes you spend exercising and how it makes you feel. Pay attention to which kinds of things act as triggers that tempt you to blow your diet, things like feeling frustrated or sad or tired or even happy. This will give you valuable information about yourself and your habit of using food for things other than true hunger.

Assignment #2
Eat six healthy meals each day.

Start eating the meals you selected in Assignment #8 of the preparatory period, the ones you placed on your refrigerator. These meals are designed to keep your calorie intake where it should be. Try to eat each of the six meals at approximately three-hour intervals throughout the day. By the way, getting behind on your eating schedule is actually worse than getting a little ahead. Are you surprised by that statement? You shouldn't be. Remember, the worst thing you can do is deprive your body of the fuel it requires.

Assignment #3
Continue the practice of organizing and preparing the following day's meals.

As you become better organized and more familiar with the calorie counts for each of the meals you have selected, this nightly process shouldn't take more than five or ten minutes. Every night, get breakfast for the next morning ready and pack that lunch!

Assignment #4
Eat breakfast within an hour of rising each day.

Eating breakfast at home before work is a great way for this assignment to develop into the habit you need it to be. But if you just can't get up in time, be sure to have something prepared to grab and take with you to eat in the car, or first thing when you get to work.

Assignment #5
Drink 16 ounces of water one hour prior to each of your six meals per day.

This assignment will accomplish two things. You'll start drinking the amount of water you should have been drinking on a daily basis all along, and you'll reduce the hunger you will likely begin to feel about an hour before each meal.

Assignment #6
Enjoy two TGIW meals this week.

It's important to enjoy a couple of really nice meals each week ... but only two! Calculate your TGIW meal calorie allotment, and make every effort to not go over this number!

Assignment #7
Practice Hara Hachi Bu.

During all of your regularly scheduled meals this week, practice paying attention to the sensation of fullness you experience while you eat. Because you are eating at a calorie deficit, many times as you finish the meal, you will probably be about 80 percent full. Most especially, practice Hara Hachi Bu during your two TGIW meals.

Assignment #8
Limit alcohol.

You might have noticed that the meal selections in Appendix A do not include alcoholic beverages. During the twenty-one day period of "The Tortoise Takes Off" you must not drink alcohol except at your TGIW meals. In fact, during this period of time, alcohol intake should be limited to a maximum of one alcoholic beverage at each of the two TGIW meals each week. Remember, the calories of any alcoholic beverages consumed should be counted as DOUBLE their actual caloric value. Here are some tips to help limit the effects of alcohol consumption:

1. Any alcoholic beverages must be consumed along with food, never alone on an empty stomach.
2. It's best to drink a maximum of one alcoholic beverage every 60 minutes.
3. For each alcoholic beverage consumed, make sure to drink a large glass of water before having another alcoholic drink.
4. Dilute the alcohol in cocktails with no-calorie mixers, like club soda, mineral water, diet soda, or water.
5. Rather than drinking larger quantities of mediocre wine, beer, or other alcoholic beverages, why not enjoy only one drink of something really special.

Assignment #9
Do LIFB aerobics for twenty minutes, three days this week.

Add the appropriate amount of calories to the meal just before or just after the exercise. On "Fool Your Body" days, these calories may be added to your TGIW meal at any time during the day.

Assignment #10
Perform the Tortoise Diet strength-training program described in Chapter Five one time this week. Focus on learning to perform each exercise with correct form.

Add the appropriate amount of calories to the meal just before or just after the exercise. On "Fool Your Body" days, these calories may be added to your TGIW meal at any time during the day.

Assignment #11
Sometime near the end of Week One, complete assignments #9, #10, and #11 from the preparatory period again.

It's time to start getting ready for the next week of challenges.

Assignment #12
On the last day of Week One, measure your waist with a tape measure and weigh yourself, or step on your body fat scale to determine your body fat percentage and current body weight.

Calculate your fat weight and lean weight. Jot this information in your journal and then plot it on your graph. Tortoise Diet members should simply log on and type their current weight and body fat percentage from the scale or their waist measurement onto their personal Web page. Compare these new numbers to the ones you recorded before you started Week One. If you have faithfully completed all of your assignments, it's likely you'll be pleased with your initial progress. Remember, you will not calculate your initial PWLR until after the completion of Week Three.

Congratulations! You've made it through Week One! How did things go? Hopefully you're starting to get the hang of some of these new habits, and you're beginning to see and feel some progress. If things didn't go quite as perfectly as you would have liked, that's okay. Changing habits is always a challenge at first, and it's pretty normal for these new behaviors to feel difficult at first.

Before we proceed to the assignments for Week Two, it's time for a serious word about our perception of success and failure. Learning to follow the Tortoise Diet is very similar to many of life's challenges. Many people decide way too early whether they are going to be a success or a failure at a certain endeavor. Let me say right now, there is only one way to fail. **If you quit, you have failed.** Anything short of quitting is not failure. You have spent many years developing the habits you have now. You cannot expect to change all of your poor health habits into good health habits in one week, three weeks, or even three months. Just keep working until these new, healthy habits eventually feel easy and natural. You have the option to repeat Week One before continuing on. **If fact, at any time during "The Tortoise Takes Off," or at any point thereafter, you can go back and repeat a week, or even go back to the beginning and start over.**

WEEK TWO

Your goal for Week Two of the Training Assignments is to successfully complete the following three assignments.

Assignment #1
Repeat all of the assignments from Week One.

I liken "The Tortoise Takes Off" period to a construction project, because it is all about building new habits. The skills learned during the previous week will form the foundation and support for the next layer of new habits. The exercise assignments are slightly changed, otherwise, all the same assignments from Week One should be continued in Week Two.

Assignment #2
Do LIFB aerobics for twenty minutes, four days this week. Again, perform the Tortoise Diet strength-training program one day this week.

Add the appropriate amount of calories to the meal just before or just after the exercise. On "Fool Your Body" days, these calories may be added to your TGIW meal anytime during the day.

Assignment #3
Take a good multiple vitamin each day.

Also, consider taking additional Calcium and Vitamin E. Check with your doctor to see if you have underlying medical conditions that could be adversely affected by vitamin supplementation.

WEEK THREE

Your goal for Week Three of the Training Assignments is to successfully complete the following six assignments.

Assignment #1
Repeat all the assignments from Week One, as well as those from Week Two. The exercise assignments are, again, slightly changed.

Similar to the start of the previous week, you are adding new habits while continuing to work on previously learned skills.

Assignment #2
Do LIFB aerobics for forty minutes, four days this week. Perform the Tortoise Diet strength-training program on two different days this week, allowing 48-72 hours of rest between sessions.

Add the appropriate amount of calories to the meal just before or after the exercise. On "Fool Your Body" days, these calories may be added to your TGIW meal anytime during the day.

This week you'll begin the complete "Walking & Weights" exercise program. If you choose to perform LIFB and strength-training exercises on separate days, you will be exercising on six of the seven days of the week, with one rest day. If you would like, it is acceptable to do both types of exercise on the same day and take either one additional day to rest each week or add one more LIFB exercise session. Because the strength-training exercise sessions have been increased to twice each week, you'll have to organize a weekly exercise plan to make sure adequate rest is allowed between sessions.

Assignment #3
Limit salt.

Become aware of how much salt you eat and start a program of reducing the amount. Begin to experiment with other ways to flavor your food.

Assignment #4
Get more sleep.

Although I haven't yet mentioned the importance of getting a good night's rest, there is an important physiologic reason why this is certainly a good practice. If you don't get enough sleep your body circulates high levels of a stress hormone called cortisol which raises your blood sugar and increases your hunger. This is why when you're tired in the afternoon that chocolate cookie looks so good to you. Therefore, **snooze a little more and you will definitely lose a little more.**

You may not have a choice about the time you have to get up in the morning for work, school, or your other responsibilities, but you generally do have a choice about when you go to bed. Your assignment for this week is to increase your sleep by half an hour if you typically wake up tired.

Assignment #5
At the end of Week Three, calculate your initial Personal Weight Loss Ratio (PWLR). Every week thereafter, recalculate the ratio, based on your current numbers.

Now that initial water loss has stabilized, it is time to calculate your initial Personal Weight Loss Ratio. If you are a Tortoise Diet member, log on and your calculation will be done for you. If you prefer to perform the calculation yourself, refer to the information in Chapter Four and make sure to jot down your results in your journal.

Assignment #6
Remind yourself of your goals and the commitments you've made to achieve good health and long-term weight loss.

Your last assignment for the final week of "The Tortoise Takes Off" is to remind yourself of your commitment to achieve good health and permanent weight loss! By now some of the habits you're developing may be getting a little easier, and that's really great. No doubt some of them remain challenging, however, and you may feel like you're not making much progress. Trust me, if you're still working at it you are making progress. Flip through the pages of your journal to learn from your experiences. Congratulate yourself for the number of times you have followed through on your commitment to exercise. Review the meals you have eaten and be amazed at the number of healthy choices you have learned to truly enjoy. Look at the numbers plotted on your graph and see how far you've come toward achieving your goals in just three short weeks. This is a good time to give yourself a pat on the back and a little "hang in there" encouragement. Remember, the only way to fail is to quit. Everything else is progress, one step at a time.

MAKING YOUR OWN PLAN

By now you have made a good start at learning to practice most of the essential twenty-five good health habits! By learning to incorporate these new habits into your daily life, you have started to build a solid foundation that will enable you to meet your goals for improved health and for permanent weight loss. You are now ready to begin the next level. This phase, entitled "Making Your Own Plan," begins the "real life" portion of the Tortoise Diet. During "Making Your Own Plan" you will learn how to further build on the skills you have learned and create a livable program of healthy eating and exercise that can last a lifetime.

All the new habits you have begun to practice during the twenty-one days of the "Tortoise Takes Off" should be continued. The big difference as you enter this next phase is, rather than being limited to eating the meals outlined in Appendix A, you will now begin to branch out a little. You will now make your own food choices and develop your own personalized meal plans, based on the Healthy Foods List (Appendix B), the Recipe section (Appendix C), and any other healthy foods you select. Because permanent weight loss requires a lifetime plan, selecting healthy foods that fit your specific calorie requirements is an important skill to develop. Of course, you may continue to include any of the meals you've already learned to enjoy from Appendix A.

"Making Your Own Plan" does present a big challenge, however. Because the meals you had to choose from during the first three weeks were all nicely set out for you in specific nutrient combinations and calorie totals, you didn't have to think too much. Part of learning to develop your own personalized menus will involve not only the calorie totals of the foods, but also the types of foods to include and how they should be combined. It's a bit of a juggling act, at first, learning to pay attention to all the important components of a healthy eating plan while also keeping calories in check. For successful weight loss, you also have to develop meals that keep you feeling full and satisfied. It sounds complicated, but the Assignments of Week Four will teach you how to do it. Developing the ability to make all of the twenty-five habits become second nature to you is the goal of "Making Your Own Plan." Just a reminder that you should feel free to go back and repeat any of the previous weeks before going on, if you need to.

WEEK FOUR

Your goal for Week Four of the Training Assignments is to successfully complete the following eleven assignments.

Assignment #1
Repeat all the assignments from Week One, Week Two, and Week Three.

Continuing to practice these skills will allow them to become habits. Keep working at it!

Assignment #2
Eat the number of calories your Weight Loss Calorie Plan allows.

In assignment #7 of the preparatory period, prior to beginning Week One, you calculated the number of calories your Weight Loss Calorie Plan allowed for each of your six daily meals. As you review the Healthy Foods List (Appendix B), pay attention to the calorie totals of foods you select to be sure your new food choices add up to the correct amount of calories for each particular meal. If you do this, you'll end up with the correct daily total as well. It may take some effort at first, and it does sound cumbersome to look up calorie counts for all of the foods you plan to include. Before long, though, as you develop your own personalized favorite healthy meals and snacks and start to eat them regularly, it will become very easy. Write these foods and their calorie counts down on a piece of paper and stick them on the refrigerator. Jot down the meals you eat and their calorie counts in your journal. Soon you'll have the calorie counts of all your favorites memorized and you won't have to keep looking them up.

Assignment #3
Count calories carefully and truthfully.

Becoming familiar with the calorie counts of your favorite foods is the easy part. This assignment goes one step further and requires that you pay attention to measuring portion sizes and make sure to count all those extra little bites! To accurately stay within your calorie range and keep that "just right" calorie deficit, you've got to be truthful! If you get a little sloppy and those extra calories start creeping onto your plate, your weight loss efforts will be hindered.

Assignment #4
Learn to know how you "feel" when you have eaten the allotted number of calories for your TGIW meals.

Staying within your calorie limits during TGIW meals is a challenge. In real life, you will be confronted with many occasions when you will not have a clue how many calories are in a meal. If your TGIW allotment is 1000 calories, for example, you must develop the ability to recognize how you "feel" when you take in approximately 1000 calories. You need to know when it is time to put down the fork. Keeping calorie intake under control during TGIW meals is one of the most important habits to acquire, to insure your weight-loss success.

Assignment #5
Eat seven to 10 servings of vegetables, fruits and legumes each day.

You must now select foods on your own from those listed in Appendix B and Appendix C that fulfill this daily requirement. If you have favorite foods that are not listed, be sure to look them up in your calorie-counter book to evaluate whether they will make a good addition to your healthy eating plan. The most beneficial suggestion I can make is to continue, for the most part, to eat the same foods you've learned to like from the meal plans in Appendix A. Make an effort, though, to experiment with unfamiliar colorful and healthy foods. This is a perfect time to make your own "Top 40" list if you haven't already done so.

Assignment #6
Make sure to eat plenty of fiber-filled foods.

Keep in mind the importance of fiber to your weight loss success. In addition to vegetables, fruits, and legumes, include 100 percent "whole-grain" pasta and bread choices. Try to eliminate white flour and refined sugar from your diet. Make sure the bread products in your house, including waffles, pancakes, muffins, pita bread, tortillas, and pastas are all made with 100 percent whole-grain flour. Be sure to check the labels to ensure that the first ingredient is actually "whole" grain. If you're not doing so already, try to eat a serving of oatmeal on most days.

Assignment #7
Always combine protein with complex carbohydrates at each meal or snack.

Every meal and snack you select should include protein and complex carbohydrates, and maybe a little heart-healthy fat. Combining these foods at every meal will help keep you full and satisfied, keep blood sugar levels stable, and will help limit calorie intake.

Assignment #8
Decrease saturated fat.

You can minimize the amount of saturated fat in your daily diet by emphasizing foods containing heart-healthy fats. Examples of these foods are nuts, seeds, olives, and avocados. Limit these foods to small servings since the calories add up quickly. Salmon is also an especially good choice for heart-healthy fat. White meat and all types of fish, while not necessarily high in heart-healthy fat, are low in saturated fat. Always broil, bake, roast or barbeque meats, without added fat. Limit the intake of red meat to a maximum of two servings per week, and switch to low fat or, better yet, nonfat dairy products.

Note: There's no need to count your intake of protein, carbohydrate, and fat grams. Following Assignments #5 through #8 will go a long way toward providing the percentage of total daily calories of these nutrients recommended earlier in the book.

Assignment #9
Perform LIFB aerobics for 40 to 60 minutes per session, on a minimum of four days each week. Continue to perform the Tortoise Diet strength-training exercise routine two times each week.

Add the appropriate amount of calories to the meal just before or after the exercise. On "Fool Your Body" days, these calories may be added to your TGIW meal anytime during the day.

Assignment #10
Pay attention to your weight loss graphs and monitor your current weekly PWLR against your initial PWLR.

Completing this important assignment will allow you to determine how well you are staying on track toward achieving your target fat weight and target lean weight. If your PWLR remains greater than zero and larger than your initial PWLR, your current exercise routine is going well. If, however, your current PWLR has dropped either below your initial PWLR, or it has "gone negative," it's time to push yourself a little harder by lifting heavier weights.

Assignment #11
Adjust your Weight Loss Calorie Plan as you lose weight, to ensure that "just right" calorie deficit for fat loss.

Keep in mind if you are more than twenty-five pounds over your target body weight when you start the Tortoise Diet, your Weight Loss Calorie Plan should be adjusted each time you enter a new twenty-five pound weight category. Whenever the daily calorie total is adjusted, you must also remember to recalculate the amount of calories you're allotted for each of your six daily meals.

MAKING YOUR OWN PLAN FOR A LIFETIME

By the time you have completed Week One through Week Four of the Training Assignments, you will have made excellent progress toward making the twenty-five good health habits a part of your new life! Every one of the twenty-five habits has been addressed during these initial four weeks of the program. It's now up to you to keep going. "Making Your Own Plan" should now be followed for a lifetime!

Review all the assignments frequently, repeat if necessary, and keep on working until the habits become second nature to you.

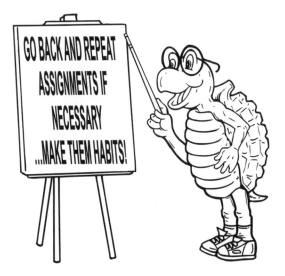

"Each week's assignments will build upon those learned during the previous week, until eventually all twenty-five are included in your daily practice. Step by step, slowly but steadily, you will make progress."

CHAPTER ELEVEN
A LIFETIME PLAN

YOU'RE IN THIS FOR THE LONG HAUL

It will be a tremendous achievement for you to reach your target body weight and body fat percentage. Practicing the new habits you have learned, like daily exercise, eating healthy foods and being an outstanding Energy Manager must continue for a lifetime. You've got to be in this for the long haul! The long haul, however, will have many challenges ahead.

IF YOU BLOW YOUR DIET

It's important for you to understand exactly what happens when you "blow your diet." Let's say that you require 2000 calories each day just to maintain your present weight. I'm not talking about the amount of calories to lose weight, just the amount of calories to keep you at your present weight. If, in one day, you go crazy and eat all 2,000 of those calories, plus another 900 calories, and you also choose not to exercise ... what happens? On this day, with no calorie deficit and an extra 900 calories, you may gain about 1/4 pound, since a pound of fat is about 3,500 calories. In other words, your fat-loss goals will have been set back by about three days. Should you quit the Tortoise Diet and call yourself a failure? The answer is an emphatic NO! You are not a failure; you have just experienced a moment of "life happens!" Three days is not the end of the world, and you shouldn't view it as such.

PRACTICING TGIW RESTRAINT

TGIW meals can be home-cooked family favorites, entertaining or being entertained by friends, or dining out. Experiment with "How Low Can You Go?" techniques when cooking at home to protect yourself from calorie overload. When eating away from home, however, you've got to be careful because calories can add up very quickly. I know that many of my own TGIW meals are eaten in a restaurant. I'm assuming that will be true for you as well, so we definitely need to talk more about developing a strategy to use when you walk through the front door of your favorite eating establishment. Here are some of the techniques I recommend to be able to enjoy a restaurant meal, without going overboard.

1. Eat the foods you really enjoy, but don't usually eat at home. After all, bread and butter, salad with full-fat dressing, or a potato may not be that special, so why waste calories on such ordinary things? Instead, find something special on the menu, like the fresh-caught fish of the day served with a delicate sauce, or something else you are not likely to make at home. In non-restaurant situations, such as socializing with friends and family, the same principle applies. For instance, when I'm visiting my parents it's a sure bet that I'll skip the ordinary mashed potatoes and gravy every time to be sure to have room for one of my Mom's homemade peanut butter twists. If I prioritize my foods this way, I'm able to enjoy them with minimal over-eating, and still appreciate the efforts of my host/hostess.

2. Watch portion sizes! Because restaurant portions are often two to three times as large as what you eat at home, don't eat everything you're served. To keep portions under control, share an entrée with a dining partner. If you do decide to order an entire meal, make sure to have at least some of the food boxed up to go, **for someone else to enjoy on the following day.** Leftovers are a bad idea because they can tempt you to eat yet another TGIW meal again the next day. Another option is to order an appetizer and an interesting soup or salad as a meal, to be able to enjoy several wonderful things without eating too much. If you do order an appetizer, be careful. An excellent choice for an appetizer, for instance, is a jumbo shrimp cocktail. A really lousy choice is a breaded and deep-fried fat-bomb onion!

3. Try to stay away from the bread basket. These calories can add up very quickly, especially if you add butter, and the bread is not likely to be a whole-grain choice. If you do eat bread, thoroughly enjoy a little of it, estimate the calories, then push the basket away or ask the waiter to remove it from the table.

4. Be careful with salad dressing! People think they are being virtuous by ordering a big salad, but then load it up with fat calories galore. A typical ladle of full-fat dressing at a salad bar contains over 300 calories! Sprinkling the salad with cheese and croutons adds even more, so use dressings and high-fat toppings sparingly. If low-fat or non-fat dressings are available, use them. One way to enjoy the taste of the full-fat dressings, however, without going too crazy is to order them served on the side. Try my technique of dipping a fork into the dressing and shaking a little bit onto the salad. A couple of shakes are enough to flavor the salad without adding huge amounts of calories and fat.

5. Select meat, chicken or seafood selections that are baked, broiled or steamed. You can even request that butter or oil not be used in the preparation of your food, not only with meat, but also with vegetables. If something on the menu sounds delicious, but is served with a lovely high-calorie sauce, ask for the sauce to be served on the side and then use the fork technique just described to judiciously enjoy the chef's creation. Avoid food preparations that include breading and deep fat frying. Any foods that have been deep fat fried will have soaked up a lot of fat calories. If you must try them, be sure to remove as much of the breading as possible.

6. If this is not a TGIW occasion, limit your calorie intake for this meal to a maximum of 35 percent of your daily total. Make sure to eat your regularly scheduled meals and snacks prior to the meal and to drink your 16 ounce glass of water just before the meal, so you won't be really hungry when you sit down. Since this is not a TGIW meal, ordering an alcoholic beverage is pretty much out of the question if you want to stay within your calorie allotment. Begin the meal by ordering a broth based vegetable or legume soup, a shrimp cocktail, or a green salad as soon as possible, so you can fill up on some nutritious food first. Scan the menu for some type of lean-protein entree that can be simply prepared without added fat or sauce, such as roasted chicken or broiled fish.

At fast food restaurants, choose a salad with a low-fat dressing, or select the grilled chicken breast sandwich on whole-grain bread, un-toasted with no mayo.

7. Always choose diet soda over regular soda. Regular soda is loaded with pure sugar that will add unnecessary calories and will only set you up for a blood sugar crash. If you order tea, sweeten it with a sugar replacement such as Splenda, or just add some lemon for flavor. Other good beverage choices are club soda or mineral water with a twist of lime.

8. Drink lots of water! Water will help fill you up faster, and can help to counteract the effects of a typically salty restaurant meal, and also any alcohol you consume.

9. Make sure to practice your Hara Hachi Bu skills, and don't boo boo!

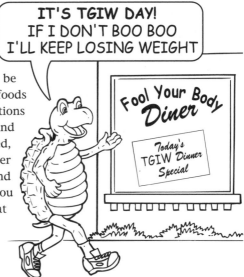

These are a few suggestions to help limit the calories consumed at a TGIW meal. Don't be afraid to question your waiter about the way foods are prepared and to request foods and preparations that meet your needs. The more you understand how your restaurant foods have been prepared, the better you will be able to control the number of calories in your meal. Eventually you may find that your favorite restaurants are ones where you know you can order a wonderful meal that doesn't exceed your calorie allotment.

PORTION CONTROL

Another challenge is that tendency in all of us to slip in an extra bite here, and extra spoonful there, and a second helping all too often. To counteract this tendency it is essential that you learn to correctly practice portion control. If your serving sizes are larger than they should be, or if the extra bites start to add up, you'll end up eating more calories than you think you are. Be honest with yourself because you are the only one who will be hurt if you "fudge." Calories can add up quickly, especially when you're not the one who is cooking. Developing the ability to closely estimate the calorie totals of your meals will allow you to stay on track and be able to enjoy yourself without compromising all your hard work. Healthy vegetables, slathered with melted butter, an extra couple of tablespoons of dressing on your salad, or a spoonful of ice cream to top off dessert may make the difference between a day of successful fat-loss and a day of making absolutely no progress toward your goals.

Another portion control challenge is correctly estimating the portion size of the food you are eating. At home, or during other circumstances where you can exert some control over the food preparation and the portion size of your meal, I strongly encourage you, especially at first, to actually use measuring spoons, measuring cups and a small kitchen food scale to accurately determine the number of calories contained in your meal. Read nutritional labels on the packages of your favorite foods. Divide the entire contents of the package into the number of servings the label says it contains. Look at that individual serving amount. Measure it into a cup or your hand. Then put it on a plate or into a bowl so you can learn to visualize what a true serving size looks like. It may even be a good idea for you to individually wrap or package the entire container into single portions, for easier calorie control. The more you familiarize yourself with what the correctly sized portion for your calorie needs looks like in a controlled environment, the better you'll be able to estimate your calorie intake in other situations when food preparation is not under your direct control.

Become familiar with the following guidelines so you can eyeball common foods and approximate the appropriate serving size.

Serving size	Approximate size of that serving
3 oz of cooked meat, fish, or poultry (without bones or skin, 4 oz weight before cooking)	A deck of cards (including the thickness) or, the size of your palm, or, the size of a mayonnaise jar lid
1 ounces of meat	The size of a matchbox
1 cup of pasta, fruit or cut vegetables	The size of your clenched fist
One bagel	The size of a hockey puck
1 medium piece of fruit	The size of a tennis ball
1 cup dried cereal	The size of a baseball
1 medium potato	The size of a computer mouse
2 TBS of salad dressing	The amount held in a 1/8 cup coffee scoop
2 TBS peanut butter	The size of a ping pong ball
1 TBS peanut butter	The size of a walnut in its shell
1 ounces cheese	The size of four dice or the size of your entire thumb
A bunch of grapes	The size of a light bulb
1 teaspoon butter or mayo	The size of the tip of your thumb
One slice of bread	The size and thickness of a CD in its case

Remember Charlie and the challenge he had with his cereal? He also had a problem with peanut butter and toast. Certainly, a slice of whole-wheat toast and a tablespoon of peanut butter is a healthy 200-calorie snack. However, we now know that a one-tablespoon serving of peanut butter, at about 100 calories, is the size of a walnut in its shell. We also know that two tablespoons of peanut butter, at 200 calories, is the size of a ping-pong ball. It seems as though for a while Charlie liked ping pong balls better than walnuts, because he was eating two pieces of toast and putting a ping pong ball size of peanut butter on each one. That made a total of 400 calories of peanut butter plus 200 calories of toast for his little snack! Charlie really liked his "healthy" "Top 40" list snack, and for a while he was really enjoying his new way to GAIN weight! We finally had to have a little talk about the difference between walnuts and ping-pong balls!

VACATIONS AND OTHER FOOD FESTS

Good news, it's vacation time! We all look forward to these well-deserved times of relaxation, and we're entitled to let loose and enjoy ourselves after working so hard. But what happens to our new, healthy eating and daily exercise routines when we're removed from our usual environment? Large quantities of exotic foods, fruity drinks, and delicious desserts run rampant through the days and nights of a vacation get away. Cruises, for example, may be the ultimate example of temptation. After you've paid good money to have wonderful food available non-stop, you've certainly got to do your best to get your money's worth, right? But what you may not realize is that it's entirely possible to gain five pounds on a 10-day vacation, if you're not careful.

Figuring out how to avoid gaining weight on a vacation is a challenge, but with a little planning you'll sail right through without blowing all your efforts, while still being able to enjoy yourself. Here are my suggestions to help with your weight loss goals while on your well-deserved vacation.

1. First, don't panic and try to starve yourself into a bathing suit before you leave. Placing time-pressure on yourself to hurry up and lose weight only sets up a deprivation mind-set that always leads to failure. Instead, find the most flattering and comfortable outfits for the person you are, and concentrate on planning for an enjoyable vacation.

2. To make sure you are as ready as possible for a vacation, try to follow your Weight Loss Calorie Plan TO THE LETTER for a three-week period prior to the date you are scheduled to leave. Make sure to do your strength-training exercises with your full effort. Also, increase your LIFB minutes. Exercising for as long as you have the energy and time for is always a way you can speed up the loss of fat weight. Just don't go overboard and injure yourself, risking being unable to enjoy your vacation. Another thing, make sure your TGIW meals absolutely do not exceed your calorie allotment. No cheating allowed!

3. Maintaining many of your new Tortoise Diet good health habits on vacation will actually be possible. Advance planning and some simple preparation will help you avoid the pitfalls of poor-food-choice snacking. Many of the snacks you rely on every day at home can be tucked into your car or your luggage. Most anywhere you go, there will be a grocery store and you'll be able to stock up on these and other nutritious and filling foods. Use some of these foods to replace a restaurant meal whenever possible. Eating breakfast, lunch and dinner out in a restaurant while on vacation is not only expensive in terms of money, but also in terms of calories! During the day, consider continuing your habit of eating small, frequent meals, just like you do at home. Many hotels now have small refrigerators. Ignore any tempting fattening foods found in them and place a few healthy food snacks of your own inside. If you'd like to go one step further, bring along a few kitchen items from home that will make it possible to more easily follow your usual eating plan.

4. Bring along comfortable shoes and clothing that will allow you to continue your exercise program, or at least to keep active. Make every attempt to continue your healthy habit of performing LIFB exercise by trying to walk as much as you can each day. Perhaps this would be the time to plan on an evening of dancing or a walk on the beach? Many hotels provide a gym with exercise equipment and weights or a swimming pool, which you could utilize to keep up your usual exercise routine for 40-60 minutes each day. The more exercise you can fit in each day, the more you'll be able to add some calories and splurge a little.

5. Use this vacation time to recharge, regroup, and reconsider your goals. Relaxation is an important component of a healthy life. Bring along some self-indulgent items ... some new bath salts, a mud masque, a juicy novel, a journal that you never seem to have time to write your short stories in, or a digital camera you've always wanted to learn how to use. Be sure to spend some quiet and reflective time during your vacation, pausing to breathe, to smell the air, to give and receive long foot-rubs, and to take long and relaxing walks. Allowing yourself to focus on things outside of your usual daily responsibilities is what a vacation is all about. Recharge those batteries. You've been working hard! Use the time away to get some perspective on your life and your achievements. Spend a lot of time laughing and paying attention to your loved ones. Dream a little bit and plan an exciting goal for yourself when you get home. Last, but not least, do a little bit more snoozin' than you're used to.

The key to limiting weight gain on vacations is continuing as best you can to practice your new healthy habits. If you're going to visit family and friends on vacation, know that family gatherings are notorious for encouraging that HARA HACHI BOO BOO tendency in all of us. To counteract this, remember to sample the wonderful, traditional, homemade treats first, savoring each bite, and try to stop eating before you've gone overboard. Always keep in mind while on vacations that pounds go on a lot easier than they come off.

GET BACK ON THAT HORSE!

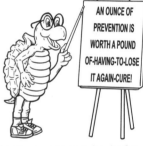

If you notice the scale inching its way up, instead of being depressed and giving up ... it's time to say "whoa" and get back on that horse! If you do find yourself slipping back into old habits, I would recommend you take the following steps:

1. Refocus on your long-term goals for good health and for reaching your target body fat percentage. Review your journal and look at your chart. Think about how much effort you've already made to get to where you are. Remember how good you were feeling and the sense of empowerment you experienced when the pounds were slipping away.

2. Continue (or re-start the practice if you've drifted away from it) to write in your journal each day. Record your food intake and your exercise. Keep track of the events of your days and how you are feeling about them. This may give you some insight as to why you have been eating too much of the wrong types of foods, and will help you to see what "triggers" have caused you to lose your motivation.

3. Re-dedicate yourself to planning and preparing healthy foods. Get back into the habit of shopping for and stocking the kitchen with nutrient-dense foods. Return to some old favorites from Appendix A and review Appendix B again to select a routine breakfast, lunch and some snacks that you really like. Get rid of any leftovers or junky foods that have sneaked back into your kitchen. Cut, chop and individually package your food so you can "grab and go" as you leave the house each day.

4. Enlist someone to help you get back on track. Tell someone who cares about you that you're struggling a little bit. Ask someone to walk with you so you'll get re-motivated to exercise. Surround yourself with people who want to see you succeed.

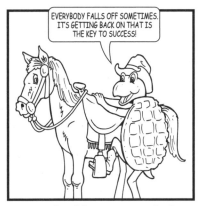

EVERYBODY FALLS OFF SOMETIMES. IT'S GETTING BACK ON THAT IS THE KEY TO SUCCESS!

5. Consider following to the letter (and to the calorie) one of the menu plans that you have used previously with some success, to get yourself mentally back on track. Being a little more exact and not allowing yourself quite so many marginally healthy choices throughout the day should help keep hunger at bay and help you get back in the groove. Making absolutely sure your calorie intake is correct should start to push those numbers downward again.

6. Focus on exercise. Re-dedicate yourself to your weekly program. Make sure you are doing your LIFB exercise at the proper heart rate. If you haven't been doing your weights, get started again. Rejuvenate your efforts by mixing things up and trying some new activities. Re-energize yourself! Remember, however, to take a break completely from exercise one day each week.

7. Review your charts to determine where you might be drifting off course. Make sure that your lean weight is where it should be.

8. Realize that stalled progress or a loss of motivation is pretty normal. You're working hard to change deeply ingrained habits, and it's not easy! You haven't failed. This is a lifetime process, so don't give up!

The one constant is that life won't always go according to plan. Living the Tortoise Diet lifestyle requires a total overhaul of your basic approach toward food, activity and health. Instead of being an all or nothing situation, learn to take each day one at a time, to make ongoing, small decisions. Work slowly but steadily at reaching your goals, regrouping if you need to, but always refocusing again on the things that are important in your life.

REACHING THE FINISH LINE

If you've worked hard, persevered, overcome the obstacles, gotten back on that horse, and proudly reached the finish line ... things will get really exciting! First of all, you'll feel great! What an achievement, to have lost all of the body fat you needed to lose! You'll feel stronger and more energetic and, even better, you'll be able to eat more! If you no longer need to lose body fat, there's no need for a calorie deficit. This means you can start eating the number of calories you calculated for your Lifetime Calorie Plan instead of the number of calories in your Weight Loss Calorie Plan. Also, during your weight loss you have only been able to add about half of the calories to your eating plan for any exercise performed. Why only half the calories? Because about half of the energy was coming from your fat storage warehouse. Now that your storage warehouse is gone, you can now start adding 100 percent of the calories burned during exercise to your Lifetime Calorie Plan!

To see how exciting this is, let's take the example of a woman who has arrived at her target body weight and target body fat percentage goals. Her Lifetime Calorie Plan has been calculated to be 2100 calories per day. While she was in the category of 0-25 pounds over her target body weight, 400 calories was subtracted from her Lifetime Calorie Plan to create a calorie deficit. Following her Weight Loss Calorie Plan of 1700 calories, plus replacing only some of the calories she burned off each day during exercise, has allowed her to reach her goals. Now that she has reached her target numbers, she no longer requires a calorie deficit. She can add back those 400 calories and begin eating 2100 calories each day to maintain her target body weight. If she continues to exercise for about an hour a day, another 300 calories or so can be added. In other words, if she continues her new healthy eating and exercise habits, she can now eat about 2,400 calories per day and not gain weight! Life will be good when you reach your goals!

"What an achievement, to have lost all of the body fat you needed to lose! You'll feel stronger and more energetic and, even better, you'll be able to eat more!"

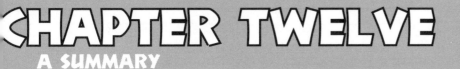

CHAPTER TWELVE
A SUMMARY

I DON'T HAVE THE_____(FILL IN THE BLANK)

If you are convinced that the Tortoise Diet is an exciting and livable plan that can work for you, congratulations! I'm excited for you! Some of you, however, may be gearing up with some good excuses. Maybe you're saying I can't follow the Tortoise Diet because I don't have the _____ (fill in the blank). You may think you don't have the ability to cook, you don't have the energy to exercise after a hard day of work, you don't have enough people in your life to support you, or any of a number of other "don't haves." Whatever you don't have really doesn't matter though, because there is only one thing you DO need to have to begin the process of successfully changing your life. **You need to have desire.**

Unfortunately, the perfect time to change your life may never come, and that zipper on your fat suit won't ever magically unzip itself. If you have desire, the only requirements to begin changing your unhealthy habits into better ones already belong to you. Just as I did, you must first and foremost face up to who you are now, compared with who you would really like to be. Once you've decided that it's time to try to become the person you envision, the next step is to ask yourself "How bad do I want it?" If you want things enough to put forth the effort and make the necessary sacrifices, and if you honestly have the desire to improve your health and lose weight permanently, the concepts shared in this book were designed specifically for you.

You're not alone if your reaction to the "moving the mountain" project of changing your life is to feel overwhelmed! Trust me when I say that the hardest part is simply to begin. If you start the Tortoise Diet and give it some effort, and if you're satisfied with slow but steady progress, I think you'll find that success will sneak up on you! It happens over time, in ways you may not realize until you take the time to pause and reflect on how much you've changed. The commitment to change the way you view food and exercise, coupled with changing habits, will allow you to not only lose weight, but to steadily increase that feeling deep within yourself of being confident and in control. This self-confidence will be accompanied by increased enthusiasm and energy. You will feel healthier, stronger, and proud of your accomplishments.

HOW MANY GOOD HABITS ARE ENOUGH?

Every single one of the twenty-five habits is extremely important! If you decide to practice just a few good habits, it may not be enough! I'll be the first to admit that some of the twenty-five good habits are harder than others. Realize, however, that making the effort to make all of these new habits a reality in your life has an incredible payoff. Very few people in the Western world live at their target body weight and target body fat percentage, and get to enjoy the feeling of strength, boundless energy, self-confidence, and satisfaction that goes along with that achievement. I want each and every one of you reading this book to know it can really happen for you!

I encourage you to use this book as you would a class textbook. It's impossible to read an instructional book like the Tortoise Diet only once and expect to absorb all the information it contains. Study this book and refer back to it often. If this were a college textbook you would expect to take an entire semester of study to learn its contents. View your weight loss in the same way. Use the assignments in Chapter Ten to make steady progress, but don't hesitate to go back and repeat weeks. Know right up front that you will have slip-ups. Don't get frustrated and quit! Get back on that horse! Keep working at it until the skills you are learning start to feel natural.

NOT A DIET ANYMORE

When your bad health habits have been changed into the twenty-five good health habits, it's not a diet any more! Instead, the Tortoise Diet will have become a satisfying and healthy way of life. It is my sincere hope that you'll make that subtle but very powerful mental transformation. Good habits are so easy to live with. You can happily live a lifetime enjoying good health and permanent weight loss by eating nutritious healthy food and getting regular exercise. This is truly the way to "Win the Race to Lose!"

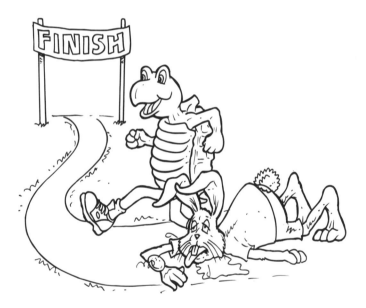

If you struggle with your weight, I hope you use the Tortoise Diet to change your life. I know, from my own life, it has that power. Make the twenty-five good health habits a part of your life and change will happen ... slow and steady ... like The Tortoise.

All the Best!

Patty

APPENDIX A
MEAL PLANS & DINNERS

125 CALORIE MEAL PLANS

1. Green salad, dressed with balsamic vinegar or lemon juice. Top with ½ cup of any combination of chopped tomatoes, onions, carrot, mushrooms, peppers, radishes and celery; plus 3 ounces water or vacuum packed albacore tuna mixed with 1 tablespoon non-fat mayo.

2. 120 calorie portion whey or soy-based protein powder, blended with water and ice.

3. 4 ounces thin-sliced, deli-style turkey OR ham wrapped into a large lettuce leaf; plus a dill pickle slice. Add mustard and non-fat mayo, as desired.

4. 1 WASA cracker (rye, sesame or whole-wheat variety) OR 1 RyKrisp rectangle; plus 1 ounce low-fat cheddar OR Swiss cheese.

5. 2 carrots; plus 8 almonds.

6. ¾ cup plain non-fat yogurt topped with ½ cup berries.

7. 2 ounces water or vacuum packed albacore tuna mixed with 1 tablespoon non-fat mayo; plus 1 tomato, sliced.

8. ½ cup non-fat cottage cheese; plus ⅓ cup cooked green peas.

9. 1 apple; plus 1 slice 2% cheese "single."

10. 1 hard-boiled egg; plus 4 ounces non-fat milk.

11. 4 cups air-popped popcorn (no oil); plus 4 ounces non-fat milk.

12. ½ cup non-fat refried beans topped with 3 tablespoons salsa and 2 tablespoons non-fat sour cream.

13. 1 cucumber and 1 large tomato chopped and mixed with one minced clove of garlic, 3 tablespoons chopped olives and 1 teaspoon extra-virgin olive oil. Add chopped basil, parsley or cilantro, as desired.

14. ½ cup Egg Beaters, scrambled or micro-waved, 1 tablespoon grated Parmesan and a total of 1 cup chopped tomato, onion, mushrooms and spinach.

15. 8-ounces V-8 juice; plus 1 (1ounce) part-skim mozzarella cheese stick.

16. 2 cups cooked butternut squash with 1 tablespoon no-sugar maple syrup and 1 tablespoon chopped walnuts.

(125 CALORIE MEAL PLANS CONT.)

17. 1 cup blueberries with ½ cup non-fat milk.

18. ¾ cup Minestrone, White Bean or Lentil Soup, or Turkey Chili. (Recipes in Appendix C)

19. 3 stalks of celery; spread with 1 tablespoon peanut butter.

20. 1 slice whole-wheat cinnamon-raisin toast; spread with 2 tablespoons non-fat cream cheese.

21. 3 ounces cooked shrimp, served with slices of fresh lemon and 3 tablespoons cocktail sauce.

22. 2 tablespoons hummus; plus 2 carrots and 2 stalks celery.

23. ¾ cup non-fat/no-sugar pudding.

150 CALORIE MEAL PLANS

1. 1 cup Minestrone, White Bean or Lentil Soup, or Turkey Chili. (Recipes in Appendix C)

2. 120 calorie portion whey or soy based protein shake blended with water, ice and ½ cup berries.

3. ⅔ cup non-fat cottage cheese; plus 1 tomato, sliced.

4. 1 (1 ounce) part-skim mozzarella cheese stick; plus 1 orange.

5. 2 carrots; plus 12 almonds.

6. 1 hard-boiled egg; plus 1 orange.

7. 1 cup non-fat/no-sugar pudding.

8. 5 cups air-popped popcorn (no oil); plus 5 ounces non-fat milk.

9. 1 cup plain non-fat yogurt topped with ½ cup berries.

10. 2 non-fat Fruit Newtons: plus ½ cup non-fat milk.

11. 3 ounces water or vacuum packed albacore tuna mixed with 2 tablespoons non-fat mayo; plus 1 WASA cracker (whole-wheat, rye or sesame variety).

12. 1 apple; plus 2 teaspoons peanut butter.

13. 4 tablespoons hummus; plus 1 carrot and 2 stalks of celery.

(150 CALORIE MEAL PLANS CONT.)

14.   2 slices whole-wheat reduced-calorie bread OR 1 slice whole-grain bread; plus 1 slice 2% cheese "single."

15.   100 calorie serving of a whole-grain, high-fiber, low sugar cereal with 5 ounces non-fat milk.

16.   ½ cup black beans and ¼ cup non-fat refried beans topped with 2 teaspoons non-fat sour cream and 2 tablespoons salsa.

17.   12 ounces V-8 juice; plus one 1 (1 ounce) part-skim mozzarella cheese stick.

18.   2 ounces thin-sliced, deli-style turkey with 1 ounce low-fat cheddar cheese wrapped in a large lettuce leaf. Add mustard and non-fat mayo, as desired.

19.   1 cup non-fat/no-sugar hot chocolate; plus 1 slice whole-grain cinnamon-raisin toast spread with 1 tablespoon non-fat cream cheese.

20.   Large green salad, dressed with balsamic vinegar. Top salad with 1 ½ cups of any combination of chopped tomato, onion, carrots, cauliflower, broccoli, mushrooms and cucumber. Top salad with either 2 ounces grilled chicken breast OR 3 ounces grilled shrimp.

21.   ¾ cup Egg Beaters, scrambled or micro-waved, topped with 2 tablespoons chopped olives, 2 tablespoons salsa and 2 tablespoons non-fat sour cream.

22.   ⅔ cup non-fat cottage cheese; plus ⅓ cup green peas.

23.   5 Ak-Mak cracker rectangles spread with 1 wedge of low-fat "Laughing Cow" cheese.

24.   ¾ cup cooked oatmeal with ½ cup non-fat milk. Add cinnamon and 1 tablespoon no-sugar maple syrup.

25.   ⅔ cup plain non-fat yogurt topped with 1 cup chopped fruit.

26.   1 slice Banana Bread. (½ of Recipe in Appendix C)

175 CALORIE MEAL PLANS

1.   1 cup plain, non-fat yogurt topped with ¾ cup berries.

2.   120 calorie portion whey or soy based protein shake blended with water, ice and ¾ cup berries.

3.   ¾ cup non-fat cottage cheese with 1 sliced tomato and 2 tablespoons chopped olives.

4.   1 (1 ounce) part-skim mozzarella cheese stick; plus 1 orange; plus 1 carrot.

5.   2 carrots; plus 15 almonds.

(175 CALORIE MEAL PLANS CONT.)

6. 1 hard-boiled egg; plus 1 banana.

7. 1 meatless burger patty, topped with 2 slices each of onion and tomato. Add lettuce, mustard and non-fat mayo as desired.

8. 3 ounces thin-sliced, deli-style turkey with 1 ounce low-fat cheddar cheese, wrapped in a large lettuce leaf. Spread with mustard and non-fat mayo, as desired.

9. 1 cup Split Pea Soup. (Recipe in Appendix C)

10. 1 apple with 1 tablespoon peanut butter.

11. 3 ounces water or vacuum packed albacore tuna mixed with 1 tablespoons non-fat mayo on either 2 WASA crackers (whole-wheat, rye or sesame variety) OR 2 RyKrisp rectangles.

12. 3 tablespoons hummus mixed with 2 tablespoons chopped olives, with 2 carrots and 2 stalks celery.

13. 5 cups air-popped popcorn (no oil); plus 1 (1 ounce) part-skim mozzarella cheese stick.

14. 100 calorie serving of a whole-grain, high-fiber, low sugar cereal with 1 cup non-fat milk.

15. 12 ounces V-8 juice; plus 1 ounce part-skim mozzarella cheese stick; plus 1 carrot.

16. ½ cup black beans with ¼ cup non-fat refried beans topped with 2 tablespoons non-fat sour cream and 2 tablespoons salsa.

17. 2 stalks celery spread with 1 tablespoon peanut butter; plus 2 carrots.

18. Large green salad, dressed with balsamic vinegar. Top salad with 1 cup of any combination of chopped tomato, onion, carrots, cauliflower, broccoli, mushrooms, and cucumber. Top salad with either 3 ounces grilled chicken breast OR 4 ounces grilled shrimp.

19. 1 cup non-fat/no-sugar hot chocolate; plus 1 slice cinnamon-raisin toast spread with 1 wedge low-fat "Laughing Cow" cheese and 1 teaspoon all-fruit/no-sugar jam.

20. ¾ cup non-fat cottage cheese; plus ½ cup green peas.

21. 2 non-fat Fruit Newtons; plus ¾ cup non-fat milk.

22. 1 slice 2% milk cheese "single" on 1 slice whole-grain bread with 2 slices of tomato and 1 entire cucumber, sliced.

23. 2 wedges low-fat "Laughing Cow" cheese and ONE of the following choices: 4 Ak-mak crackers, OR 3 RyKrisp rectangles, OR 6 reduced-fat Triscuit crackers.

24. ⅔ cup Egg Beaters, scrambled or micro-waved with 1 ounce low-fat cheese. Top with 2 tablespoons salsa and 1 tablespoon non-fat sour cream.

(175 CALORIE MEAL PLANS CONT.)

25. ¾ cup cooked oatmeal with 4 ounces non-fat milk. Add cinnamon and 2 tablespoons no-sugar maple syrup.

26. 1 cup non-fat/no-sugar pudding with 1 tablespoon non-fat/no-sugar whipped topping.

27. 1 cup plain non-fat yogurt with ¾ cup chopped fruit.

28. ¾ cup cooked oatmeal with 6 ounces non-fat milk. Add cinnamon and 1 tablespoon no-sugar maple syrup.

200 CALORIE MEAL PLANS

1. ¾ cup Split Pea Soup (Recipe in Appendix C); plus either 2 WASA crackers (whole-wheat, rye or sesame varieties) OR 2 RyKrisp rectangles.

2. ½ of a whole-wheat pita filled with 1 tablespoon chopped olives, 1 ounce crumbled low-fat feta cheese and a total of 1 cup of chopped onion, tomato, peppers and cucumber.

3. ⅔ cup non-fat cottage cheese with 2 tablespoons chopped olives and 2 tomatoes, sliced.

4. 1 (1ounce) part-skim mozzarella cheese stick; plus 1 orange; plus 2 carrots.

5. 2 carrots; plus 18 almonds.

6. 1 hard-boiled egg; plus 1 slice whole-grain toast with 1 tablespoon all-fruit/no-sugar jam.

7. 1 ⅓ cups Minestrone, White Bean, or Lentil Soup, or Turkey Chili (Recipes in Appendix C) OR A 200 calorie serving (check label) of a canned or packaged vegetable and legume-based soup.

8. 4 ounces thin-sliced, deli-style turkey OR ham with 1 ounce low-fat cheddar cheese, wrapped in a large lettuce leaf. Add mustard and non-fat mayo, as desired.

9. 1 cup non-fat plain yogurt topped 1 cup berries.

10. 1 apple with 1 tablespoon peanut butter.

11. 4 ounces water or vacuum packed albacore tuna mixed with 1 tablespoon non-fat mayo on either 2 WASA (whole-wheat, rye, or sesame variety) OR 2 RyKrisp rectangles.

12. 120 calorie portion whey or soy based protein shake blended with water, ice and either 1 cup berries OR 1 banana.

13. 6 cups air-popped popcorn (no oil); plus 1 (1 ounce) part-skim mozzarella cheese stick.

(200 CALORIE MEAL PLANS CONT.)

14. 3 ounces tofu, stir-fried in 1 teaspoon extra-virgin olive oil, soy sauce and ginger. Also stir-fry 2 cups Oriental mixed vegetables.

15. ⅔ cup Egg Beaters, scrambled or micro-waved with 1 ounce low-fat cheddar, Swiss or feta cheese and 1 cup total of tomato, mushrooms, and spinach.

16. ⅔ cup black beans and ⅓ cup non-fat refried beans topped with 2 tablespoons non-fat sour cream and 2 tablespoons salsa.

17. 2 stalks celery; spread with 1 ⅔ tablespoons peanut butter.

18. Large green salad, dressed with balsamic vinegar and 1 teaspoon extra-virgin olive oil Top salad with ½ cup of any combination of chopped tomato, onion, carrots, cauliflower, broccoli, mushrooms and cucumber. Top salad with either 3 ounces grilled chicken breast OR 4 ounces grilled shrimp.

19. ⅔ cup cooked oatmeal with one of the following choices: 1 tablespoon raisins OR 1 tablespoon chopped walnuts OR 1 tablespoon mini chocolate chips; add cinnamon and 2 tablespoons no-sugar maple syrup.

20. ¾ cup non-fat cottage cheese; plus ⅔ cup green peas.

21. 12 ounces V-8 juice; plus 1 (1 ounce) part-skim mozzarella stick; plus 2 carrots.

22. 2 non-fat Fruit Newtons; plus 1 cup non-fat milk.

23. 12 ounces V-8 juice; plus 1 part-skim mozzarella sticks; plus 2 carrots.

24. 120 calorie serving of any whole-grain, high-fiber, low sugar cereal; plus 1 cup non-fat milk.

25. 1 slice whole-grain cinnamon-raisin toast spread with 2 tablespoons non-fat cream cheese; plus 1 orange.

26. ¾ cup non-fat/no-sugar pudding; plus 1 cup berries.

27. 1 cup plain non-fat yogurt topped with 1 cup chopped fruit.

28. ½ cup cooked brown rice with 1 tablespoon chopped walnuts; plus 1 cup lightly steamed broccoli florets.

29. 1 slice whole-grain bread; plus either 2 slices 2% cheese "singles" OR 1 tablespoon peanut butter.

30. 1 meatless burger patty with 1 slice 2% cheese "single." Add lettuce, mustard and non-fat mayo, as desired.

31. 1 slice Banana Bread (½ of Recipe in Appendix C) plus 4 ounces non-fat milk.

225 CALORIE MEAL PLANS

1. ¾ cup non-fat cottage cheese; plus 2 tablespoons chopped olives; plus 2 tomatoes, sliced.

2. 120 calorie portion whey or soy based shake blended with water, ice and 1 ⅓ cups berries OR 1 large banana.

3. 1 ¼ cups Split Pea Soup. (Recipe in Appendix C)

4. 1 (1 ounce) part-skim mozzarella stick; plus 2 carrots; plus 1 apple.

5. 2 carrots; plus 21 almonds.

6. 1 hard-boiled egg; plus 1 orange; plus 8 ounces non-fat milk.

7. 1 meatless burger patty with 1 slice 2% cheese "single" topped with 2 slices, tomato and onion. Add lettuce, mustard and non-fat mayo, as desired.

8. 3 ounces water or vacuum packed albacore tuna mixed with 2 tablespoons non-fat mayo and ONE of the following choices: 3 WASA (whole-wheat, rye, or sesame varieties) OR 3 RyKrisp rectangles OR 5 Ak-Mak crackers OR 6 reduced-fat Triscuit crackers.

9. 1 apple; plus 1 ⅓ tablespoons peanut butter.

10. 165 calorie serving of any whole-grain, high-fiber/low sugar cereal with 6 ounces non-fat milk.

11. ⅔ cup black beans with ½ cup non-fat refried beans topped with 1 tablespoon non-fat sour cream and 2 tablespoons salsa.

12. ½ of a whole-wheat pita filled with 3 tablespoons hummus and 1 cup total of chopped tomato, onion, cucumber.

13. 1 whole-grain English muffin, toasted. Top with ¾ cup Egg Beaters, scrambled or micro-waved.

14. 1 whole-wheat tortilla (7"), cut into wedges and baked into "chips." Top with 1 slice 2% cheese "single" and melt cheese in oven or microwave. Top with 2 tablespoons salsa and 1 tablespoon non-fat sour cream.

15. Large green salad, dressed with balsamic vinegar and 1 teaspoon extra-virgin olive oil Top salad with 1 cup of any combination of chopped tomato, onion, carrots, cauliflower, broccoli, mushrooms, and cucumber. Top salad with either 3 ounces grilled chicken breast OR 4 ounces grilled shrimp.

16. 1 cup non-fat cottage cheese; plus ⅔ cup green peas.

17. 1 cup non-fat/no-sugar pudding; plus 1 orange.

(225 CALORIE MEAL PLANS CONT.)

18. 1 cup plain non-fat yogurt with ¾ cup chopped fruit topped with 1 tablespoon chopped walnuts OR pecans.

19. 1 cup non-fat/no-sugar hot chocolate; plus 1 slice whole-grain cinnamon-raisin toast; plus 1 tablespoon peanut butter.

20. 1 cup plain non-fat yogurt topped with ¾ cup berries and 1 tablespoon chopped walnuts. Add cinnamon and 2 tablespoons no-sugar maple syrup.

21. 1 cup Egg Beaters, scrambled or micro-waved topped with 1 ounce low-fat cheddar or Swiss cheese; plus 2 tablespoons salsa and 1 tablespoon non-fat sour cream.

22. 5 ounces thin-sliced, deli-style turkey and 1 slice 2% cheese "single" with 2 slices tomato, wrapped in large lettuce leaf. Add mustard and non-fat mayo, as desired.

23. 3 ounces grilled chicken breast; plus 1 cup cooked butternut squash topped with 1 tablespoon chopped walnuts and 1 tablespoon no-sugar maple syrup.

24. ⅔ cup non-fat/no-sugar pudding; plus 2 non-fat Fruit Newtons.

25. 3.5 ounces grilled chicken; plus 1 cup green beans; plus 1 tomato, sliced.

26. 2 stalks celery spread with 2 tablespoons peanut butter.

27. 12 ounces V-8 juice; plus 1 (1ounce) part-skim mozzarella stick; plus 1 orange.

28. ½ of a whole-wheat pita filled with 2 tablespoons chopped olives, 1 ounce crumbled low-fat feta cheese and 1 cup total of chopped onion, tomato, cucumber, and red, yellow and orange peppers.

29. 1 slice whole-grain bread OR 2 slices reduced-calorie whole-grain bread with 3 ounces thin-sliced, deli-style ham and 2 slices each, tomato and onion. Add lettuce, mustard and non-fat mayo, as desired.

30. 1 cup Minestrone, White Bean, or Lentil Soup, or Turkey Chili (Recipes in Appendix C); plus ONE of the following selections: 2 WASA (whole-wheat, rye or sesame varieties) OR 2 RyKrisp rectangles OR 3 Ak-Mak crackers OR 4 reduced-fat Triscuit crackers.

31. ½ cup cooked brown rice with 1 tablespoon chopped walnuts; plus 1 ⅔ cup any combination of lightly steamed tomato, broccoli, onions, mushrooms, carrots, zucchini, and cabbage.

32. ¾ cup cooked oatmeal with ONE of the following choices: 1 tablespoon raisins OR 1 tablespoon miniature chocolate chips OR 1 tablespoon chopped walnuts. Add cinnamon and 2 tablespoons no-sugar maple syrup.

33. 3 ounces tofu, stir-fried in 1 teaspoon extra-virgin olive oil. Also stir-fry 2 ¾ cups Oriental mixed vegetables.

34. 1 slice Banana Bread (½ of Recipe in Appendix C); plus 8 ounces non-fat milk.

250 CALORIE MEAL PLANS

1. 1 cup Split Pea Soup (Recipe in Appendix C); plus 2 WASA (whole-wheat, rye, or sesame varieties) OR 2 RyKrisp rectangles.

2. 120 calorie whey or soy based shake blended with water, ice and 1 cup berries OR 1 banana; plus 6 almonds.

3. 1 apple; plus 1 ½ tablespoons peanut butter.

4. 1 (1 ounce) part-skim mozzarella stick; plus 3 carrots; plus 1 apple.

5. 3 carrots; plus 20 almonds.

6. 1 hard-boiled egg; plus 1 orange; plus 1 cup plain non-fat yogurt.

7. 1 whole-wheat tortilla (7"), cut into wedges and baked into "chips." Sprinkle with 1 ounce low-fat cheddar and melt cheese in oven or microwave. Top with 3 tablespoons salsa and 3 tablespoons non-fat sour cream.

8. 5 ounces water or vacuum packed tuna mixed with 2 tablespoons non-fat mayo; plus ONE of the following selections: 2 WASA crackers (whole-wheat, rye or sesame varieties) OR 2 RyKrisp rectangles OR 3 Ak-Mak crackers OR 4 reduced-fat Triscuit crackers.

9. ⅔ cup plain non-fat yogurt with 1 cup berries sprinkled with 100 calorie serving of a whole-wheat, high-fiber, low sugar cereal; plus 1 tablespoon no-sugar maple syrup.

10. ⅔ cup non-fat cottage cheese; plus 3 tablespoons chopped olives and 1 tomato, sliced; plus ONE of the following selections: 2 WASA (whole-wheat, rye or sesame varieties) OR 2 RyKrisp rectangles, OR 3 Ak-Mak crackers.

11. ½ cup black beans and ⅔ cup non-fat refried beans with 1 tablespoon non-fat sour cream and 3 tablespoons salsa.

12. ½ of a whole-wheat pita filled with 2 tablespoons chopped olives, 1 ounce crumbled low-fat feta cheese and a total of 1 ½ cups chopped onion, tomato, red, orange and yellow peppers.

13. 1 slice whole-grain bread OR 2 slices reduced-calorie whole-grain bread; plus either 3 ounces thin-sliced, deli-style ham OR turkey with 2 slices each, tomato and onion and lettuce. Add mustard and non-fat mayo, as desired.

14. 1 toasted whole-grain English muffin topped with ½ cup Egg Beaters, scrambled or micro-waved; plus 1 slice 2% cheese "single".

15. 12 ounces V-8 juice; plus 1 (1 ounce) part-skim mozzarella stick; plus 1 orange; plus 1 carrot.

16. 5 ounces thin-sliced, deli-style turkey; plus 1 ounce low-fat cheddar OR Swiss cheese and 2 slices of tomato, wrapped in a large lettuce leaf. Add mustard and non-fat mayo, as desired.

(250 CALORIE MEAL PLANS CONT.)

17. 1 meatless burger; plus 1 slice whole-grain bread and 1 slice each of tomato and onion. Add lettuce, mustard and non-fat mayo, as desired.

18. Large green salad, dressed with balsamic vinegar and 1 teaspoon extra-virgin olive oil. Top salad with a total of 1 ¾ cups chopped tomato, onion, carrots, cauliflower, broccoli, mushrooms, and cucumber. Top salad with either 3 ounces grilled chicken breast OR 4 ounces grilled shrimp.

19. 4 ounces tofu, any variety, stir-fried in 1 teaspoon extra-virgin olive oil. Also stir-fry 3 cups Oriental mixed

20. 1 ⅓ cups chopped fruit; plus 1 cup plain non-fat yogurt; plus 1 tablespoon chopped walnuts.

21. 2 stalks celery spread with 1 tablespoon peanut butter and 1 tablespoon raisins; plus 1 apple.

22. 175 calorie serving of a whole-grain, high fiber, low sugar cereal; plus 8 ounces non-fat milk.

23. 1 cup non-fat/no-sugar hot chocolate; plus 2 slices whole-grain cinnamon-raisin toast spread with 2 tablespoons non-fat cream cheese.

24. 1 non-fat ice cream sandwich (check label to find one that is approximately 140 calories per sandwich); plus 2 non-fat Fruit Newtons.

25. 5 ounces thin-sliced, deli-style turkey; plus 1 ounce low-fat cheddar OR Swiss cheese with 2 slices of tomato, wrapped in a large lettuce leaf. Add mustard and non-fat mayo, as desired.

26. 1 cup non-fat/no sugar pudding; plus 1 cup chopped fruit.

27. 1 cup non-fat cottage cheese; plus ¾ cup green peas.

28. 3 ounces grilled chicken breast; plus ⅔ cup cooked butternut squash topped with 1 tablespoon chopped walnuts and 2 tablespoons no-sugar maple syrup.

29. 1 cup cooked oatmeal topped with 1 tablespoon chopped walnuts and either 1 tablespoon raisins OR 1 tablespoon miniature chocolate chips. Add cinnamon and 2 tablespoons no-sugar maple syrup.

30. 1 ⅔ cup Minestrone, White Bean Soup, or Turkey Chili (Recipes in Appendix C) OR a 250 calorie serving of a canned or packaged vegetable and legume based soup (check package labels).

31. ½ cup cooked brown rice with 1 tablespoon chopped walnuts; plus 2 cups of any combination of chopped broccoli, carrots, asparagus, beets, Brussels sprouts, green beans, cauliflower, tomato, and mushrooms.

(250 CALORIE MEAL PLANS CONT.)

32. 1 slice Banana Bread (½ of Recipe in Appendix C); plus 4 ounces non-fat milk; plus 1 orange.

275 CALORIE MEAL PLANS

1. ¾ cup Split Pea Soup (Recipe in Appendix C); plus ONE of the following selections spread with 1 wedge low-fat "Laughing Cow" cheese: plus 3 WASA (whole-wheat, rye or sesame varieties) OR 3 RyKrisp rectangles OR 4 Ak-Mak crackers OR 6 reduced-fat Triscuit crackers.

2. Large green salad, dressed with balsamic vinegar and 1 teaspoon extra-virgin olive oil. Top salad with 1 ½ cups of any combination of chopped tomato, onion, carrots, cauliflower, broccoli, mushrooms, and cucumber. Top salad with either 3.5 ounces grilled chicken breast OR 5 ounces grilled shrimp.

3. ¾ cup non-fat cottage cheese; plus 2 tomatoes, sliced; plus ONE of the following selections: 2 WASA (whole-wheat, rye or sesame varieties)   OR 2 RyKrisp rectangles OR 3 Ak-Mak crackers OR 4 reduced-fat Triscuit crackers.

4. 1 slice whole-grain bread OR 2 slices reduced-calorie whole-grain bread; plus ONE of the following: 3 ounces thin-sliced, deli-style ham OR turkey OR 2 ounces grilled chicken breast OR 3 ounces water or vacuum packed albacore tuna; plus 2 slices each, tomato and onion; plus 1 slice 2% cheese "single." Add lettuce, mustard and non-fat mayo, as desired.

5. 2 carrots; plus 19 almonds; plus 1 orange.

6. 1 apple; plus 1 ⅔ tablespoons peanut butter.

7. 120 calorie portion whey or soy based protein shake blended with water, ice and 1 cup berries OR 1 large banana; plus 10 almonds.

8. ⅔ cup black beans and ⅔ cup non-fat refried beans with 2 tablespoons non-fat sour cream and 3 tablespoons salsa.

9. 1 cup plain non-fat yogurt with 1 cup berries; plus an 80 calorie serving of a whole-grain, high-fiber, low sugar cereal sprinkled on top.

10. 5 ounces tofu, any variety, stir-fried in 1 teaspoon extra-virgin olive oil, ginger and low-sodium soy sauce. Also stir-fry 3 cups Oriental mixed vegetables.

11. 1 cup non-fat/no-sugar pudding; plus 1 ⅓ cups chopped fruit.

12. 4 ounces grilled chicken; plus 2 cups of any combination of cooked spinach, broccoli, green beans, zucchini, cauliflower, squash, tomatoes, and mushrooms.

(275 CALORIE MEAL PLANS CONT.)

13. ¾ cup cooked oatmeal with 1 tablespoon chopped walnuts and either 1 tablespoon raisins OR 1 tablespoon miniature chocolate chips with cinnamon and 2 tablespoons no-sugar maple syrup; plus ½ cup non-fat milk.

14. 1 toasted whole-wheat English muffin topped with ⅔ cup Egg Beaters, scrambled or micro-waved; plus 1 orange.

15. 1 hard-boiled egg; plus 1 orange; plus 1 cup plain non-fat yogurt with 2 tablespoons no-sugar maple syrup.

16. 12 ounces V-8 juice; plus 1 (1 ounce) part-skim mozzarella stick; plus 1 apple; plus 1 carrot.

17. 3 celery stalks spread with 2 tablespoons peanut butter; plus 1 tablespoon raisins.

18. 1 orange; plus 1 meatless burger patty with 1 slice 2% cheese "single" with 1 slice tomato and 1 slice onion. Add lettuce, mustard and non-fat mayo, as desired.

19. ½ of a whole-wheat pita filled with 1 tablespoon chopped olives and 1 ounce crumbled low-fat feta cheese and a total of 1 cup chopped onion, tomato, cucumber, red, orange and yellow peppers; plus 1 orange.

20. ¾ cup non-fat cottage cheese; plus ½ cup green peas; plus 1 slice whole-grain bread.

21. 1 ⅓ cups Egg Beaters, scrambled or micro-waved, topped with 1 ounce low-fat cheddar OR Swiss cheese with 2 tablespoons salsa and 1 tablespoon non-fat sour cream.

22. 1 cup non-fat/no-sugar hot chocolate; plus 2 slices whole-wheat cinnamon-raisin bread with 1 wedge low-fat "Laughing Cow" cheese.

23. 6 ounces thin-sliced, deli-style ham or turkey; plus 1 ounce low-fat cheddar OR Swiss cheese and 1 sliced tomato wrapped in a large lettuce leaf. Add mustard and non-fat mayo, as desired.

24. 1 whole-wheat tortilla (7") filled with 1 slice 2% cheese "single" and a total of 1 cup chopped tomato and onion, 4 tablespoons salsa and 3 tablespoons non-fat sour cream.

25. 1 whole-wheat tortilla (7"), cut into wedges and baked into "chips." Sprinkle with 1 ounce low-fat cheddar and melt cheese in oven or microwave. Top with 3 tablespoons salsa and 3 tablespoons non-fat sour cream.

26. Spinach Egg Pie (Recipe in Appendix C): ⅓ of entire recipe; plus 1 slice whole-grain toast with 1 teaspoon all-fruit/no-sugar jam.

27. 200 calorie serving of any whole-grain, high-fiber, low sugar cereal with 8 ounces non-fat milk.

28. 1 ⅓ cups Minestrone, White Bean or Lentil Soup, or Turkey Chili (Recipe in Appendix C); plus ONE of the following selections: 2 WASA (whole-wheat, rye or sesame varieties) OR 2 RyKrisp rectangles OR 3 Ak-Mak crackers OR 4 reduced-fat Triscuit crackers.

(275 CALORIE MEAL PLANS CONT.)

29. ⅔ cup cooked brown rice with 1 tablespoon chopped walnuts; plus 1 ½ cups of any combination of lightly steamed tomato, onions, spinach, mushrooms, carrots, cauliflower, zucchini, and broccoli.

30. 1 slice Banana Bread (½ of Recipe in Appendix C); plus 6 ounces non-fat milk; plus 1 orange.

300 CALORIE MEAL PLANS

1. 1 cup Split Pea Soup (Recipe in Appendix C); plus ONE of the following selections: 3 WASA (whole-wheat, rye or sesame varieties) OR 3 RyKrisp rectangles OR 5 Ak-Mak crackers OR 7 reduced-fat Triscuit crackers.

2. Large green salad, dressed with balsamic vinegar and 1 teaspoon extra-virgin olive oil. Top salad with a total of 2 cups chopped tomato, onion, carrots, cauliflower, broccoli, mushrooms, and cucumber. Top salad with 4 ounces grilled chicken breast OR 5 ounces grilled shrimp.

3. ⅔ cup non-fat cottage cheese; plus 2 tomatoes, sliced; plus ONE of the following choices: 3 WASA (whole-wheat, rye or sesame varieties) OR 3 RyKrisp rectangles OR 5 Ak-Mak crackers.

4. 12 ounces V-8 juice; plus 1 (1 ounce) part-skim mozzarella cheese stick; plus 1 orange; plus ONE of the following selections: 2 WASA (whole-wheat, rye or sesame varieties) OR 2 RyKrisp rectangles, OR 4 Ak-Mak crackers OR 5 reduced-fat Triscuit crackers.

5. 2 carrots; plus 22 almonds; plus 1 orange.

6. 1 apple; plus 2 tablespoons peanut butter.

7. 1 meatless burger patty on 1 whole-grain hamburger bun with 2 slices each, tomato and onion. Add lettuce, mustard and non-fat mayo, as desired.

8. ½ cup black beans and ½ cup non-fat refried beans; plus 1 ounce grated low-fat cheese with 2 tablespoons non-fat sour cream and 2 tablespoons salsa.

9. 1 cup plain non-fat yogurt with 1 cup berries; plus a 50 calorie serving of a whole-grain, high-fiber, low sugar cereal with 1 tablespoon chopped nuts sprinkled on top.

10. ½ of a whole-wheat pita filled with 3 tablespoons hummus and a total of 1 cup chopped tomato, onion, peppers, cucumber; plus 1 ounce crumbled low-fat feta cheese.

11. 1 toasted whole-wheat English muffin topped with ¾ cup Egg Beaters, scrambled or micro-waved; plus 1 orange.

12. 1 hard-boiled egg; plus 1 orange; plus 1 ⅓ cups plain, non-fat yogurt with 2 tablespoons no-sugar maple syrup.

(300 CALORIE MEAL PLANS CONT.)

13. 5 ounces water or vacuum packed albacore tuna mixed with 2 tablespoons non-fat mayo on 1 slice whole-grain bread with 1 slice each, tomato and onion. Add lettuce, as desired.

14. 4 ounces tofu stir-fried in 1 teaspoon extra-virgin olive oil, ginger and reduced sodium soy sauce. Also stir-fry 2 ¾ cups Oriental mixed vegetables with 1 tablespoon chopped walnuts OR cashews.

15. 4 ounces grilled chicken; plus 3 cups of any combination of cooked broccoli, spinach, tomatoes, cauliflower, zucchini, green beans, carrots, mushrooms and peppers.

16. 6 ounces thin-sliced, deli-style turkey OR ham on 1 slice whole-wheat bread with 2 slices each of tomato, cucumber and onion. Add lettuce, mustard and non-fat mayo, as desired.

17. ¾ cup cooked oatmeal with 1 grated apple, 1 tablespoon chopped walnuts and 4 ounces non-fat milk. Add cinnamon and 2 tablespoons no-sugar maple syrup.

18. 4 ounces grilled chicken; plus 3 cups of any combination of cooked broccoli, spinach, tomato, cauliflower, zucchini, green beans, carrots, and peppers.

19. 1 cup non-fat/no-sugar hot chocolate; plus 2 slices whole-wheat cinnamon-raisin bread with 3 tablespoons non-fat cream cheese and 1 tablespoon all-fruit/no-sugar jam.

20. 1 whole-wheat tortilla (7") filled with 1 ounce grated low-fat cheese, ¼ cup black beans, ½ cup chopped tomato and onion, 2 tablespoons salsa and 2 tablespoons non-fat sour cream.

21. Omelet made with 1 cup Egg Beaters, 1 ounce low-fat cheddar OR Swiss OR feta cheese, 2 tablespoons chopped olives and a total of 2 cups chopped onion, tomato, spinach and mushrooms.

22. 150 calorie serving of a whole-grain, high-fiber, low sugar cereal with 8 ounces non-fat milk; plus 1 orange.

23. 4 stalks celery spread with 2 tablespoons peanut butter; plus 1 tablespoon raisins.

24. ¾ cup non-fat cottage cheese; plus 1 apple; plus 1 cup of any combination of lightly cooked spinach, broccoli, tomato, zucchini, mushrooms and cauliflower with 1 tablespoon chopped walnuts.

25. 1½ whole-wheat tortillas (7"), cut into wedges and baked into "chips." Sprinkle with 1 ounce low-fat cheddar and melt cheese in oven or microwave. Top with 2 tablespoons salsa and 2 tablespoons non-fat sour cream.

26. 1 cup non-fat/no-sugar pudding; plus 1 cup chopped fruit; plus 1 tablespoon chopped nuts.

27. Spinach Egg Pie (Recipe in Appendix C): ½ of the entire recipe; plus 1 orange.

(300 CALORIE MEAL PLANS CONT.)

28. 1 cup Minestrone, White Bean or Lentil Soup, or Turkey Chili. (Recipe in Appendix C); plus 1 (1 ounce) part-skim mozzarella cheese stick; plus 1 orange.

29. 120 calorie portion whey or soy based protein shake blended with water, ice and 1 cup berries OR 1 banana; plus 13 almonds.

30. 2 slices Banana Bread. (½ of Recipe in Appendix C)

325 CALORIE MEAL PLANS

1. 1 ¼ cups Split Pea Soup; plus one of the following selections: 3 WASA (whole wheat, rye or sesame varieties) OR 3 RyKrisp rectangles OR 4 Ak-Mak crackers OR 7 reduced-fat Triscuit crackers.

2. 3 ounces grilled chicken; plus ½ cup cooked brown rice plus 1 ½ cups of one of the following vegetables, lightly steamed: spinach, broccoli, tomatoes, or green beans carrots, mushrooms.

3. ¾ cup non-fat cottage cheese plus 2 tomatoes, sliced; plus one of the following: 3 WASA (whole wheat, rye or sesame varieties) OR 3 RyKrisp rectangles OR 5 Ak-Mak crackers OR 7 reduced-fat Triscuit crackers.

4. 6 ounces tofu, stir fried in 1 teaspoon extra-virgin olive oil, ginger and reduced sodium soy sauce. Also stir fry 2 cups Oriental mixed vegetables; plus 1 tablespoon chopped walnuts or cashews.

5. 2 slices whole-grain bread; plus 2 slices each of tomato and onion. Top with one of the following choices: 3 ounces water or vacuum packed albacore tuna OR 3 ounces thin-sliced, deli-style turkey or ham OR 2 ounces grilled chicken breast. Lettuce, mustard and non-fat mayo, as desired.

6. 12 ounces V-8 juice; plus 1 (1 ounce) part-skim mozzarella cheese stick; plus 1 orange; plus one of the following: 3 WASA (whole wheat, rye or sesame varieties) OR 3 RyKrisp rectangles OR 5 Ak-Mak crackers OR 6 reduced-fat Triscuit crackers.

7. 1 meatless burger patty on 1 slice whole grain bread; plus 1 slice 2% cheese "single," plus 2 slices each of tomato and onion. Lettuce, mustard and non-fat mayo, as desired.

8. ⅔ cup black beans; plus ½ cup non-fat refried beans; plus 1 ounce grated low-fat cheese; plus 3 tablespoons non-fat sour cream; plus 3 tablespoons salsa.

9. 1 hard boiled egg; plus 1 orange; plus 1 slice whole grain toast; plus 1 wedge low-fat "Laughing Cow" cheese; plus 1 tablespoon all-fruit/no-sugar jam.

10. 4 stalks celery spread with 1 ⅔ tablespoons peanut butter and 1 tablespoon raisins; plus 1 apple.

(325 CALORIE MEAL PLANS CONT.)

11. 325 calorie serving of a high protein/low sugar energy bar (check labels).

12. 24 almonds; plus 2 carrots; plus 1 apple.

13. ½ of a whole wheat pita, filled with 3 tablespoons hummus; plus a total of 1 cup chopped tomato, onion and cucumber; plus 2 tablespoons chopped olives; plus 1 apple.

14. ½ of a whole-wheat pita filled with a total of 2 cups chopped onion, tomatoes, cucumber, red, orange and yellow peppers; plus 2 tablespoons chopped olives; plus 1 ounce crumbled low-fat feta cheese; plus 2 tablespoons hummus.

15. 1 cup cooked oatmeal; plus 1 tablespoon chopped walnuts; plus either 1 tablespoon raisins OR 1 tablespoon miniature chocolate chips; plus 6 ounces non-fat milk. Add cinnamon and 2 tablespoons no-sugar maple syrup.

16. 1 ⅓ cups plain non-fat/no-sugar yogurt with 1 cup berries; plus either a 100 calorie serving of a high-fiber/low sugar whole-grain cereal sprinkled on top OR 2 tablespoons chopped walnuts.

17. 1 slice Banana Bread (1/12 of Recipe in Appendix C); plus 9 ounces non-fat milk; plus 1 apple.

350 CALORIE MEAL PLANS

1. 1 cup Split Pea Soup (Recipe in Appendix C); plus ONE of the following selections spread with 1 wedge low-fat "Laughing Cow" cheese: 4 WASA (whole-wheat, rye or sesame varieties) OR 4 RyKrisp rectangles OR 5 Ak-Mak crackers OR 8 reduced-fat Triscuit crackers.

2. 1 ⅓ cups plain non-fat yogurt with 1 cup berries and either a 100 calorie serving of a whole-grain, high-fiber, low sugar cereal OR 2 tablespoons chopped walnuts OR pecans. Top with 2 tablespoons no-sugar maple syrup.

3. 1 cup non-fat cottage cheese; plus 2 tomatoes, sliced; plus ONE of the following selections: 3 WASA crackers (whole-wheat, rye or sesame varieties) OR 3 RyKrisp rectangles OR 5 Ak-Mak crackers OR 6 reduced-fat Triscuit crackers.

4. 2 slices whole-grain bread with 2 slices each, tomato and onion, and ONE of the following selections: 4 ounces water or vacuum packed albacore tuna OR 4 ounces thin-sliced, deli-style ham OR turkey. Add lettuce, mustard and non-fat mayo, as desired.

5. 3 carrots; plus 25 almonds; plus 1 orange.

6. 1 meatless burger patty on 1 whole-grain hamburger bun with 1 slice 2% cheese "single" and 2 slices each, tomato and onion. Add lettuce, mustard and non-fat mayo, as desired.

(350 CALORIE MEAL PLANS CONT.)

7. 1 whole-wheat tortilla (7") filled with 1 ounce grated low-fat cheese, ½ cup black beans, ½ cup chopped tomato and onion, 3 tablespoons salsa and 2 tablespoons non-fat sour cream.

8. 120 calorie portion whey or soy based protein shake blended with water, ice and 1 cup berries OR 1 banana; plus 20 almonds.

9. 2 carrots; plus 1 apple; plus 1 tablespoon peanut butter on 1 slice whole-wheat bread.

10. 5 ounces tofu stir-fried in 1 teaspoon extra-virgin olive oil, ginger and reduced sodium soy sauce. Also stir-fry 2 cups Oriental mixed vegetables with 2 tablespoons chopped cashews OR walnuts.

11. 4 ounces grilled chicken; plus ½ cup cooked brown rice; plus 1 cup of any combination of lightly-cooked broccoli, spinach, tomato, cauliflower, zucchini, green beans and peppers.

12. 1 ⅓ cups Minestrone, White Bean or Lentil Soup, or Turkey Chili (Recipes in Appendix C); plus 1 (1 ounce) part-skim mozzarella cheese stick; plus 1 orange.

13. 200 calorie serving of a whole-grain, high-fiber, low sugar cereal with 8 ounces non-fat milk; plus 1 orange.

14. 1 cup cooked oatmeal with 1 tablespoon chopped walnuts and 1 grated apple; plus 6 ounces non-fat milk. Top with cinnamon and 2 tablespoons no-sugar maple syrup.

15. 12 ounces V-8 juice; plus 1 (1 ounce) part-skim mozzarella cheese stick; plus 1 orange; plus ONE of the following selections: 4 WASA (whole-wheat, rye or sesame varieties) OR 4 RyKrisp rectangles OR 6 Ak-Mak crackers, or 8 reduced-fat Triscuit crackers.

16. 1 whole-grain waffle or pancake (⅓ of Recipe in Appendix C) with 1 cup plain non-fat yogurt and 1 cup berries. Top with 2 tablespoons no-sugar maple syrup.

17. 2 slices toasted whole-wheat cinnamon-raisin bread with 1 tablespoon peanut butter; plus 1 cup non-fat/no-sugar hot chocolate.

18. ½ of a whole-wheat pita filled with 2 tablespoons chopped olives, 1 ounce crumbled low-fat feta cheese, 3 tablespoons hummus and a total of 1 ½ cups chopped onion, tomatoes, cucumber, red, orange and yellow peppers.

19. ⅔ cup cooked edamame; plus ½ cup cooked brown rice; plus 2 ½ cups of any combination of lightly-cooked spinach, broccoli, tomato, cauliflower, green beans and onions.

20. ¾ cup non-fat cottage cheese; plus 1 apple; plus 2 ½ cups of any combination of lightly steamed spinach, broccoli, tomato, zucchini, mushrooms, onions and cauliflower with 1 tablespoon chopped walnuts.

21. Omelet made with 1 cup Egg Beaters, 1 ½ ounces low-fat cheddar OR Swiss cheese, 3 tablespoons chopped olives and a total of 2 cups chopped onion, tomato, spinach, and mushrooms.

(350 CALORIE MEAL PLANS CONT.)

22. 1 toasted whole-wheat English muffin topped with ¾ cup Egg Beaters, scrambled or micro-waved with 1 slice 2% cheese "single"; plus 1 orange.

23. 1 hard-boiled egg; plus 1 orange; plus 1 slice whole-wheat bread; plus ⅔ cup plain non-fat yogurt with 2 tablespoons no-sugar maple syrup.

24. Large green salad, dressed with balsamic vinegar and 1 teaspoon extra-virgin olive oil. Top salad with a total of 2 cups chopped tomato, onion, carrots, cauliflower, broccoli, mushrooms, and cucumber. Top salad with either 5 ounces grilled chicken breast OR 7 ounces grilled shrimp.

25. 2 whole-wheat tortillas (7"), cut into wedges and baked into "chips." Sprinkle with 1 ounce low-fat cheddar and melt cheese in oven or microwave. Top with 2 tablespoons salsa and 1 tablespoon non-fat sour cream.

26. 1 cup non-fat/no-sugar pudding with 1 cup chopped fruit and 1 tablespoon chopped nuts; plus 1 non-fat Fruit Newton.

27. Spinach Egg Pie (½ of Recipe in Appendix C); plus 1 orange; plus 4 ounces non-fat milk.

28. 2 slices Banana Bread (1/12 of Recipe in Appendix C); plus 5 ounces non-fat milk.

375 CALORIE MEAL PLANS

1. 1 toasted whole-wheat English muffin topped with ¾ cup Egg Beaters, scrambled or micro-waved, with 1 ounce low-fat cheddar, Swiss or feta cheese; plus 1 orange.

2. 1 ⅓ cups plain non-fat yogurt with 1 cup berries; plus a 100 calorie serving of a whole-grain, high-fiber, low sugar cereal with 1 tablespoon chopped walnuts OR pecans. Top with 1 tablespoon no-sugar maple syrup.

3. 3 ounces grilled chicken breast; plus ½ cup cooked brown rice; plus 2 ½ cups of any combination of lightly steamed broccoli, spinach, tomato, cauliflower, zucchini, green beans, carrots, onions and peppers.

4. 2 slices whole-grain bread with 2 slices each, tomato and onion, with ONE of the following selections: 3 ounces grilled chicken breast OR 4 ounces water or vacuum packed albacore tuna OR 4 ounces thin-sliced, deli-style ham OR turkey. Add lettuce, mustard and non-fat mayo, as desired.

5. 3 carrots; plus 28 almonds; plus 1 orange.

6. 3 carrots; plus 1 apple; plus 1 tablespoon peanut butter on 1 slice whole-wheat bread.

(375 CALORIE MEAL PLANS CONT.)

7. 1 meatless burger patty on 1 slice whole-grain bread with 1 slice 2% cheese "single" and 2 slices each, tomato and onion; plus 1 orange. Add lettuce, mustard and non-fat mayo, as desired.

8. 1 ½ cups Split Pea Soup (Recipe in Appendix C); plus ONE of the following selections: 3 WASA (whole-wheat, rye or sesame varieties) OR 3 RyKrisp rectangles OR 4 Ak-Mak crackers OR 6 reduced-fat Triscuit crackers.

9. 120 calorie portion whey or soy based protein shake blended with water, ice and 1 cup berries OR 1 banana; plus 22 almonds.

10. 1 ½ cups Minestrone, White Bean or Lentil Soup, or Turkey Chili (Recipes in Appendix C); plus 1 (1 ounce) part-skim mozzarella cheese stick; plus 1 orange.

11. 1 hard-boiled egg; plus 1 orange; plus 1 slice whole-wheat bread; plus 1 cup plain non-fat yogurt with 2 tablespoons no-sugar maple syrup.

12. 1 cup non-fat/no-sugar pudding with 1 cup chopped fruit and 1 tablespoon chopped nuts; plus an 85 calorie portion of a whole-grain, high-fiber, low sugar cereal sprinkled on top.

13. ½ of a whole-wheat pita filled with 4 tablespoons hummus, 3 tablespoons chopped olives, 1 ounce crumbled low-fat feta cheese and a total of ½ cup chopped tomato, onion, cucumber and peppers.

14. 1 whole-grain waffle or pancake (⅓ of Recipe in Appendix C) with 1 cup plain non-fat yogurt and 1 ⅓ cups berries. Top with 2 tablespoons no-sugar maple syrup.

15. 1 cup cooked oatmeal with 1 tablespoon chopped walnuts and 1 grated apple; plus 8 ounces non-fat milk. Add cinnamon and 2 tablespoons sugar-free maple syrup.

16. 12 ounces V-8 juice; plus 1 (1 ounce) part-skim mozzarella cheese stick; plus 1 apple; plus ONE of the following selections: 4 WASA (whole-wheat, rye or sesame varieties) OR 4 RyKrisp rectangles OR 6 Ak-Mak crackers, or 8 reduced-fat Triscuit crackers.

17. 230 calorie serving of a whole-grain, high-fiber, low sugar cereal with 8 ounces non-fat milk; plus 1 orange.

18. 2 slices toasted whole-wheat cinnamon-raisin bread with 1 ½ tablespoons peanut butter; plus 1 cup non-fat/no-sugar hot chocolate.

19. Large green salad, dressed with balsamic vinegar and 1 teaspoon extra-virgin olive oil. Top salad with 2 cups of any combination of chopped tomato, onion, carrots, cauliflower, broccoli, mushrooms, and cucumber. Top salad with either 5 ounces grilled chicken breast OR 6 ounces grilled shrimp.

(375 CALORIE MEAL PLANS CONT.)

20. 2 whole-wheat tortillas (7"), cut into wedges and baked into "chips." Sprinkle with 1 ounce low-fat cheddar and melt cheese in oven or microwave. Top with 2 tablespoons salsa and 2 tablespoons non-fat sour cream.

21. 1 whole-wheat tortilla (7") filled with ⅔ cup black beans, 1 ounce shredded low-fat cheddar cheese, ¼ cup chopped tomato and onion, 3 tablespoons salsa and 2 tablespoons non-fat sour cream.

22. 1 whole-wheat tortilla (7") filled with 1 cup Egg Beaters, scrambled or micro-waved, 1 ounce low-fat cheddar, Swiss, or feta cheese; plus 2 tablespoons non-fat sour cream and 2 tablespoons salsa.

23. 1 cup non-fat cottage cheese; plus 1 apple; plus 2 cups of any combination of lightly steamed spinach, broccoli, tomato, zucchini, mushrooms, cauliflower, onion and green beans with 1 tablespoon chopped walnuts.

24. 5 ounces tofu stir-fried in 1 teaspoon extra-virgin olive oil, ginger and reduced sodium soy sauce. Also stir-fry 2 ¾ cups Oriental mixed vegetables with 2 tablespoons chopped cashews OR walnuts.

25. Spinach Egg Pie (½ of Recipe in Appendix C); plus 1 slice whole-grain toast with 1 tablespoon all-fruit/no-sugar jam.

26. 120 calorie portion whey or soy based protein shake blended with water, ice and 1 cup berries OR 1 banana; plus 22 almonds.

27. 2 slices Banana Bread (½ of Recipe in Appendix C); plus 6 ounces non-fat milk.

400 CALORIE MEAL PLANS

1. 1 ¼ cup Split Pea Soup (Recipe in Appendix C); plus 1 ounce low-fat cheddar OR Swiss cheese; plus ONE of the following selections: 3 WASA (whole-wheat, rye or sesame varieties) OR 3 RyKrisp rectangles OR 4 Ak-Mak crackers.

2. 6 ounces tofu stir-fried in 1 teaspoon extra-virgin olive oil, ginger and reduced sodium soy sauce. Also stir-fry 3 cups Oriental mixed vegetables with 2 tablespoons chopped cashews OR walnuts.

3. 1 meatless burger patty on 1 whole-grain hamburger bun with 1 slice 2% cheese "single" and 2 slices each, tomato and onion; plus 1 orange. Add lettuce, mustard and non-fat mayo as desired.

4. 4 ounces grilled chicken; plus ½ cup cooked brown rice; plus 2 ½ cups of any combination of lightly steamed broccoli, spinach, tomato, cauliflower, zucchini, green beans, and peppers.

(400 CALORIE MEAL PLANS CONT.)

5.   2 carrots; plus 10 almonds; plus 1 orange; plus 12 reduced-fat Triscuit crackers.

6.   2 carrots; plus 1 apple; plus 1 ½ tablespoons peanut butter on 1 slice whole-wheat bread.

7.   1 cup non-fat/no-sugar pudding with 1 cup chopped fruit and 1 tablespoon chopped walnuts OR pecans; plus 2 non-fat Fruit Newtons.

8.   1 whole-wheat tortilla (7") with ¾ cup black beans, ½ cup non-fat refried beans, 2 tablespoons non-fat sour cream and 3 tablespoons salsa.

9.   1 ⅓ cup plain non-fat yogurt with 1 cup berries and ONE of the following selections: a 150 calorie serving of a whole-grain, high-fiber, low sugar cereal sprinkled on top OR 1 whole-grain pancake or waffle (⅓ of Recipe in Appendix C) topped with 2 tablespoons no-sugar maple syrup.

10. 2 slices whole-grain bread with 2 slices each, tomato and onion, plus ONE of the following selections: 3 ounces grilled chicken OR 4 ounces water or vacuum packed albacore tuna OR 4 ounces thin-sliced, deli-style ham OR turkey. Add lettuce, mustard and non-fat mayo, as desired.

11. 1 hard-boiled egg; plus 1 orange; plus 1 slice whole-wheat bread; plus 1 ⅓ cups plain non-fat yogurt with 2 tablespoons no-sugar maple syrup.

12. 180 calories whey or soy based protein shake blended with water, ice and 1 cup berries OR 1 banana; plus 18 almonds.

13. ½ of a whole-wheat pita filled with 3 tablespoons hummus, 2 tablespoons chopped olives, 1 ounce low-fat feta cheese and a total of 1 ⅓ cups chopped tomato, onion, cucumber and peppers; plus 1 orange.

14. 1 toasted whole-wheat English muffin filled with cup Egg Beaters, scrambled or micro-waved with 1 ounce either low-fat cheddar or Swiss cheese; plus 1 orange.

15. 1 cup cooked oatmeal with 1 tablespoon chopped walnuts and 1 grated apple; plus 6 ounces non-fat milk. Top with cinnamon and 2 tablespoons no-sugar maple syrup.

16. 12 ounces V-8 juice; plus 1 (1 ounce) part-skim mozzarella cheese stick; plus 1 orange; plus ONE of the following selections: 5 WASA (whole-wheat, rye or sesame varieties) OR 5 RyKrisp rectangles OR 8 Ak-Mak crackers OR 10 reduced-fat Triscuit crackers.

17.   Spinach Egg Pie (⅔ of Recipe in Appendix C); plus 1 orange.

18. 1 whole-wheat tortilla (7") filled with 1 ounce grated low-fat cheese, ⅔ cup black beans, 1 cup chopped tomato and onion, 3 tablespoons salsa and 2 tablespoons non-fat sour cream.

(400 CALORIE MEAL PLANS CONT.)

19. Large green salad, dressed with balsamic vinegar and 1 teaspoon extra-virgin olive oil. Top salad with 2 cups of any combination of chopped tomato, onion, carrots, cauliflower, broccoli, mushrooms, and cucumber. Top salad with and 1 ounce low-fat cheddar or Swiss cheese and either 4 ounces grilled chicken breast OR 6 ounces grilled shrimp.

20. 2 whole-wheat tortillas (7"), cut into wedges and baked into "chips." Sprinkle with 1 ounce low-fat cheddar cheese and ¼ cup black beans and place in oven or microwave. Top with 2 tablespoons salsa and 2 tablespoons non-fat sour cream.

21. 1 cup non-fat cottage cheese; plus 1 apple; plus 2 ¾ cups of any combination of lightly steamed spinach, broccoli, tomatoes, zucchini, mushrooms, onion, green beans, and cauliflower with 1 tablespoons chopped walnuts.

22. 2 slices Banana Bread (½ of Recipe in Appendix C); plus 1 apple.

23. Omelet made with 1 cup Egg Beaters and 1 ounce low-fat cheddar, Swiss or feta cheese, either 3 ounces Canadian bacon OR 4 ounces thin-sliced, deli-style ham and a total of 1 cup chopped tomato, onion, mushrooms and spinach with 2 tablespoons chopped olives.

24. 250 calorie serving of a whole-grain, high-fiber, low sugar cereal with 8 ounces non-fat milk; plus 1 orange.

25. 2 slices toasted whole-wheat cinnamon-raisin bread with 1 ½ tablespoons peanut butter; plus 1 cup non-fat/no-sugar hot chocolate.

26. 1 cup Minestrone, White Bean or Lentil Soup, or Turkey Chili (Recipes in Appendix C); plus 1 (1 ounce) part-skim mozzarella cheese stick; plus 1 orange; plus ONE of the following selections: 3 WASA (whole-wheat, rye or sesame varieties) OR 3 RyKrisp rectangles OR 5 Ak-Mak crackers OR 6 reduced-fat Triscuit crackers.

27. 1 cup non-fat cottage cheese; plus 2 tomatoes, sliced; plus ONE of the following selections spread with 1 wedge low-fat "Laughing Cow" cheese: 3 WASA (whole-wheat, rye or sesame varieties) OR 3 RyKrisp rectangles OR 5 Ak-Mak crackers OR 7 reduced-fat Triscuit crackers.

425 CALORIE MEAL PLANS

1. 1 ½ cup Split Pea Soup (Recipe in Appendix C); plus one of the following selections: 2 WASA (whole wheat, rye or sesame varieties) OR 2 RyKrisp rectangles OR 3 Ak-Mak crackers OR 4 reduced-fat Triscuit crackers; plus 1 apple.

2. ⅔ cup non-fat cottage cheese; plus 2 cups of any combination of lightly steamed spinach, broccoli, tomatoes, zucchini, mushrooms, cauliflower; plus 1 tablespoon chopped walnuts; plus 1 apple; plus 3 WASA (whole wheat, rye or sesame varieties) OR 3 RyKrisp rectangles OR 4 Ak-Mak crackers OR 6 reduced-fat Triscuit crackers.

(425 CALORIE MEAL PLANS CONT.)

3. 1 ⅓ cup cooked oatmeal; plus 1 tablespoon chopped walnuts; plus 1 tablespoon raisins; plus one apple grated into the oatmeal; plus 4 ounces non-fat milk. Add cinnamon and 1 tablespoon no-sugar maple syrup.

4. Omelet made with 1 cup Egg Beaters, topped with 1 ounce low-fat cheddar or Swiss; plus a total of 1 cup chopped tomato, onion, mushrooms, spinach; plus either 3 ounces Canadian bacon OR 4 ounces thin-sliced, deli-style ham; plus 2 tablespoons grated parmesan cheese.

5. 120 calorie portion whey or soy based protein shake, blended with water and ice; plus 1 cup berries OR 1 banana; plus 29 almonds.

6. Spinach Egg Pie (½ of Recipe in Appendix C); plus 1 slice whole wheat toast spread with 1 teaspoon all-fruit/no-sugar jam; plus 1 orange.

7. 1 meatless burger patty on 1 whole-grain hamburger bun; plus 1 slice 2% cheese "single" and 2 slices each tomato and onion; plus 1 apple.

8. 1 cup non-fat/no-sugar pudding; plus 1 ⅓ cups chopped fruit; plus 1 tablespoon chopped nuts; plus 2 non-fat Fruit Newtons.

9. 1 cup plain non-fat/no-sugar yogurt; plus 1 ½ cups berries; plus one of the following: a 200 calorie serving of a high-fiber/low sugar whole-grain cereal sprinkled on top OR 1 whole-grain pancake or waffle (Recipe in Appendix C); plus 2 tablespoons no-sugar maple syrup.

10. Large green salad, dressed with balsamic vinegar and 1 teaspoon extra-virgin olive oil. Top salad with a total of 2 ½ cups chopped tomato, onion, carrots, cauliflower, broccoli, mushrooms, cucumber, etc. Top salad with 6 ounces grilled chicken breast OR 8 ounces grilled shrimp.

11. 1 apple; plus 2 carrots; plus 1 ⅔ tablespoons peanut butter; plus 1 slice whole-wheat bread.

12. 16 almonds; plus 1 orange; plus 2 carrots; plus 10 reduced-fat Triscuit crackers.

13. ½ of a whole wheat pita filled with 4 tablespoons hummus, 2 tablespoons chopped olives, a total of 1 cup chopped tomato, onion, cucumber, peppers; plus 1 ounce low-fat feta cheese; plus 1 apple.

14. 1 hard boiled egg; plus 1 slice whole-wheat bread; plus 1 orange; plus 1 ½ cups plain, non-fat/no sugar yogurt, drizzled with 2 tablespoons no-sugar maple syrup.

15. 2 slices Banana Bread (½ of Recipe in Appendix C); plus 4 ounces non-fat milk; plus 1 orange.

16. 4 ounces grilled chicken; plus ½ cup cooked brown rice; plus 2 ¾ cups of an combination of lightly steamed broccoli, spinach, tomatoes, cauliflower, zucchini, green beans, carrots, peppers.

(425 CALORIE MEAL PLANS CONT.)

17. 12 ounces V-8 juice; plus 2 (1 ounce each) part-skim mozzarella cheese sticks; plus 1 orange; plus one of the following: 4 WASA (whole wheat, rye or sesame varieties) OR 4 RyKrisp rectangles OR 5 Ak-Mak crackers or 8 reduced-fat Triscuit crackers.

18. 1 ¾ cups Minestrone, White Bean or Lentil Soup, or Turkey Chili (Recipes in Appendix C); plus 1 (1 ounce) part-skim mozzarella cheese stick; plus 1 apple.

19. 2 slices toasted whole-wheat cinnamon-raisin bread spread with 2 tablespoons peanut butter.

20. 2 slices whole-grain bread; plus 2 slices each tomato and onion. Top with ONE of the following choices: 3 ounces grilled chicken OR 4 ounces water or vacuum packed albacore tuna OR 4 ounces thin-sliced, deli-style ham or turkey. Lettuce, mustard and non-fat mayo, as desired.

21. 2 whole wheat tortillas (7"), cut into wedges and baked into "chips." Sprinkle with 1 ½ ounces low-fat cheddar and melt the cheese in the oven or microwave. Top with 2 tablespoons salsa and 2 tablespoons non-fat sour cream.

22. One whole-grain waffle or pancake (⅓ of Recipe in Appendix C) with 1 ⅓ cups plain non-fat/no sugar yogurt; plus 1 ⅓ cup berries. Top with 2 tablespoons no-sugar maple syrup.

23. 1 whole-wheat tortilla filled with 1 ounce grated low-fat cheddar; ½ cup black beans, ⅓ cup non-fat refried beans, ¼ cup chopped tomato and onion; plus 3 tablespoons salsa and 3 tablespoons non-fat sour cream.

24. 1 toasted whole-wheat English muffin topped with 1 cup scrambled Egg Beaters; plus 2 slices 2% cheese "singles" plus 1 orange.

25. 175 calorie serving of a whole-grain, high-fiber, low sugar cereal with 6 ounces non-fat milk; plus 1 orange; plus 1 slice whole-wheat toast spread with 2 teaspoons all-fruit/no-sugar jam.

26. 1 toasted whole-wheat English muffin topped with 1 cup scrambled or micro-waved Egg Beaters; plus 2 slices 2% cheese "singles" plus 1 orange.

450 CALORIE MEAL PLANS

1. 1 ⅓ cups Split Pea Soup (Recipe in Appendix C); plus 1 apple; plus ONE of the following selections spread with 1 wedge low-fat "Laughing Cow" cheese: 3 WASA (whole-wheat, rye or sesame varieties) OR 3 RyKrisp rectangles OR 4 Ak-Mak crackers OR 5 reduced-fat Triscuit crackers.

2. 2 whole-wheat tortillas (7"), cut into wedges and baked into "chips." Sprinkle with 2 ounces low-fat cheddar and melt cheese in oven or microwave. Top with 2 tablespoons salsa and 2 tablespoons non-fat sour cream.

(450 CALORIE MEAL PLANS CONT.)

3. 1 cup non-fat cottage cheese; plus 1 ½ cups of any combination of lightly steamed spinach, broccoli, tomatoes, zucchini, mushroom, onions and cauliflower; plus ⅔ cup cooked brown rice; plus 1 apple.

4.   5 ounces grilled chicken; plus ½ cup cooked brown rice; plus 2 ⅓ cups of any combination of lightly steamed broccoli, spinach, tomato, cauliflower, zucchini, green beans, onion, carrots and peppers.

5. 2 slices whole-grain bread with 1 tablespoon peanut butter and 1 teaspoon all-fruit/no-sugar jam; plus 2 carrots; plus 1 apple.

6.   Spinach Egg Pie (⅔ of Recipe in Appendix C); plus 1 slice whole-wheat bread and 2 teaspoons all-fruit/no-sugar jam.

7. 1 ⅓ cups cooked oatmeal with 1 tablespoon chopped walnuts, 1 tablespoon raisins and 1 grated apple; plus 5 ounces non-fat milk.   Add cinnamon and 2 tablespoons sugar-free maple syrup.

8. 1 cup cooked edamame; plus ½ cup cooked brown rice; plus 2 cups Oriental mixed vegetables stir-fried in ginger and low-sodium soy sauce; plus 1 tablespoons chopped walnuts.

9. 1 cup plain non-fat yogurt with 1 ½ cup berries; plus ONE of the following selections: a 175 calorie serving of a whole-grain, high-fiber, low sugar cereal sprinkled on top OR 1 whole-grain pancake or waffle (⅓ of Recipe in Appendix C) with 1 tablespoon chopped walnuts and 2 tablespoons no-sugar maple syrup.

10. 12 ounces V-8 juice; plus 1 (1 ounce) part-skim mozzarella cheese stick; plus 1 orange; plus ONE of the following selections, spread with 1 wedge low-fat "Laughing Cow" cheese: 4 WASA (whole-wheat, rye or sesame varieties) OR 4 RyKrisp rectangles OR 6 Ak-Mak crackers OR 8 reduced-fat Triscuit crackers.

11. 1 hard-boiled egg; plus 1 orange; plus 2 slices whole-wheat bread with 1 tablespoon peanut butter.

12. 2 cups Minestrone, White Bean or Lentil soup, or Turkey Chili (Recipes in Appendix C); plus 1 (1 ounce) part-skim mozzarella cheese stick; plus 1 orange.

13. 1 whole-wheat pita filled with 3 tablespoons hummus, 2 tablespoons chopped olives, 1 ounce low-fat feta cheese and a total of 2 cups chopped tomato, onion, cucumber and peppers.

14. 1 toasted whole-wheat English muffin topped with 1 cup Egg Beaters, scrambled or micro-waved and 1 slice 2% cheese "single" plus 1 cup Minestrone, White Bean or Lentil Soup, or Turkey Chili. (Recipes in Appendix C)

15. 1 meatless burger patty on 1 whole-grain hamburger bun with 1 slice 2% cheese "single" and 3 slices each, tomato and onion. Add lettuce, mustard and non-fat mayo, as desired. Plus 1 apple.

(450 CALORIE MEAL PLANS CONT.)

16. 2 whole-grain waffles or pancakes (⅓ of Recipe in Appendix C) with ¾ cup plain non-fat yogurt and 1 cup berries. Top with 2 tablespoons no-sugar maple syrup.

17. 2 slices whole-wheat bread with 4 ounces thin-sliced, deli-style turkey OR ham, 1 ounce low-fat cheese and 3 slices each tomato and onion. Add lettuce, mustard and non-fat mayo, as desired.

18. 2 slices toasted whole-wheat cinnamon-raisin bread with 1⅓ tablespoons peanut butter; plus 1 orange; plus 1 cup non-fat/no sugar hot chocolate.

19. Large green salad, dressed with balsamic vinegar and 1 teaspoon extra-virgin olive oil. Top salad with 2 ½ cups of any combination of chopped tomato, onion, carrots, cauliflower, broccoli, mushrooms, and cucumber. Top salad with 1 ounce low-fat cheddar or Swiss cheese and either 5 ounces grilled chicken breast OR 6 ounces grilled shrimp.

20. 2 slices whole-grain bread with 1 slice 2% cheese "single" and 2 slices each, tomato and onion; and ONE of the following choices: 3.5 ounces grilled chicken OR 5 ounces water or vacuum packed albacore tuna OR 5 ounces thin-sliced, deli-style ham. Add lettuce, mustard and non-fat mayo, as desired.

21. 1 whole-wheat tortilla filled with 1 ounce grated low-fat cheese, ½ cup black beans, ⅓ cup non-fat refried beans, ½ cup chopped tomato and onion, 2 tablespoons chopped olives, 2 tablespoons salsa and 2 tablespoons non-fat sour cream.

22. Omelet made with 1 cup Egg Beaters, 1 ounce low-fat cheese, and either 3 ounces Canadian bacon OR 4 ounces thin-sliced, deli-style ham and a total of 2 cups chopped tomato, onion, mushrooms and spinach.

23. 200 calorie serving of a whole-grain, high-fiber, low sugar cereal with 6 ounces non-fat milk; plus 1 orange; plus 1 slice whole-wheat toast spread with 1 tablespoon all-fruit/no-sugar jam.

24. 5 ounces tofu stir-fried in 1 teaspoon extra-virgin olive oil, ginger and reduced sodium soy sauce. Also stir-fry 3 cups of Oriental mixed vegetables and add 1 tablespoon chopped cashews; plus ½ cup cooked brown rice.

25. 2 carrots; plus 1 apple; plus 2 tablespoons peanut butter on 1 slice whole-wheat bread.

26. 1 cup non-fat/no-sugar pudding with 1 cup chopped fruit and 2 tablespoons chopped walnuts OR pecans; plus 2 non-fat Fruit Newtons.

475 CALORIE MEAL PLANS

1. 2 slices toasted whole-wheat cinnamon-raisin bread with 1 tablespoons peanut butter; plus 1 orange; plus 1 cup non-fat/no-sugar hot chocolate.

(475 CALORIE MEAL PLANS CONT.)

2. 2 carrots; plus 1 apple; plus 2 tablespoons peanut butter on 1 slice whole-wheat bread.

3. ¾ cup non-fat cottage cheese; plus 2 tomatoes, sliced; plus ONE of the following selections: 5 WASA (whole-wheat, rye or sesame varieties) OR 5 RyKrisp rectangles OR 7 Ak- Mak crackers OR 10 reduced-fat Triscuit crackers; plus 1 tablespoon peanut butter.

4. 5 ounces grilled chicken; plus ½ cup cooked brown rice; plus 3 cups of any combination of lightly steamed broccoli, spinach, tomato, cauliflower, zucchini, green beans, and peppers.

5. 2 carrots; plus 13 almonds; plus 1 orange; plus 15 reduced-fat Triscuit crackers.

6. Spinach Egg Pie (¾ of Recipe in Appendix C); plus 1 orange; plus 4 ounces non-fat milk.

7. 1 meatless burger patty on 1 whole-grain hamburger bun with 2 slices 2% cheese "singles" and 2 slices each, tomato and onion. Add lettuce, mustard and non-fat mayo, as desired. Plus 1 orange.

8. 1 whole-wheat tortilla (7") filled with ⅔ cup black beans, ½ cup non-fat refried beans, 1 ounce low-fat cheddar cheese, 2 tablespoons minced onion, 3 tablespoons non-fat sour cream and 3 tablespoons salsa.

9. 2 whole-grain pancakes or waffles (⅔ of Recipe in Appendix C) with ¾ cup plain non-fat yogurt and 1 cup berries. Top with 2 tablespoons no-sugar maple syrup.

10. 1 hard-boiled egg; plus 2 slices whole-wheat bread; plus 1 orange; plus 1 cup plain non-fat yogurt with 2 tablespoons no-sugar maple syrup.

11. 2 whole-wheat tortillas (7"), cut into wedges and baked into "chips." Sprinkle with 1 ounce low-fat cheddar and melt cheese in oven or microwave. Top with mashed ⅓ of an avocado, and 3 tablespoons salsa and 2 tablespoons non-fat sour cream.

12. 2 slices whole-grain bread with 1 slice 2% cheese "single" and 2 slices each, tomato and onion, and ONE of the following selections: 3 ounces grilled chicken OR 4 ounces water or vacuum packed albacore tuna OR 4 ounces thin-sliced, deli-style ham OR turkey. Add lettuce, mustard and non-fat mayo, as desired. Plus 1 orange.

13. 1 whole-wheat pita filled with 3 tablespoons hummus, 1 tablespoon chopped olives, 2 ounces crumbled low-fat feta cheese and a total of 1 cup chopped tomato, onion, cucumber and peppers.

14. 1 toasted whole-wheat English muffin filled with 1 cup Egg Beaters, scrambled or micro-waved, and 1 ounce low-fat cheddar OR Swiss cheese; plus 1 cup Minestrone, White Bean or Lentil Soup, or Turkey Chili. (Recipes in Appendix C)

15. 1 ⅓ cups Split Pea Soup (Recipe in Appendix C); plus ONE of the following selections spread with 1 wedge low-fat "Laughing Cow" cheese: 3 WASA (whole-wheat, rye or sesame varieties) OR 3 RyKrisp rectangles OR 4 Ak-Mak crackers OR 6 reduced-fat Triscuit crackers; plus 1 apple.

(475 CALORIE MEAL PLANS CONT.)

16. 12 ounces V-8 juice; plus 2 (1 ounce each) part-skim mozzarella cheese sticks; plus 1 orange; plus ONE of the following selections: 5 WASA (whole-wheat, rye or sesame varieties) OR 5 RyKrisp rectangles OR 8 Ak-Mak crackers OR 11 reduced-fat Triscuit crackers.

17. 1 ⅓ cups cooked oatmeal with 1 tablespoon chopped walnuts, 1 tablespoon raisins, 1 grated apple and 8 ounces non-fat milk. Top with cinnamon and 2 tablespoons no-sugar maple syrup.

18. 5 ounces tofu stir-fried in 1 teaspoon extra-virgin olive oil, ginger and reduced sodium soy sauce. Also stir-fry 2 cups Oriental mixed vegetables with 2 tablespoons chopped cashews or walnuts.

19. Large green salad, dressed with balsamic vinegar and 1 teaspoon extra-virgin olive oil. Top salad with a total of 2 cups chopped tomato, onion, carrots, cauliflower, broccoli, mushrooms and cucumber. Top salad with 1 ounce low-fat cheese and either 5 ounces grilled chicken breast OR 7 ounces grilled shrimp.

20. 1 ½ cups Minestrone, White Bean or Lentil Soup, or Turkey Chili (Recipes in Appendix C); plus 1 (1 ounce) part-skim mozzarella cheese stick; plus 1 orange; plus ONE of the following selections: 3 WASA crackers (whole-wheat, rye or sesame varieties) OR 3 RyKrisp rectangles OR 4 Ak-Mak crackers OR 6 reduced fat Triscuit crackers.

21. ¾ cup non-fat cottage cheese; plus ¾ cup cooked brown rice; plus 1 apple; plus 2 cups of any combination of lightly steamed spinach, broccoli, tomato, zucchini, mushroom and cauliflower.

22. Omelet made with 1 cup Egg Beaters, 1 ounce low-fat cheddar OR Swiss cheese, either 3 ounces Canadian bacon OR 5 ounces thin-sliced, deli-style ham, and a total of 1 ½ cups chopped onion, tomato, spinach and mushrooms; plus 1 orange.

23. 200 calorie serving of a whole-grain, high-fiber, low sugar cereal with 8 ounces non-fat milk; plus 1 orange; plus 1 slice whole-wheat toast spread with 1 tablespoon all-fruit/no-sugar jam.

24. 1 cup non-fat/no-sugar pudding with 1 ⅓ cups chopped fruit and 2 tablespoons chopped nuts; plus 2 non-fat Fruit Newtons.

500 CALORIE MEAL PLANS

1. 1 ½ cups Split Pea Soup (Recipe in Appendix C); plus 1 apple; plus ONE of the following selections spread with 1 wedge low-fat "Laughing Cow" cheese: 3 WASA (whole-wheat, rye or sesame varieties) OR 3 RyKrisp rectangles OR 5 Ak-Mak crackers OR 7 reduced-fat Triscuit crackers.

(500 CALORIE MEAL PLANS CONT.)

2. 1½ cups cooked oatmeal with 1 tablespoon chopped walnuts, 1 tablespoon raisins OR pecans, 1 grated apple and 8 ounces non-fat milk. Add cinnamon and 2 tablespoons no-sugar maple syrup.

3. 1 meatless burger patty on 1 whole-grain hamburger bun with 2 slices 2% cheese "singles" and 2 slices each, tomato and onion. Add lettuce, mustard and non-fat mayo, as desired. Plus 1 apple.

4.   4 ounces grilled chicken; plus ⅔ cup cooked brown rice; plus 1 apple; plus 2 cups of any combination of lightly steamed broccoli, spinach, tomatoes, cauliflower, zucchini, green beans and peppers.

5. 2 carrots; plus 26 almonds; plus 1 orange; plus 10 reduced-fat Triscuit crackers.

6. Spinach Egg Pie (⅔ of Recipe in Appendix C); plus 1 orange; plus 1 slice whole-wheat toast, spread with 1 teaspoon all-fruit/no-sugar jam.

7. Omelet made with 1 cup Egg Beaters, 1 ounce low-fat cheddar OR Swiss cheese, either 3 ounces Canadian bacon OR 5 ounces thin-sliced, deli-style ham and a total of 2 cups chopped onion, tomato, mushroom, peppers and spinach; plus 1 orange.

8. 12 ounces V-8 juice; plus 2 carrots; plus 2 (1 ounce) part-skim mozzarella cheese sticks; plus ONE of the following selections: 6 WASA (whole-wheat, rye or sesame varieties) OR 6 RyKrisp rectangles OR 9 Ak-Mak crackers OR 12 reduced-fat Triscuit crackers.

9. 2 slices whole-grain bread with ONE of the following choices: 3 ounces grilled chicken breast OR 5 ounces water or vacuum packed albacore tuna OR 5 ounces thin-sliced, deli-style ham; plus 1ounces low-fat cheddar OR Swiss OR part-skim mozzarella cheese with 2 slices each, tomato and onion. Add lettuce, mustard and non-fat mayo, as desired. Plus 1 apple.

10. Large green salad, dressed with balsamic vinegar and 2 teaspoons extra-virgin olive oil. Top salad with 1 ½ cups chopped tomato, onion, carrots, cauliflower, broccoli, mushrooms, and cucumber. Top salad with either 6 ounces grilled chicken breast OR 8 ounces grilled shrimp. Add 1 ounce low-fat cheddar OR Swiss OR part-skim mozzarella cheese.

11. 1 hard-boiled egg; plus 1 orange; plus 2 slices whole-wheat bread; plus 1 tablespoon all-fruit, no-sugar jam; plus 1 cup plain non-fat yogurt with 2 tablespoons no-sugar maple syrup.

12. 2 whole-grain pancakes or waffles (⅔ of Recipe in Appendix C); plus 1 cup plain non-fat yogurt topped with 1 cup berries and 2 tablespoons no-sugar maple syrup.

13. 1 whole-wheat pita filled with 2 tablespoons hummus, 2 ounces crumbled low-fat feta cheese, 3 tablespoons chopped olives and a total of 2 cups chopped tomato, onion, cucumber and peppers.

14. 1 toasted whole-wheat English muffin topped with 1 cup Egg Beaters, scrambled or micro-waved, and 1 slice 2% cheese "single" plus 1 1/3 cups Minestrone, White Bean or Lentil Soup, or Turkey Chili. (Recipes in Appendix C)

(500 CALORIE MEAL PLANS CONT.)

15. 2 slices toasted whole-wheat cinnamon-raisin bread with 2 tablespoons peanut butter; plus 1 orange; plus 1 cup non-fat no-sugar hot chocolate.

16. 225 calorie serving of a whole-grain, high-fiber, low sugar cereal with 8 ounces non-fat milk; plus 1 orange; plus 1 slice whole-grain toast and 1 tablespoon all-fruit/no-sugar jam.

17. 1 ½ cups cooked oatmeal with 2 tablespoons chopped walnuts, 1 tablespoon miniature chocolate chips and 1 tablespoon raisins; plus 1 apple.

18. 1 cup non-fat/no-sugar pudding with 1 ½ cups chopped fruit and 2 tablespoons chopped walnuts OR pecans; plus 2 non-fat Fruit Newtons.

19. 2 whole-wheat tortillas (7"), cut into wedges and baked into "chips." Sprinkle with 1 ounce low-fat cheddar and melt cheese in oven or microwave. Top with mashed ½ of an avocado, 3 tablespoons salsa and 1 tablespoon non-fat sour cream.

20. 1 ½ cups Minestrone, White Bean or Lentil soup, or Turkey Chili (Recipes in Appendix C); plus 1 part-skim mozzarella cheese stick; plus 1 orange; plus ONE of the following selections: 4 WASA (whole-wheat, rye or sesame varieties) OR 4 RyKrisp rectangles OR 6 Ak-Mak crackers OR 8 reduced fat Triscuit crackers.

21. 1 cup non-fat cottage cheese; plus ⅔ cup cooked brown rice; plus 1 apple; plus 2 ¾ cups of any combination of lightly-steamed spinach, broccoli, tomato, zucchini, mushrooms and cauliflower.

22. 6 ounces tofu stir-fried with 1 teaspoon extra-virgin olive oil, ginger and reduced sodium soy sauce. Also stir-fry 2 ⅓ cups Oriental mixed vegetables and 2 tablespoons chopped walnuts OR cashews; plus ½ cup cooked brown rice.

23. 1 whole-wheat tortilla (7") filled with 1 ounce grated low-fat cheddar cheese, ⅔ cup black beans, ½ cup non-fat refried beans, ½ cup chopped tomato and onion, 4 tablespoons salsa and 2 tablespoons non-fat sour cream.

24. 1 apple; plus 3 carrots; plus 2 tablespoons peanut butter on 1 slice whole-wheat bread.

525 CALORIE MEAL PLANS

1. 1 ⅓ cups Split Pea Soup (Recipe in Appendix C); plus 1 apple; plus ONE of the following selections spread with 2 wedges low-fat "Laughing Cow" cheese: 4 WASA (whole-wheat, rye or sesame varieties) OR 4 RyKrisp rectangles OR 7 Ak-Mak crackers OR 9 reduced-fat Triscuit crackers.

2. 2 whole-wheat tortillas (7"), cut into wedges and baked into "chips." Sprinkle with 1 ounce low-fat cheddar and melt cheese in oven or microwave. Top with mashed ½ of an avocado, 4 tablespoons salsa and 3 tablespoons non-fat sour cream.

(525 CALORIE MEAL PLANS CONT.)

3. 1 meatless burger patty on 1 whole-grain hamburger bun with 1 slice 2% cheese "single" and 2 slices each, tomato and onion. Add lettuce, mustard and non-fat mayo, as desired. Plus 1 apple; plus ⅔ cup Minestrone, White Bean or Lentil Soup, or Turkey Chili. (Recipe in Appendix C)

4. 5 ounces grilled chicken; plus ⅔ cup cooked brown rice; plus 3 cups of any combination of lightly steamed broccoli, spinach, tomato, cauliflower, zucchini, green beans, onions and peppers.

5. 26 almonds; plus 1 orange; plus 15 reduced-fat Triscuit crackers.

6. 2 slices toasted whole-wheat cinnamon-raisin bread with 2 tablespoons peanut butter; plus 1 orange; plus 1 cup non-fat/no-sugar hot chocolate.

7. 2 whole-grain pancakes or waffles. (⅔ of Recipe in Appendix C); plus 1⅓ cups plain non-fat yogurt and 1 cup berries with 2 tablespoons no-sugar maple syrup.

8. 1 toasted whole-wheat English muffin topped with 1 cup Egg Beaters, scrambled or micro-waved, with 1 slice 2% cheese "single" plus 1 ⅓ cups Minestrone, White Bean or Lentil Soup, or Turkey Chili. (Recipes in Appendix C)

9. 2 slices whole-grain bread with ONE of the following choices: 4 ounces grilled chicken breast OR 6 ounces water or vacuum packed albacore tuna OR 6 ounces thin-sliced, deli-style ham OR turkey; plus 1 slice 2% cheese "single" and 2 slices each, tomato and onion. Add lettuce, mustard and non-fat mayo, as desired.

10. Large green salad, dressed with balsamic vinegar and 2 teaspoons extra-virgin olive oil. Top salad with 2 cups chopped tomato, onion, carrots, cauliflower, broccoli, mushrooms, and cucumber. Top salad with 6 ounces grilled chicken breast OR 8 ounces grilled shrimp. Add 1 ounce low-fat cheddar OR Swiss OR part-skim mozzarella cheese.

11. 1 hard-boiled egg; plus 1 orange; plus 2 slices whole-wheat toast spread with 2 tablespoons non-fat cream cheese and 1 tablespoon all-fruit/no-sugar jam; plus 1 cup plain non-fat yogurt with 2 tablespoons no-sugar maple syrup.

12. 1 whole-wheat tortilla (7") filled with 1 ounce grated low-fat cheddar cheese, 1 cup black beans, ½ cup non-fat refried beans, 1 cup chopped tomato and onion, 2 tablespoons salsa and 2 tablespoons non-fat sour cream.

13. 1 whole-wheat pita filled with 3 tablespoons hummus, 2 ounces crumbled low-fat feta cheese, 3 tablespoons chopped olives and a total of 1 ½ cups chopped tomato, onion, cucumber and peppers.

14. 1 ¾ cups cooked oatmeal with 2 tablespoons chopped walnuts, 1 tablespoon miniature chocolate chips and 1 tablespoon raisins; plus 1 orange.

15. 1 ¾ cups cooked oatmeal with 2 tablespoons chopped walnuts OR pecans, 1 grated apple and 6 ounces non-fat milk. Add cinnamon and 2 tablespoons no-sugar maple syrup.

(525 CALORIE MEAL PLANS CONT.)

16. 250 calorie serving of a whole-grain, high-fiber, low sugar cereal with 8 ounces non-fat milk; plus 1 orange; plus 1 slice whole-grain toast with 1 tablespoon all-fruit/no-sugar jam.

17. 1 cup non-fat cottage cheese; plus 1 tomato, sliced; plus 2 slices whole-grain bread with 1 tablespoon peanut butter and 2 teaspoons all-fruit/no-sugar jam.

18. Spinach Egg Pie (⅔ of Recipe in Appendix C); plus 1 orange; plus 1 slice whole-wheat toast with 2 tablespoons non-fat cream cheese and 2 teaspoons all-fruit/no-sugar jam.

19. 6 ounces tofu stir-fried with 1 teaspoon extra-virgin olive oil, ginger and reduced sodium soy sauce. Also stir-fry 1 ½ cups Oriental mixed vegetables with 2 tablespoons chopped walnuts OR cashews; plus ¾ cup cooked brown rice.

20. 1 ½ cups Minestrone, White Bean or Lentil soup, or Turkey Chili. (Recipes in Appendix C); plus 1 (1 ounce) part-skim mozzarella cheese stick; plus 1 orange; plus ONE of the following selections: 4 WASA (whole-wheat, rye or sesame varieties) OR 4 RyKrisp rectangles OR 7 Ak-Mak crackers OR 9 reduced-fat Triscuit crackers.

21. 1 cup non-fat cottage cheese; plus 1 slice whole-wheat bread; plus 1 apple; plus 2 cups of any combination of lightly steamed spinach, broccoli, tomato, zucchini, mushrooms and cauliflower with 2 tablespoons chopped walnuts.

22. 1 cup Egg Beaters, scrambled or micro-waved; 1 ounce low-fat cheddar OR Swiss cheese; either 4 ounces Canadian bacon OR 6 ounces thin- sliced, deli-style ham and a total of 2 cups chopped onion, tomato, mushroom, peppers and spinach; plus 1 slice whole-grain toast.

550 CALORIE MEAL PLANS

1. 1 ⅓ cups Split Pea Soup (Recipe in Appendix C); plus 1 apple; plus ONE of the following selections spread with 2 wedges low-fat "Laughing Cow" cheese: 4 WASA (whole-wheat, rye or sesame varieties) OR 4 RyKrisp rectangles OR 7 Ak-Mak crackers OR 9 reduced-fat Triscuit crackers.

2. 2 whole-wheat tortillas (7"), cut into wedges and baked into "chips." Sprinkle with 1 ½ ounces low-fat cheddar and melt cheese in oven or microwave. Top with mashed ½ of an avocado, 3 tablespoons salsa and 2 tablespoons non-fat sour cream.

3. 2 meatless burger patties on 1 whole-grain hamburger bun with 1 slice 2% cheese "single" and 2 slices each, tomato and onion. Add lettuce, mustard and non-fat mayo, as desired. Plus 1 apple.

4. 6 ounces grilled chicken; plus ¾ cup cooked brown rice; plus 2 cups of any combination of lightly steamed broccoli, spinach, tomato, cauliflower, zucchini, green beans and peppers.

5. 6 ounces tofu stir-fried with 1 teaspoon extra-virgin olive oil, ginger and reduced sodium soy sauce. Also stir-fry 2 ⅓ cups Oriental mixed vegetables with 2 tablespoons chopped walnuts OR cashews; plus ¾ cup cooked brown rice.

(550 CALORIE MEAL PLANS CONT.)

6. 2 slices toasted whole-wheat cinnamon-raisin bread with 2 ⅓ tablespoons peanut butter; plus 1 orange; plus 1 cup non-fat/no-sugar hot chocolate.

7. 2 whole-grain pancakes or waffles (Entire 300 calorie Recipe in Appendix C); plus 1 ⅓ cups plain non-fat yogurt and 1 cup berries; plus 2 tablespoons no-sugar maple syrup.

8. 1 whole-wheat tortilla (7") filled with ⅔ cup black beans, ⅔ cup non-fat refried beans, 1 ounce low-fat cheddar cheese, 1 cup chopped onion and tomato, 3 tablespoons non-fat sour cream and 4 tablespoons salsa.

9. 2 slices whole-grain bread with ONE of the following choices: 2 ounces grilled chicken breast OR 3 ounces water or vacuum packed albacore tuna OR 3 ounces thin-sliced, deli-style ham OR turkey with 1 ounce low-fat cheddar OR Swiss OR part-skim mozzarella cheese and 2 slices each, tomato and onion. Add lettuce, mustard and non-fat mayo, as desired. Plus 1 cup Minestrone, White Bean or Lentil Soup, or Turkey Chili. (Recipes in Appendix C)

10. Large green salad, dressed with balsamic vinegar and 2 teaspoons extra-virgin olive oil. Top salad with 2 cups chopped tomato, onion, carrots, cauliflower, broccoli, mushrooms, and cucumber. Top salad with either 6 ounces grilled chicken breast OR 8 ounces grilled shrimp. Add 1 ounce low-fat cheddar OR Swiss OR part-skim mozzarella cheese.

11. 1 hard-boiled egg; plus 1 orange; plus 2 slices whole-wheat bread with 1 tablespoon peanut butter; plus ⅔ cup plain non-fat yogurt with 2 tablespoons no-sugar maple syrup.

12. 1 toasted whole-wheat English muffin topped with 1 cup Egg Beaters, scrambled or micro-waved, and 2 slices 2% cheese "singles" plus 1 ½ cups either Minestrone, White Bean or Lentil soup, or Turkey Chili. (Recipes in Appendix C)

13. 1 whole-wheat pita filled with 3 tablespoons hummus, 3 tablespoons chopped olives, 2 ounces crumbled low-fat feta cheese and a total of 2 cups chopped tomato, onion, cucumber and peppers.

14. ¾ cup cooked edamame; plus 1 cup cooked brown rice; plus 2 cups lightly steamed spinach, broccoli, tomato, carrots, mushrooms, zucchini or green beans with 2 tablespoons chopped walnuts OR pecans.

15. 1½ cups cooked oatmeal with 2 tablespoons chopped walnuts OR pecans, 1 grated apple and 8 ounces non-fat milk. Add cinnamon and 2 tablespoons no-sugar maple syrup.

16. 275 calorie serving of a whole-grain, high-fiber, low sugar cereal with 8 ounces non-fat milk; plus 1 orange; plus 1 slice whole-grain toast spread with 1 tablespoon all-fruit/no-sugar jam.

17. 1 cup non-fat cottage cheese; plus 2 tomatoes, sliced; plus 2 slices whole-grain bread with 1 tablespoon peanut butter.

18. Spinach Egg Pie (⅔ of Recipe in Appendix C); plus 1 orange; plus 1 slice whole-wheat toast spread with 1 wedge reduced fat "Laughing Cow" cheese and 2 teaspoons all-fruit/no-sugar jam.

(550 CALORIE MEAL PLANS CONT.)

19. 12 ounces V-8 juice; plus 2 carrots; plus 2 (1 ounce each) part-skim mozzarella cheese sticks; plus 5 ounces thin-sliced, deli-style ham or turkey; plus ONE of the following selections: 3 WASA (whole-wheat, rye or sesame) OR 3 RyKrisp rectangles OR 4 Ak-Mak crackers OR 6 reduced-fat Triscuit crackers.

20. 1½ cups Minestrone, White Bean or Lentil Soup, or Turkey Chili (Recipes in Appendix C); plus 1 (1 ounce) part-skim mozzarella cheese stick; plus 1 orange; plus ONE of the following selections: 5 WASA (whole-wheat, rye or sesame varieties) OR 5 RyKrisp rectangles OR 8 Ak-Mak crackers OR 10 reduced-fat Triscuit crackers.

21. 1 cup non-fat cottage cheese; plus ⅔ cup cooked brown rice; plus 1 apple; plus 2 ½ cups of any combination of lightly steamed spinach, broccoli, tomato, zucchini, mushrooms and cauliflower.

22. 1 cup Egg Beaters, scrambled or micro-waved, 1 ounce low-fat cheddar OR Swiss cheese, either 4 ounces Canadian bacon OR 6 ounces thin-sliced, deli-style ham and 2 cups chopped onion, tomato, mushroom, peppers and spinach; plus 1 slice whole-grain toast.

23. 1 apple; plus 2 carrots; plus 2 tablespoons peanut butter on 2 slices whole-wheat bread.

24. 1 cup non-fat pudding with 2 cups chopped fruit and 2 tablespoons chopped walnuts OR pecans; plus 2 non-fat Fruit Newtons.

575 CALORIE MEAL PLANS

1. 1 ½ cups Split Pea Soup (Recipe in Appendix C); plus 1 apple; plus ONE of the following selections spread with 2 wedges low-fat "Laughing Cow" cheese: 4 WASA (whole-wheat, rye or sesame varieties) OR 4 RyKrisp rectangles OR 7 Ak-Mak crackers OR 10 reduced-fat Triscuit crackers.

2. 2 ½ whole-wheat tortillas (7"), cut into wedges and baked into "chips." Sprinkle with 1 ounce low-fat shredded cheddar and melt cheese in oven or microwave. Top with mashed ½ of an avocado, 2 tablespoons salsa and 2 tablespoons non-fat sour cream.

3. 2 meatless burger patties on 1 whole-grain hamburger bun with 1 slice 2% cheese "single" and 2 slices each, tomato and onion. Add lettuce, mustard and non-fat mayo, as desired. Plus 1 apple; plus 1 carrot.

4. 6 ounces grilled chicken; plus ½ cup cooked brown rice; plus 2 ½ cups of any combination of lightly steamed broccoli, spinach, tomato, cauliflower, zucchini, green beans and peppers.

5. 1 cup non-fat/no-sugar pudding with 2 cups chopped fruit and 2 tablespoons chopped walnuts OR pecans; plus 3 non-fat Fruit Newtons.

6. 2 slices toasted whole-wheat cinnamon-raisin bread with 2 ½ tablespoons peanut butter; plus 1 orange; plus 1 cup no-sugar/non-fat hot chocolate.

(575 CALORIE MEAL PLANS CONT.)

7. 2 whole-grain pancakes or waffles (Entire 300 calorie Recipe in Appendix C); plus 1 ⅔ cup plain non-fat yogurt, 1 cup berries and 2 tablespoons no-sugar maple syrup.

8. 1 whole-wheat tortilla (7") filled with ⅔ cup black beans, ⅔ cup non-fat refried beans, 1 ½ ounces low-fat cheddar cheese, 1 cup chopped onion and tomato, 3 tablespoons non-fat sour cream and 4 tablespoons salsa.

9. 2 slices whole-grain bread with ONE of the following choices: 2.5 ounces grilled chicken breast OR 3.5 ounces water or vacuum packed albacore tuna OR 3.5 ounces thin-sliced, deli-style ham OR turkey, 1 ounce low-fat cheddar OR Swiss OR part-skim mozzarella cheese and 2 slices each, tomato and onion. Add lettuce, mustard and non-fat mayo, as desired. Plus 1 cup Minestrone, White Bean or Lentil Soup, or Turkey Chili. (Recipes in Appendix C)

10. Large green salad, dressed with balsamic vinegar and 2 teaspoons extra-virgin olive oil. Top salad with a total of 2 cups chopped tomato, onion, carrots, cauliflower, broccoli, mushrooms, and cucumber. Top salad with either 5 ounces grilled chicken breast OR 7 ounces grilled shrimp. Add 1 ounce low-fat cheddar OR Swiss OR part-skim mozzarella cheese; plus 1 slice whole-grain bread.

11. 1 hard-boiled egg; plus 1 orange; plus 2 slices whole-wheat bread with 1 tablespoon peanut butter; plus 1 cup plain non-fat yogurt with 2 tablespoons no-sugar maple syrup.

12. 1 toasted whole-wheat English muffin topped with 1 cup Egg Beaters, scrambled or micro-waved, and 2 slices 2% cheese "singles" plus 1 orange; plus 1 cup Minestrone, White Bean or Lentil soup, or Turkey Chili. (Recipes in Appendix C)

13. 1 whole-wheat pita filled with 2 tablespoons hummus, 2 tablespoons chopped olives, 2 ounces crumbled low-fat feta cheese and a total of 2 cups chopped tomato, onion, cucumber and peppers; plus 1 apple.

14. ¾ cup cooked edamame; plus 1 cup cooked brown rice; plus 2 ½ cups lightly steamed spinach, broccoli, tomato, carrots, mushrooms, zucchini or green beans with 2 tablespoons chopped walnuts OR pecans.

15. 2 cups cooked oatmeal with 2 tablespoons chopped walnuts OR pecans, 1 grated apple and 8 ounces non-fat milk. Add cinnamon and 2 tablespoons no-sugar maple syrup.

16. 5 ounces tofu stir-fried with 1 teaspoon extra-virgin olive oil, ginger and reduced sodium soy sauce. Also stir-fry 3 ½ cups Oriental mixed vegetables with 2 tablespoons chopped walnuts OR cashews; plus 3/4 cup cooked brown rice.

17. 1 cup non-fat cottage cheese; plus 1 tomato, sliced; plus 1 orange; plus 2 slices whole-grain bread with 1 tablespoon peanut butter.

18. 1 apple; plus 2 carrots; plus 2 slices whole-wheat bread with 2 tablespoons peanut butter and 2 teaspoons all-fruit/no-sugar jam.

(575 CALORIE MEAL PLANS CONT.)

19. 12 ounces V-8 juice; plus 2 carrots; plus 2 (1 ounce each) part-skim mozzarella cheese sticks; plus either 6 ounces thin-sliced, deli-style turkey OR ham; plus ONE of the following selections: 3 WASA (whole-wheat, rye or sesame) OR 3 RyKrisp rectangles OR 4 Ak-Mak crackers OR 6 reduced-fat Triscuit crackers.

20. 2 cups Minestrone, White Bean or Lentil soup, or Turkey Chili (Recipes in Appendix C); plus 1 (1 ounce) part-skim mozzarella cheese stick; plus 1 orange; plus ONE of the following selections: 4 WASA (whole-wheat, rye or sesame varieties) OR 4 RyKrisp rectangles OR 6 Ak-Mak crackers OR 8 reduced-fat Triscuit crackers.

21. 1 cup non-fat cottage cheese; plus ½ cup cooked brown rice; plus 1 apple; plus 2 ½ cups of any combination of lightly steamed spinach, broccoli, tomato, zucchini, mushrooms, onion and cauliflower with 1 tablespoon chopped walnuts.

22. 1 cup Egg Beaters, scrambled or micro-waved, 1 ½ ounces low-fat cheddar OR Swiss cheese, either 4 ounces Canadian bacon OR 6 ounces thin-sliced, deli-style ham and 1 ½ cups chopped onion, tomato, mushroom, peppers and spinach; plus 1 slice whole-grain toast.

23. Spinach Egg Pie (⅔ of Recipe in Appendix C); plus 1 orange; plus 1 toasted whole-wheat English muffin spread with 2 tablespoons non-fat cream cheese and 2 teaspoons all-fruit/no-sugar jam.

24. 300 calorie serving of a whole-grain, high-fiber, low sugar cereal with 8 ounces non-fat milk; plus 1 orange; plus 1 slice whole-grain toast with 1 tablespoon all-fruit/no-sugar jam.

DINNERS

DINNER #1   SALMON WITH MANGO SALSA

Salad made with all types of leafy greens: lettuce, spinach and cabbage.
Top salad with any combination of chopped carrots, onions, tomatoes, cucumbers, mushrooms, radishes or peppers.
Dress salad with a splash of balsamic vinegar or lemon juice.

Prepare any of the following vegetables, lightly steamed, grilled, or roasted: spinach, zucchini, tomato, mushrooms, broccoli, cauliflower, carrots, onions, green beans, asparagus, peppers or Brussels sprouts.

Salmon: baked, broiled or grilled.
Flavor salmon with lemon juice, cilantro, thyme, ginger, orange juice or lime juice.

Top cooked salmon and salad with Mango Salsa. (Recipe in Appendix C)

CALORIE TOTAL	PORTION SIZE	FOOD ITEM	CALORIE TOTAL	PORTION SIZE	FOOD ITEM
350	2 cups	Green salad	375	2 cups	Green salad
	1 cup	Chopped salad vegetables		1 ½ cups	Chopped salad vegetables
	3 ounces	Salmon (cooked)		3 ounces	Salmon (cooked)
	1 ½ cups	Steamed vegetables		1 ½ cups	Steamed vegetables
	⅓ recipe	Mango Salsa		½ recipe	Mango Salsa
400	2 cups	Green salad	425	2 cups	Green salad
	½ cup	Chopped salad vegetables		1 cup	Chopped salad vegetables
	4 ounces	Salmon (cooked)		4 ounces	Salmon (cooked)
	1 ½ cups	Steamed vegetables		2 cups	Steamed vegetables
	½ recipe	Mango Salsa		½ recipe	Mango Salsa
450	2 cups	Green salad	475	2 cups	Green salad
	1 cup	Chopped salad vegetables		½ cup	Chopped salad vegetables
	4 ounces	Salmon (cooked)		5 ounces	Salmon (cooked)
	2 ½ cups	Steamed vegetables		1 ½ cups	Steamed vegetables
	½ recipe	Mango Salsa		½ recipe	Mango Salsa
500	2 cups	Green salad	525	2 cups	Green salad
	½ cup	Chopped salad vegetables		1 cup	Chopped salad vegetables
	5 ounces	Salmon (cooked)		5 ounces	Salmon (cooked)
	2 cups	Steamed vegetables		2 ½ cups	Steamed vegetables
	½ recipe	Mango Salsa		½ recipe	Mango Salsa

(DINNER #1 SALMON WITH MANGO SALSA CONT.)

CALORIE TOTAL	PORTION SIZE	FOOD ITEM	CALORIE TOTAL	PORTION SIZE	FOOD ITEM
550	2 cups	Green salad	575	2 cups	Green salad
	½ cup	Chopped salad vegetables		½ cup	Chopped salad vegetables
	6 ounces	Salmon (cooked)		6 ounces	Salmon
	2 cups	Steamed vegetables		2 ½ cups	Steamed vegetables
	½ recipe	Mango Salsa		½ recipe	Mango Salsa
600	2 cups	Green salad	625	2 cups	Green salad
	1 cup	Chopped salad vegetables		1 cup	Chopped salad vegetables
	6 ounces	Salmon (cooked)		6 ounces	Salmon (cooked)
	2 cups	Steamed vegetables		2 ½ cups	Steamed vegetables
	⅔ recipe	Mango Salsa		⅔ recipe	Mango Salsa

DINNER #2   BAKED CHICKEN OR TURKEY

Salad made with all types of leafy greens: lettuce, spinach and cabbage.
Top salad with any combination of chopped carrots, onions, tomatoes, cucumbers, mushrooms, radishes or peppers.
Dress salad with a splash of balsamic vinegar or lemon juice.

Prepare any of the following vegetables, lightly steamed, grilled, or roasted: spinach, zucchini, tomato, mushrooms, broccoli, cauliflower, carrots, onions, green beans, asparagus, peppers or Brussels sprouts.

Chicken or turkey (skin removed, white meat), roasted, baked or grilled.
Season with herbs, as desired.

CALORIE TOTAL	PORTION SIZE	FOOD ITEM	CALORIE TOTAL	PORTION SIZE	FOOD ITEM
350	2 cups	Green salad	375	2 cups	Green salad
	½ cup	Chopped salad vegetables		1 cup	Chopped salad vegetables
	5 ounces	Chicken or Turkey breast (cooked)		5 ounces	Chicken or Turkey breast (cooked)
	2 cups	Steamed vegetables		2 cups	Steamed vegetables
400	2 cups	Green salad	425	2 cups	Green salad
	1 cup	Chopped salad vegetables		1 cup	Chopped salad vegetables
	5 ounces	Chicken or Turkey breast (cooked)		6 ounces	Chicken or Turkey breast (cooked)
	2 ½ cups	Steamed vegetables		2 cups	Steamed vegetables
450	2 cups	Green salad	475	2 cups	Green salad
	½ cup	Chopped salad vegetables		½ cup	Chopped salad vegetables
	6 ounces	Chicken or Turkey breast (cooked)		6 ounces	Chicken or Turkey breast (cooked)
	2 ½ cups	Steamed vegetables		3 cups	Steamed vegetables

(DINNER #2 BAKED CHICKEN OR TURKEY CONT.)

CALORIE TOTAL	PORTION SIZE	FOOD ITEM	CALORIE TOTAL	PORTION SIZE	FOOD ITEM
500	2 cups	Green salad	525	2 cups	Green salad
	½ cup	Chopped salad vegetables		1 cup	Chopped salad vegetables
	6 ounces	Chicken or Turkey breast (cooked)		6 ounces	Chicken or Turkey breast (cooked)
	2 cups	Steamed vegetables		2 cups	Steamed vegetables
	½ cup	Cooked brown rice		½ cup	Cooked brown rice
550	2 cups	Green salad	575	2 cups	Green salad
	½ cup	Chopped salad vegetables		½ cup	Chopped salad vegetables
	6 ounces	Chicken or Turkey breast (cooked)		6 ounces	Chicken or Turkey breast (cooked)
	1 ½ cups	Steamed vegetables		2 cups	Steamed vegetables
	¾ cup	Cooked brown rice		¾ cup	Cooked brown rice
600	2 cups	Green salad	625	2 cups	Green salad
	½ cup	Chopped salad vegetables		½ cup	Chopped salad vegetables
	6 ounces	Chicken or Turkey breast (cooked)		6 ounces	Chicken or Turkey breast (cooked)
	2 ½ cups	Steamed vegetables		3 cups	Steamed vegetables
	¾ cup	Cooked brown rice		¾ cup	Cooked brown rice

DINNER #3   PITA PIZZA

Salad made with all types of leafy greens: lettuce, spinach and cabbage.
Top salad with any combination of chopped carrots, onions, tomatoes, cucumbers, mushrooms, radishes or peppers.
Dress salad with a splash of balsamic vinegar or lemon juice.

Pita Pizza (Recipe in Appendix C).

Top with any of the following vegetables: chopped zucchini, tomato, mushrooms, peppers, eggplant, onion or spinach. Add other toppings, as directed.

350	2 cups	Green salad	375	2 cups	Green salad
	½ cup	Chopped salad vegetables		½ cup	Chopped salad vegetables
	1 whole	Whole-wheat pita round		1 whole	Whole-wheat pita round
	½ cup	Tomato sauce		½ cup	Tomato sauce
	1 ½ cups	Chopped vegetables		1 ½ cups	Chopped vegetables
	2 TBS	Grated Parmesan cheese		3 TBS	Grated Parmesan cheese
400	2 cups	Green salad	425	2 cups	Green salad
	½ cup	Chopped salad vegetables		½ cup	Chopped salad vegetables
	1 whole	Whole-wheat pita round		1 whole	Whole-wheat pita round
	½ cup	Tomato sauce		½ cup	Tomato sauce
	2 cups	Chopped vegetables		1 ½ cups	Chopped vegetables
	3 TBS	Grated Parmesan cheese		1 TBS	Grated Parmesan cheese
	1 ounce	Grated part-skim mozzarella		1 ounce	Grated part-skim mozzarella

167

(DINNER #3 PITA PIZZA CONT.)

CALORIE TOTAL	PORTION SIZE	FOOD ITEM	CALORIE TOTAL	PORTION SIZE	FOOD ITEM
450	2 cups	Green salad	475	2 cups	Green salad
	½ cup	Chopped salad vegetables		½ cup	Chopped salad vegetables
	1 whole	Whole-wheat pita round		1 whole	Whole-wheat pita round
	½ cup	Tomato sauce		½ cup	Tomato sauce
	1 ½ cups	Chopped vegetables		2 cups	Chopped vegetables
	2 TBS	Grated Parmesan cheese		3 TBS	Grated Parmesan cheese
	1 ounce	Grated part-skim mozzarella		1 ounce	Grated part-skim mozzarella
500	2 cups	Green salad	525	2 cups	Green salad
	½ cup	Chopped salad vegetables		½ cup	Chopped salad vegetables
	1 whole	Whole-wheat pita round		1 whole	Whole-wheat pita round
	½ cup	Tomato sauce		½ cup	Tomato sauce
	1 cup	Chopped vegetables		1 ½ cups	Chopped vegetables
	2 TBS	Grated Parmesan cheese		2 TBS	Grated Parmesan cheese
	1 ounce	Grated part-skim mozzarella		1 ounce	Grated part-skim mozzarella
	2 ounces	Canadian bacon		2 ounces	Canadian bacon
550	2 cups	Green salad	575	2 cups	Green salad
	½ cup	Chopped salad vegetables		½ cup	Chopped salad vegetables
	1 whole	Whole-wheat pita round		1 whole	Whole-wheat pita round
	½ cup	Tomato sauce		½ cup	Tomato sauce
	1 ½ cups	Chopped vegetables		2 cups	Chopped vegetables
	3 TBS	Grated Parmesan cheese		3 TBS	Grated Parmesan cheese
	1 ounce	Grated part-skim mozzarella		1 ounce	Grated part-skim mozzarella
	2 ounces	Canadian bacon		2 ounces	Canadian bacon
600	2 cups	Green salad	625	2 cups	Green salad
	½ cup	Chopped salad vegetables		½ cup	Chopped salad vegetables
	1 whole	Whole-wheat pita round		1 whole	Whole-wheat pita round
	½ cup	Tomato sauce		½ cup	Tomato sauce
	2 ½ cups	Chopped vegetables		2 ½ cups	Chopped vegetables
	3 TBS	Grated Parmesan cheese		2 TBS	Grated Parmesan cheese
	1 ounce	Grated part-skim mozzarella		1 ounce	Grated part-skim mozzarella
	2 ounces	Canadian bacon		3 ounces	Canadian bacon

DINNER #4   TURKEY MEATLOAF

Salad made with all types of leafy greens: lettuce, spinach and cabbage.
Top salad with any combination of chopped carrots, onions, tomatoes, cucumbers,
mushrooms, radishes or peppers.
Dress salad with a splash of balsamic vinegar or lemon juice.

Roasted vegetables:
Cut into bite-sized pieces any combination of the following vegetables: carrots, onions,
Brussels sprouts, squash, tomatoes, cauliflower. Bake in oven until they are fork-soft.

Turkey Meatloaf (Recipe in Appendix C).

CALORIE TOTAL	PORTION SIZE	FOOD ITEM	CALORIE TOTAL	PORTION SIZE	FOOD ITEM
350	2 cups	Green salad	375	2 cups	Green salad
	½ cup	Chopped salad vegetables		½ cup	Chopped salad vegetables
	1/6 of recipe	Turkey Meatloaf		1/6 of recipe	Turkey Meatloaf
	1 ½ cups	Roasted vegetables		2 cups	Roasted vegetables
400	2 cups	Green salad	425	2 cups	Green salad
	½ cup	Chopped salad vegetables		1 cup	Chopped salad vegetables
	1/6 of recipe	Turkey Meatloaf		1/6 of recipe	Turkey Meatloaf
	2 ¾ cups	Roasted vegetables		3 cups	Roasted vegetables
450	2 cups	Green salad	475	2 cups	Green salad
	½ cup	Chopped salad vegetables		1 cup	Chopped salad vegetables
	1/5 of recipe	Turkey Meatloaf		1/5 of recipe	Turkey Meatloaf
	2 ½ cups	Roasted vegetables		3 cups	Roasted vegetables
500	2 cups	Green salad	525	2 cups	Green salad
	½ cup	Chopped salad vegetables		1 cup	Chopped salad vegetables
	¼ of recipe	Turkey Meatloaf		¼ of recipe	Turkey Meatloaf
	2 cups	Roasted vegetables		2 cups	Roasted vegetables
550	2 cups	Green salad	575	2 cups	Green salad
	½ cup	Chopped salad vegetables		½ cup	Chopped salad vegetables
	¼ of recipe	Turkey Meatloaf		¼ of recipe	Turkey Meatloaf
	3 cups	Roasted vegetables		3 ½ cups	Roasted vegetables
600	2 cups	Green salad	625	2 cups	Green salad
	½ cup	Chopped salad vegetables		1 cup	Chopped salad vegetables
	1 teaspoon	Extra-virgin olive oil for salad		1 teaspoon	Extra-virgin olive oil for salad
	¼ of recipe	Turkey Meatloaf		¼ of recipe	Turkey Meatloaf
	3 ½ cups	Roasted vegetables		3 ½ cups	Roasted vegetables

DINNER #5 CHICKEN ARTICHOKE CASSEROLE

Salad made with all types of leafy greens: lettuce, spinach and cabbage.
Top salad with any combination of chopped carrots, onions, tomatoes, cucumbers, mushrooms, radishes or peppers.
Dress salad with a splash of balsamic vinegar or lemon juice.

Prepare any of the following vegetables, lightly steamed, grilled, or roasted: spinach, zucchini, tomato, mushrooms, broccoli, cauliflower, carrots, onions, green beans, asparagus, peppers or Brussels sprouts.

Chicken Artichoke Casserole (Recipe in Appendix C).
Saute spinach in 1 teaspoon extra-virgin olive oil and minced garlic.

CALORIE TOTAL	PORTION SIZE	FOOD ITEM	CALORIE TOTAL	PORTION SIZE	FOOD ITEM
350	2 cups	Green salad	375	2 cups	Green salad
	½ cup	Chopped salad vegetables		½ cup	Chopped salad vegetables
	¼ recipe	Chicken Artichoke Casserole		¼ recipe	Chicken Artichoke Casserole
	1 cup	Sautéed spinach		1 cup	Sautéed spinach
	½ cup	Steamed vegetables		3/4 cup	Steamed vegetables
400	2 cups	Green salad	425	2 cups	Green salad
	½ cup	Chopped salad vegetables		½ cup	Chopped salad vegetables
	¼ recipe	Chicken Artichoke Casserole		¼ recipe	Chicken Artichoke Casserole
	1½ cups	Sautéed spinach		2 cups	Sautéed spinach
	1 cup	Steamed vegetables		1 cup	Steamed vegetables
450	2 cups	Green salad	475	2 cups	Green salad
	½ cup	Chopped salad vegetables		½ cup	Chopped salad vegetables
	⅓ recipe	Chicken Artichoke Casserole		⅓ recipe	Chicken Artichoke Casserole
	1 cup	Sautéed spinach		1 cup	Sautéed spinach
	1 cup	Steamed vegetables		1 ½ cups	Steamed vegetables
500	2 cups	Green salad	525	2 cups	Green salad
	½ cup	Chopped salad vegetables		½ cup	Chopped salad vegetables
	⅓ recipe	Chicken Artichoke Casserole		⅓ recipe	Chicken Artichoke Casserole
	1 cup	Sautéed spinach		2 cups	Sautéed spinach
	2 cups	Steamed vegetables		2 cups	Steamed vegetables
550	2 cups	Green salad	575	2 cups	Green salad
	½ cup	Chopped salad vegetables		½ cup	Chopped salad vegetables
	⅓ recipe	Chicken Artichoke Casserole		⅓ recipe	Chicken Artichoke Casserole
	2 cups	Sautéed spinach		2 cups	Sautéed spinach
	2 ½ cups	Steamed vegetables		3 cups	Steamed vegetables
600	2 cups	Green salad	625	2 cups	Green salad
	½ cup	Chopped salad vegetables		½ cup	Chopped salad vegetables
	½ recipe	Chicken Artichoke Casserole		½ recipe	Chicken Artichoke Casserole
	2 cups	Sautéed spinach		2 cups	Sautéed spinach
	1 ½ cups	Steamed vegetables		2 cups	Steamed vegetables

DINNER #6   TERIYAKI CHICKEN

Spinach Salad with Sweet Orange Vinaigrette. (Recipe in Appendix C)

Skewered vegetables: place any combination of onions, tomatoes, mushrooms and peppers on skewers.

Teriyaki Chicken (Recipe in Appendix C).

Chicken and vegetables can be cooked either on the barbecue or under the broiler in the oven.

CALORIE TOTAL	PORTION SIZE	FOOD ITEM	CALORIE TOTAL	PORTION SIZE	FOOD ITEM
350	⅓ recipe	Spinach Salad	375	⅓ recipe	Spinach Salad
	¼ recipe	Teriyaki Chicken		¼ recipe	Teriyaki Chicken
	1 ½ cups	Skewered vegetables		2 cups	Skewered vegetables
400	⅓ recipe	Spinach Salad	425	½ recipe	Spinach Salad
	¼ recipe	Teriyaki Chicken		¼ recipe	Teriyaki Chicken
	2 ½ cups	Skewered vegetables		2 cups	Skewered vegetables
450	½ recipe	Spinach Salad	475	½ recipe	Spinach Salad
	⅓ recipe	Teriyaki Chicken		⅓ recipe	Teriyaki Chicken
	1 cup	Skewered vegetables		1 ½ cups	Skewered vegetables
500	½ recipe	Spinach Salad	525	½ recipe	Spinach Salad
	⅓ recipe	Teriyaki Chicken		⅓ recipe	Teriyaki Chicken
	2 cups	Skewered vegetables		2 ½ cups	Skewered vegetables
550	⅓ recipe	Spinach Salad	575	½ recipe	Spinach Salad
	½ recipe	Teriyaki Chicken		½ recipe	Teriyaki Chicken
	2 cups	Skewered vegetables		2 cups	Skewered vegetables
600	½ recipe	Spinach Salad	625	½ recipe	Spinach Salad
	½ recipe	Teriyaki Chicken		½ recipe	Teriyaki Chicken
	2 ½ cups	Skewered vegetables		3 cups	Skewered vegetables

DINNER #7 MEXICAN SAUTÉ

Salad made with all types of leafy greens: lettuce, spinach and cabbage.
Top salad greens with Mexican Sauté. (Recipe in Appendix C)
Then top salad with remaining items, listed below.

May substitute 2 ounces shredded chicken breast for the chopped olives and low fat cheddar, for each calorie level, if desired.

If adding calories for exercise, try some Guacamole! (Recipe and calories in Appendix C)

CALORIE TOTAL	PORTION SIZE	FOOD ITEM	CALORIE TOTAL	PORTION SIZE	FOOD ITEM
350	3 cups	Salad greens	375	3 cups	Salad greens
	½ recipe	Mexican Sauté		½ recipe	Mexican Sauté
	1 cup	Black beans		1 cup	Black beans
	½ cup	Non-fat refried beans		½ cup	Non-fat refried beans
	2 TBS	Non-fat sour cream		1 TBS	Non-fat sour cream
	3 TBS	Salsa		2 TBS	Salsa
	2 TBS	Chopped olives		2 TBS	Chopped olives
				1 ounce	Shredded low-fat cheddar
400	3 cups	Salad greens	425	3 cups	Salad greens
	½ recipe	Mexican Sauté		½ recipe	Mexican Sauté
	½ cup	Black beans		¾ cup	Black beans
	½ cup	Non-fat refried beans		½ cup	Non-fat refried beans
	2 TBS	Non-fat sour cream		2 TBS	Non-fat sour cream
	2 TBS	Salsa		2 TBS	Salsa
	2 TBS	Chopped olives		2 TBS	Chopped olives
	1 ounce	Shredded low-fat cheddar		1 ounce	Shredded low-fat cheddar
450	3 cups	Salad greens	475	3 cups	Salad greens
	½ recipe	Mexican Sauté		½ recipe	Mexican Sauté
	1 cup	Black beans		1 cup	Black beans
	½ cup	Non-fat refried beans		½ cup	Non-fat refried beans
	2 TBS	Non-fat sour cream		2 TBS	Non-fat sour cream
	2 TBS	Salsa		4 TBS	Salsa
	2 TBS	Chopped olives		3 TBS	Chopped olives
	1 ounce	Shredded low-fat cheddar		1 ounce	Shredded low-fat cheddar
500	3 cups	Salad greens	525	3 cups	Salad greens
	½ recipe	Mexican Sauté		½ recipe	Mexican Sauté
	1 cup	Black beans		1 cup	Black beans
	½ cup	Non-fat refried beans		¾ cup	Non-fat refried beans
	3 TBS	Non-fat sour cream		2 TBS	Non-fat sour cream
	4 TBS	Salsa		3 TBS	Salsa
	4 TBS	Chopped olives		3 TBS	Chopped olives
	1 ounce	Shredded low-fat cheddar		1 ounce	Shredded low-fat cheddar

#7 DINNER MEXICAN SAUTÉ (CONT.)

CALORIE TOTAL	PORTION SIZE	FOOD ITEM	CALORIE TOTAL	PORTION SIZE	FOOD ITEM
550	3 cups	Salad greens	575	3 cups	Salad greens
	½ recipe	Mexican Sauté		½ recipe	Mexican Sauté
	1 cup	Black beans		1 cup	Black beans
	¾ cup	Non-fat refried beans		¾ cup	Non-fat refried beans
	2 TBS	Non-fat sour cream		3 TBS	Non-fat sour cream
	3 TBS	Salsa		4 TBS	Salsa
	2 TBS	Chopped olives		3 TBS	Chopped olives
	1 ½ ounces	Shredded low-fat cheddar		1 ½ ounces	Shredded low-fat cheddar
600	3 cups	Salad greens	625	3 cups	Salad greens
	½ recipe	Mexican Sauté		½ recipe	Mexican Sauté
	1 cup	Black beans		1 cup	Black beans
	⅔ cup	Non-fat refried beans		¾ cup	Non-fat refried beans
	2 TBS	Non-fat sour cream		2 TBS	Non-fat sour cream
	3 TBS	Salsa		4 TBS	Salsa
	2 TBS	Chopped olives		3 TBS	Chopped olives
	2 ounces	Shredded low-fat cheddar		2 ounces	Shredded low-fat cheddar

#8 DINNER CHICKEN CAESAR SALAD

Make the Caesar Salad Dressing (Recipe in Appendix C) without oil, adding oil only when indicated by your Weight Loss Calorie Plan.

Use whole-wheat bread to make Skinny Homemade Croutons. (Recipe in Appendix C)

Chicken breast (skin removed): grill or barbecue with a sprinkle of garlic salt. Cut into bite-sized chunks and toss into the salad.

350	4 cups	Torn romaine	375	4 cups	Torn romaine
	4 ounces	Chicken breast (cooked)		4 ounces	Chicken breast (cooked)
	½ recipe	No-oil Caesar Salad Dressing		½ recipe	No-oil Caesar Salad Dressing
	1 slice	Whole-grain bread (for croutons)		1 ½ slices	Whole-grain bread (for croutons)
400	4 cups	Torn romaine	425	4 cups	Torn romaine
	4 ounces	Chicken breast (cooked)		5 ounces	Chicken breast (cooked)
	½ recipe	No-oil Caesar Salad Dressing		½ recipe	No-oil Caesar Salad Dressing
	1 ⅔ slices	Whole-grain bread (for croutons)		1 ½ slices	Whole-grain bread (for croutons)

#8 DINNER CHICKEN CAESAR SALAD (CONT.)

CALORIE TOTAL	PORTION SIZE	FOOD ITEM	CALORIE TOTAL	PORTION SIZE	FOOD ITEM
450	4 cups	Torn romaine	475	4 cups	Torn romaine
	5 ounces	Chicken breast (cooked)		5 ounces	Chicken breast (cooked)
	⅔ recipe	No-oil Caesar Salad Dressing		⅔ recipe	No-oil Caesar Salad Dressing
	1 ½ slices	Whole-grain bread (for croutons)		1 ¾ slices	Whole-grain bread (for croutons)
500	4 cups	Torn romaine	525	4 cups	Torn romaine
	5 ounces	Chicken breast (cooked)		6 ounces	Chicken breast (cooked)
	⅔ recipe	No-oil Caesar Salad Dressing		⅔ recipe	No-oil Caesar Salad Dressing
	2 slices	Whole-grain bread (for croutons)		1 ⅔ slices	Whole-grain bread (for croutons)
550	4 cups	Torn romaine	575	4 cups	Torn romaine
	6 ounces	Chicken breast (cooked)		6 ounces	Chicken breast (cooked)
	⅔ recipe	No-oil Caesar Salad Dressing		⅔ recipe	No-oil Caesar Salad Dressing
	1 ⅔ slices	Whole-grain bread (for croutons)		2 slices	Whole-grain bread (for croutons)
	1 teaspoon	Extra-virgin olive oil		1 teaspoon	Extra-virgin olive oil
600	4 cups	Torn romaine	625	4 cups	Torn romaine
	6 ounces	Chicken breast (cooked)		6 ounces	Chicken breast (cooked)
	⅔ recipe	No-oil Caesar Salad Dressing		⅔ recipe	No-oil Caesar Salad Dressing
	1 ¾ slices	Whole-grain bread (for croutons)		2 slices	Whole-grain bread (for croutons)
	2 teaspoons	Extra-virgin olive oil		2 teaspoons	Extra-virgin olive oil

DINNER #9 BBQ CHICKEN WITH BAKED "FRIES"

Salad made with all types of leafy greens: lettuce, spinach and cabbage.
Top salad with any combination of chopped carrots, onions, tomatoes, cucumbers, mushrooms, radishes or peppers.
Dress salad with a splash of balsamic vinegar or lemon juice.

Chicken breast (skin removed): baked, broiled or grilled. Brush with barbecue sauce during the last few minutes of cooking.

Baked "Fries" (Recipe in Appendix C).
The following portions are based on using medium red potatoes, approximately 100 calories per potato.

350	3 cups	Salad greens	375	3 cups	Salad greens
	½ cup	Chopped vegetables		½ cup	Chopped vegetables
	3 ounces	Chicken breast (cooked)		3 ounces	Chicken breast (cooked)
	1 TBS	BBQ sauce		1 TBS	BBQ sauce
	1 ½	Potatoes, baked into "fries"		1 ¾	Potatoes, baked into "fries"

#9 DINNER   BBQ CHICKEN WITH BAKED "FRIES" (CONT.)

CALORIE TOTAL	PORTION SIZE	FOOD ITEM	CALORIE TOTAL	PORTION SIZE	FOOD ITEM
400	3 cups	Salad greens	425	3 cups	Salad greens
	½ cup	Chopped vegetables		½ cup	Chopped vegetables
	3 ounces	Chicken breast (cooked)		4 ounces	Chicken breast (cooked)
	1 TBS	BBQ sauce		1 TBS	BBQ sauce
	2	Potatoes, baked into "fries"		1 ¾	Potatoes, baked into "fries"
450	3 cups	Salad greens	475	3 cups	Salad greens
	½ cup	Chopped vegetables		½ cup	Chopped vegetables
	4 ounces	Chicken breast (cooked)		4 ounces	Chicken breast (cooked)
	1 TBS	BBQ sauce		1 TBS	BBQ sauce
	2	Potatoes, baked into "fries"		2 ¼	Potatoes, baked into "fries"
500	3 cups	Salad greens	525	3 cups	Salad greens
	½ cup	Chopped vegetables		½ cup	Chopped vegetables
	5 ounces	Chicken breast (cooked)		5 ounces	Chicken breast (cooked)
	1 TBS	BBQ sauce		1 TBS	BBQ sauce
	2	Potatoes, baked into "fries"		2 ¼	Potatoes, baked into "fries"
550	3 cups	Salad greens	575	3 cups	Salad greens
	½ cup	Chopped vegetables		½ cup	Chopped vegetables
	5 ounces	Chicken breast (cooked)		6 ounces	Chicken breast (cooked)
	1 TBS	BBQ sauce		1	TBS BBQ sauce
	2 ½	Potatoes, baked into "fries"		2 ¼	Potatoes, baked into "fries"
600	3 cups	Salad greens	625	3 cups	Salad greens
	½ cup	Chopped vegetables		1 cup	Chopped vegetables
	6 ounces	Chicken breast (cooked)		6 ounces	Chicken breast (cooked)
	1 TBS	BBQ sauce		1 TBS	BBQ sauce
	2 ½	Potatoes, baked into "fries"		2 ½	Potatoes, baked into "fries"

DINNER #10   THAI CHICKEN SALAD

Recipe in Appendix C.

Boneless chicken breast (skin removed) should be baked, broiled or grilled.

350	¼ recipe	Thai Chicken Salad	375	¼ recipe	Thai Chicken Salad
				½ ounce	Cooked chicken
400	¼ recipe	Thai Chicken Salad	425	¼ recipe	Thai Chicken Salad
	1 ounce	Cooked chicken		1 ½ ounce	Cooked chicken
450	¼ recipe	Thai Chicken Salad	475	⅓ recipe	Thai Chicken Salad
	1 ounce	Cooked chicken			
	1 TBS	Chopped peanuts			

DINNER #10 THAI CHICKEN SALAD (CONT.)

CALORIE TOTAL	PORTION SIZE	FOOD ITEM	CALORIE TOTAL	PORTION SIZE	FOOD ITEM
500	⅓ recipe ½ ounce	Thai Chicken Salad Cooked chicken	525	⅓ recipe 1 ounce	Thai Chicken Salad Cooked chicken
550	⅓ recipe 1 TBS	Thai Chicken Salad Chopped peanuts	575	⅓ recipe 1 TBS	Thai Chicken Salad Chopped peanuts
600	¼ recipe ½ ounce 2 TBS	Thai Chicken Salad Cooked chicken Chopped peanuts	625	⅓ recipe 1 ounce 2 TBS	Thai Chicken Salad Cooked chicken Chopped peanuts

DINNER #11 BAKED OR GRILLED FISH

Fresh fish: baked, broiled, steamed or grilled.

Season with any type of citrus juices, garlic salt, basil, thyme, tarragon, Cajun spice, etc.

Choose any of the following types of fish (all are approximately 30 calories for each 1 ounce serving): cod, sole, halibut, orange roughy, tilapia, flounder, grouper, albacore tuna or haddock.

Sauté spinach in 1 teaspoon extra-virgin olive oil and minced garlic. Add chopped walnuts to spinach or rice.

350	4 ounces ½ cup 1 ¾ cups	Fish (cooked) Cooked brown rice Sautéed spinach	375	4 ounces ½ cup 2 cups	Fish (cooked) Cooked brown rice Sautéed spinach
400	5 ounces ½ cup 2 cups	Fish (cooked) Cooked brown rice Sautéed spinach	425	5 ounces ½ cup 2 ½ cups	Fish (cooked) Cooked brown rice Sautéed spinach
450	5 ounces ½ cup 3 cups	Fish (cooked) Cooked brown rice Sautéed spinach	475	5 ounces ½ cup 2 ½ cups 1 TBS	Fish (cooked) Cooked brown rice Sautéed spinach Chopped walnuts
500	6 ounces ½ cup 3 cups 1 TBS	Fish (cooked) Cooked brown rice Sautéed spinach Chopped walnuts	525	6 ounces ¾ cup 2 ½ cups 1 TBS	Fish (cooked) Cooked brown rice Sautéed spinach Chopped walnuts
550	6 ounces ¾ cup 2 cups 2 TBS	Fish (cooked) Cooked brown rice Sautéed spinach Chopped walnuts	575	6 ounces ¾ cup 2 ½ cups 2 TBS	Fish (cooked) Cooked brown rice Sautéed spinach Chopped walnuts
600	6 ounces 1 cup 2 cups 2 TBS	Fish (cooked) Cooked brown rice Sautéed spinach Chopped walnuts	625	6 ounces 1 cup 2 ½ cups 2 TBS	Fish (cooked) Cooked brown rice Sautéed spinach Chopped walnuts

DINNER #12   TACOS

Mexican Sauté (Recipe in Appendix C).

Chicken breast (skin removed): grilled.
Heat 7" whole-wheat tortilla in microwave, place all ingredients onto the tortilla, roll and eat.
If adding calories for exercise, try some Guacamole! (Recipe in Appendix C)

CALORIE TOTAL	PORTION SIZE	FOOD ITEM	CALORIE TOTAL	PORTION SIZE	FOOD ITEM
350	1	Whole-wheat tortilla	375	1	Whole-wheat tortilla
	½ recipe	Mexican Sauté		½ recipe	Mexican Sauté
	1 cup	Black beans		⅓ cup	Black beans
	2 TBS	Non-fat sour cream		⅓ cup	Non-fat refried beans
	3 TBS	Salsa		2 TBS	Salsa
				1 TBS	Non-fat sour cream
400	1	Whole-wheat tortilla	425	1	Whole-wheat tortilla
	½ recipe	Mexican Sauté		½ recipe	Mexican Sauté
	½ cup	Black beans		½ cup	Black beans
	⅓ cup	Non-fat refried beans		⅓ cup	Non-fat refried beans
	3 TBS	Non-fat sour cream		2 TBS	Non-fat sour cream
	3 TBS	Salsa		2 TBS	Salsa
				2 TBS	Shredded low-fat cheddar
450	1	Whole-wheat tortilla	475	1	Whole-wheat tortilla
	½ recipe	Mexican Sauté		½ recipe	Mexican Sauté
	⅓ cup	Black beans		⅓ cup	Black beans
	⅓ cup	Non-fat refried beans		⅓ cup	Non-fat refried beans
	2 TBS	Non-fat sour cream		2 TBS	Non-fat sour cream
	2 TBS	Salsa		2 TBS	Salsa
	2 ounces	Chicken breast (cooked)		2 ounces	Chicken breast (cooked)
				1 TBS	Shredded low-fat cheddar
500	1	Whole-wheat tortilla	525	1	Whole-wheat tortilla
	½ recipe	Mexican Sauté		½ recipe	Mexican Sauté
	⅓ cup	Black beans		⅓ cup	Black beans
	⅓ cup	Non-fat refried beans		⅓ cup	Non-fat refried beans
	2 TBS	Non-fat sour cream		2 TBS	Non-fat sour cream
	2 TBS	Salsa		2 TBS	Salsa
	2 ounces	Chicken breast (cooked)		3 ounces	Chicken breast (cooked)
	2 TBS	Shredded low-fat cheddar		1 TBS	Shredded low-fat cheddar
550	1	Whole-wheat tortilla	575	1	Whole-wheat tortilla
	½ recipe	Mexican Sauté		½ recipe	Mexican Sauté
	½ cup	Black beans		⅓ cup	Black beans
	⅓ cup	Non-fat refried beans		⅓ cup	Non-fat refried beans
	2 TBS	Non-fat sour cream		3 TBS	Non-fat sour cream
	2 TBS	Salsa		2 TBS	Salsa
	3 ounces	Chicken breast (cooked)		4 ounces	Chicken breast (cooked)
	1 TBS	Shredded low-fat cheddar		1 TBS	Shredded low-fat cheddar

DINNER #12 TACOS (CONT.)

CALORIE TOTAL	PORTION SIZE	FOOD ITEM	CALORIE TOTAL	PORTION SIZE	FOOD ITEM
600	1	Whole-wheat tortilla	625	1	Whole-wheat tortilla
	½ recipe	Mexican Sauté		½ recipe	Mexican Sauté
	½ cup	Black beans		¾ cup	Black beans
	⅓ cup	Non-fat refried beans		⅓ cup	Non-fat refried beans
	2 TBS	Non-fat sour cream		3 TBS	Non-fat sour cream
	2 TBS	Salsa		2 TBS	Salsa
	4 ounces	Chicken breast (cooked)		4 ounces	Chicken breast (cooked)
	1 TBS	Shredded low-fat cheddar		1 TBS	Shredded low-fat cheddar

DINNER #13 SEAFOOD PASTA

Salad made with all types of leafy greens: lettuce, spinach and cabbage.
Dress the salad with a splash of balsamic vinegar or lemon juice

Prepare any of the following vegetables, lightly steamed: tomatoes, mushrooms, spinach, broccoli, carrots and onions.

Seafood selections may be any combination of shrimp, scallops, clams or mussels. Sauté seafood with garlic, green onion and a little ginger or soy sauce.

Use whole-wheat pasta. When cooked and drained, add the vegetables and seafood, toss together, and serve. You'll feel like you get "more" by using small pasta noodles, like shells or elbow macaroni, rather than spaghetti or fettuccini.

* This is a good meal to plan when calories are to be added for exercise, as the calories from pasta can add up quickly. Be sure to measure portion sizes!

350	2 cups	Green salad	375	2 cups	Green salad
	1 cup	Cooked pasta		1 cup	Cooked pasta
	3 ounces	Seafood selection (cooked)		3 ounces	Seafood selection (cooked)
	1 cup	Steamed vegetables		1 ½ cups	Steamed vegetables
400	2 cups	Green salad	425	2 cups	Green salad
	1 cup	Cooked pasta		1 cup	Cooked pasta
	4 ounces	Seafood selection (cooked)		4 ounces	Seafood selection (cooked)
	1 ½ cups	Steamed vegetables		2 cups	Steamed vegetables
450	2 cups	Green salad	475	2 cups	Green salad
	1 ½ cups	Cooked pasta		1 ½ cups	Cooked pasta
	3 ounces	Seafood selection (cooked)		3 ounces	Seafood selection (cooked)
	1 ½ cups	Steamed vegetables		2 cups	Steamed vegetables
500	2 cups	Green salad	525	2 cups	Green salad
	1 ½ cups	Cooked pasta		1 ½ cups	Cooked pasta
	3 ounces	Seafood selection (cooked)		4 ounces	Seafood selection (cooked)
	2 ½ cups	Steamed vegetables		2 ½ cups	Steamed vegetables

DINNER #13 SEAFOOD PASTA (CONT.)

CALORIE TOTAL	PORTION SIZE	FOOD ITEM	CALORIE TOTAL	PORTION SIZE	FOOD ITEM
550	2 cups	Green salad	575	2 cups	Green salad
	1 ¾ cups	Cooked pasta		1 ¾ cups	Cooked pasta
	4 ounces	Seafood selection (cooked)		4 ounces	Seafood selection (cooked)
	2 cups	Steamed vegetables		2 ½ cups	Steamed vegetables
600	2 cups	Green salad	625	2 cups	Green salad
	2 cups	Cooked pasta		2 cups	Cooked pasta
	4 ounces	Seafood selection (cooked)		5 ounces	Seafood selection (cooked)
	2 cups	Steamed vegetables		2 cups	Steamed vegetables

NOTES

NOTES

NOTES

NOTES

NOTES

NOTES

HEALTHY FOODS LIST

PROTEIN CHOICES

**Protein should make up approximately
25% of the daily calorie total.**

NON-FAT OR LOW-FAT DAIRY

Recommendation: 2 to 3 servings per day.
May substitute low-fat soy products, if dairy is not tolerated.

	SERVING SIZE	CALORIES
1 slice 2% processed cheese "single"	1	50
1 slice non-fat processed cheese "single"	1	30
1 wedge low-fat "Laughing Cow" cheese	1 wedge	35
Low-fat buttermilk, liquid	1 cup	100
Low-fat buttermilk, powdered	1 TBS	25
Low-fat cheese (cheddar, jack, Jarlsburg, mozzarella, Swiss, etc.)	1 ounce	80
Low-fat cream cheese	2 TBS	60
Low-fat feta cheese	1 ounce	65
Non-fat cottage cheese	1 cup	160
Non-fat cream cheese	2 TBS	30
Non-fat evaporated milk	½ cup	100
Non-fat milk	1 cup	80
Non-fat plain yogurt	1 cup	110
Non-fat ricotta cheese	¼ cup	60
Non-fat sour cream	2 TBS	25
Non-fat, no-sugar fruit yogurt	1 cup	80-100
Parmesan cheese, grated	1 TBS	25
Part-skim mozzarella cheese	1 ounce	80
Part-skim ricotta cheese	¼ cup	85
Shredded low-fat cheddar cheese	1 TBS	27

LOW-FAT SEAFOOD AND POULTRY

SEAFOOD

Albacore tuna, fresh.	each 1 ounce	40
Albacore tuna, water or vacuum packed	each 1 ounce	30
Clams	each 1 ounce	40
Crab	each 1 ounce	30
Lobster	each 1 ounce	30
Salmon, fresh or frozen	each 1 ounce	65
Salmon, canned	each 1 ounce	55
Salmon, smoked	each 1 ounce	40
Sardines, canned in oil and drained	each 1 ounce	63
Scallops	each 1 ounce	35
Shrimp or prawns	each 1 ounce	35
Swordfish	each 1 ounce	45

(PROTEIN CHOICES CONT.)

	SERVING SIZE	CALORIES
Trout	each 1 ounce	50
White fish: cod, sole, haddock, halibut, roughy, tombo, tilapia, turbot, grouper, flounder, etc.	each 1 ounce	35

POULTRY

Chicken breast, no skin	each 1 ounce	47
Deli-style white meat chicken or turkey, thinly sliced	each 1 ounce	30
Egg white	1	15
Ground turkey breast (check package, no skin or dark meat)	each 1 ounce	45
Pasteurized egg product (like Egg Beaters)	¼ cup	30
Turkey breast, no skin.	each 1 ounce	45
Whole chicken egg	1 medium	80

LOW-FAT SOY

May substitute on a 1:1 basis for one or more
lean protein servings each day.

Edamame, cooked and shelled	½ cup	100
Meatless burger crumbles (like Morningstar Farms)	½ cup	60
Meatless burger patty (like Morningstar Farms)	1 patty	140
Miso	1 TBS	35
Soy milk	1 cup	80-100
Tofu, any variety	each 1 ounce	24

LOW-FAT BEANS & LEGUMES

Recommendation: a minimum of
one serving per day.

Black beans (canned)	½ cup	70
Adzuki beans (canned)	½ cup	80
Black eyed peas (canned)	½ cup	100
Cannellini beans (canned)	½ cup	100
Garbanzo beans (canned)	½ cup	80
Great northern beans (canned)	½ cup	110
Hummus spread (commercially packaged)	2 TBS	60
Kidney beans (canned)	½ cup	110
Lentils (canned)	½ cup	90
Lima beans (canned)	½ cup	93
Non-fat re-fried beans	½ cup	110
Pinto beans (canned)	½ cup	93
Split peas (dried)	½ cup	220

PROTEIN CHOICES (CONT.)

OTHER LOW-FAT PROTEIN CHOICES

	SERVING SIZE	CALORIES
High-protein energy bar	1 bar	check labels
Soy or whey protein powder mixed as a shake	1 serving	check labels

HIGHER-FAT PROTEIN CHOICES

All of the following choices should be lean and trimmed of any visible fat before cooking. The lowest calorie preparations are broiled, baked or grilled.

Recommendation: limit servings of these foods to one or two per week.

BEEF

Extra lean ground beef	each 1 ounce	75
Eye of round	each 1 ounce	62
Flank steak	each 1 ounce	68
Lean chuck/pot roast	each 1 ounce	100
Lean ground beef	each 1 ounce	80
Lean tenderloin	each 1 ounce	75
Porterhouse	each 1 ounce	61
T-bone steak	each 1 ounce	85
Top round	each 1 ounce	55
Top sirloin	each 1 ounce	70

PORK

Pork tenderloin	each 1 ounce	50
Canadian bacon	each 1 ounce	45
Deli-style ham, thinly sliced	each 1 ounce	30
Ham, roasted	each 1 ounce	60
Pork chops, broiled, bone in	each 1 ounce	60

LAMB

Lamb shank	each 1 ounce	70
Loin chop (lean)	each 1 ounce	90
Rib roast (lean)	each 1 ounce	67
Roast leg of lamb (lean)	each 1 ounce	55

COMPLEX CARBOHYDRATE CHOICES

Complex carbohydrates should make up approximately 55% of the daily calorie total.

Note: Each serving of Minestrone, White Bean, Lentil or Split Pea soup counts as two servings of vegetables and one serving of legumes.

VEGETABLES

Recommendation: 5 to 7 servings per day.

	SERVING SIZE	CALORIES
Alfalfa sprouts	1 cup	10
Artichoke	1 medium	60
Artichoke, cooked and drained	1 cup	80
Asparagus	1 cup	45
Asparagus	4 spears	15
Bamboo shoots	1 cup	25
Snap beans, green or yellow	1 cup	45
Bean sprouts	1 cup	30
Beets, cooked and sliced	1 cup	55
Beet, collard, turnip greens, cooked	1 cup	25
Bok choy	1 cup	20
Broccoli	1 cup	40
Brussels sprouts	1 cup	65
Cabbage, raw, shredded	1 cup	20
Carrots, raw	1 whole	30
Carrots, cooked	1 cup	45
Cauliflower	1 cup	25
Celery	1 stalk	5
Cucumber	1 whole	35
Eggplant	1 cup	30
Leeks	1 cup	30
Lettuces and other greens. All varieties, including kale, collards, endive, romaine, iceberg, Boston, bibb, loose leaf, etc.	1 cup	5
Mushrooms	1 cup	30
Shiitake mushrooms, cooked	1 cup	83
Onion, mature	1 whole	45
Peppers, sweet: red, orange, yellow, green	1 whole	35
Pumpkin, cooked and mashed	1 cup	50
Pumpkin, canned (no sugar added)	1 cup	85
Spaghetti sauce (jarred, look for low in sugar and low in fat)	½ cup	80
Spinach, raw, chopped	1 cup	15
Spinach, cooked and drained	1 cup	40
Squash, acorn, cooked and drained	1 cup	35
Squash, butternut, cooked and drained	1 cup	80
Tomato	1 raw	40
Tomatoes, chopped	1 cup	40
Tomatoes, canned with liquid and solids	1 cup	45
Tomatoes, stewed	1 cup	70

COMPLEX CARBOHYDRATE CHOICES (CONT.)

	SERVING SIZE	CALORIES
Tomato paste	1 cup	215
Tomato sauce	1 cup	80
Tomato juice	1 cup	40
Turnips, cooked	1 cup	30
Water chestnuts, canned	1 cup	70
Vegetable juice (like V-8)	12 ounces	70
Zucchini, sliced, raw	1 cup	20

FRUITS

Recommendation: 2 to 3 servings per day.

Apple (2 ¾" in diameter)	1	80
Applesauce, unsweetened	½ cup	50
Apricot (1.5 ounces)	1	20
Banana (7" long)	1	100
Blackberries	1 cup	75
Blueberries	1 cup	80
Melons: cantaloupe, honeydew	½ melon	60
Cherries, raw, sweet	10	50
Cherries, canned, water-pack	1 cup	100
Cranberries, fresh, chopped	1 cup	55
Dried cranberries (like Craisins)	⅓ cup	130
Dried cranberries (like Craisins)	1 TBS	25
Dates, whole	5	115
Dates, chopped	1 cup	490
Dates, chopped	1 TBS	31
Figs, dried	2	100
Grapefruit (3 ¾" in diameter)	1	80
Grapes	10	35
Grapes	1 cup	115
Kiwi, medium sized	1	45
Lemon (2 ⅛" in diameter)	1	15
Lime (2 ⅛" in diameter)	1	10
Mango	1	135
Mango, sliced	1 cup	105
Nectarine (2 ½" in diameter)	1	70
Orange (2 ½" in diameter)	1	65
Orange juice	1 cup	110
Papaya	1	120
Peach (2 ½" in diameter)	1	45
Pear (2 ½" in diameter)	1	100
Pineapple, raw, cut into chunks	1 cup	75
Pineapple, chunks or sliced, canned in juice	1 cup	125
Plum (2 ⅛" in diameter)	1	35
Prunes, dried and pitted	5	100
Prunes, stewed (fruit and liquid)	1 cup	200

COMPLEX CARBOHYDRATE CHOICES (CONT.)

	SERVING SIZE	CALORIES
Raisins	1 TBS	27
Raspberries	1 cup	70
Strawberries, sliced, raw	1 cup	50
Tangerines (2 ⅜ in diameter)	1	40
Watermelon, 1 wedge (about 1/16 of a 15" long melon)	1 wedge	110

STARCHY VEGETABLES

Recommendation: Limit to one serving per day.

Corn (5" x 1 ¾ cob)	1 ear	85
Corn kernels	1 cup	150
Peas, green	1 cup	115
Potato, baked (2 ⅓ x 4 ¾)	1	220
Potato, boiled (2 ½ diameter)	1	120
Red potato	1 medium	100
Sweet potato, baked or boiled (2" x 5")	1	160
Yukon Gold potato (5.3 ounces)	1	110

WHOLE-GRAINS

Recommendation: 3-6 servings per day.

Recommended whole-grain, high-fiber, high-protein cereals:

Fiber One, 100% Bran, All Bran, Kashi, Barbara's Bakery.

Ak-Mak whole-wheat crackers	1 rectangle	23
Bread crumbs (commercially prepared)	¼ cup	110
Bread crumbs (commercially prepared)	1 TBS	28
Brown rice, cooked	½ cup	120
Buckwheat flour, whole groats	1 cup	400
Buckwheat groats, cooked	¾ cup	120
Bulgar, cooked	1 cup	150
Bulgar, uncooked	1 cup	479
Chex All Bran Cereal	1 cup	200
Couscous, cooked	½ cup	90
Cracked wheat, whole-grain cereal, cooked	½ cup	120
Melba toast	2 rounds	25
Oat bran, cooked	1 cup	90
Oat bran, uncooked	1 cup	230
Oatmeal, cooked	1 cup	145
Oatmeal, dry	1 cup	300
Oatmeal, instant packet (no sugar added)	1	130
Pearled barley, cooked	½ cup	100
Popcorn, air popped	1 cup	20
Raisin and bran cereals (various brands)	1 cup	170
Reduced-fat wheat squares (like Wheat Thins)	1 cracker	8
Rice cake, brown (only if fiber content is 2 plus per cake)	1	50
RyKrisp cracker	1 rectangle	35

COMPLEX CARBOHYDRATE CHOICES (CONT.)

	SERVING SIZE	CALORIES
Shredded Wheat (large biscuits)	2 biscuits	165
Total cereal	¾ cup	105
Triscuit reduced-fat crackers	1 cracker	17
WASA whole-grain cracker (whole-wheat, rye or sesame varieties)	1 rectangle	35
Wheat germ	1 TBS	30
Wheaties	1 cup	180
White all purpose flour (try to use whole-grain flour)	1 cup	455
Whole-grain bagel (3 ½ in diameter)	1 whole	200
Whole-grain bread	1 slice	100
Whole-grain English muffin	1 whole	135
Whole-wheat elbow macaroni, cooked	1 cup	200
Whole-wheat flour	1 cup	410
Whole-wheat flour	1 TBS	27
Whole-wheat lasagne noodles, dry	2 ounces	180
Whole-wheat pita bread	1 entire circle	180
Whole-wheat spaghetti noodles, cooked	1 cup	200
Whole-wheat tortilla (6 ½ in diameter)	1	120
Wild rice, cooked	1 cup	165

HEART-HEALTHY FAT CHOICES
Heart-healthy fats should make up approximately 20% of the daily calorie total.

Avocado	½	125
"Fat-free" mayonnaise	1 TBS	15
"Light" mayonnaise	1 TBS	50
Almonds	13	100
Almonds, sliced	¼ cup	140
Artichokes in oil (drain before use)	1 jar (6 ounces)	100
Black olives	1	5
Bottled commercial salad dressings	2 TBS	140-160
Bottled commercial salad dressings, fat free (these have more sugar)	2 TBS	45 to 60
Bottled commercial salad dressings, reduced calorie	2 TBS	70
Canola oil	1 TBS	125
Cashews	11	100
Hazelnuts	16	100
Kalamata olives	1	9
Macadamia nuts	10	200
Non-fat cooking spray (like "PAM")	1 second spray	5
No-trans fat/non -hydrogenated buttery spread (like Smart-Balance)	1 TBS	80
Olive oil, peanut oil, sunflower oil, safflower oil	1 TBS	120
Peanut butter	1 TBS	110
Peanuts, dry roasted	17 nuts	100
Pecans	10 halves	100

(HEART-HEALTHY FAT CHOICES CONT.)

	SERVING SIZE	CALORIES
Pine nuts	1 TBS	50
Pistachio nuts	30	105
Sundried tomatoes, in oil (drain before use)	1 TBS	50
Sunflower seeds	2 TBS	95
Tahini	1 TBS	90
Walnuts	8 halves	105
Walnuts, chopped	½ cup	385
Walnuts, chopped	1 TBS	50

MISCELLANEOUS LITTLE "EXTRAS"

Recommendation: Use in very limited quantities to enhance the flavors of foods. Be sure to add the calories to your daily calorie totals

Anchovies, canned in oil (drained)	5	42
Animal crackers	12	130
Bread and butter pickles	5 slices	30
Catsup, BBQ sauce, teriyaki sauce, Worcestershire sauce	1 TBS	15
Chocolate chips, semi-sweet	10 chips	23
Chocolate chips, miniature	1 TBS	55
Chocolate syrup (like Hersheys)	2 TBS	100
Cocoa powder, unsweetened	1 TBS	11
Coconut milk	1 TBS	30
Coconut, dried, sweetened, shredded	¼ cup	115
Coconut, flaked and sweetened	1 TBS	70
Cornstarch	1 TBS	30
Cranberry sauce, jellied or whole berry	¼ cup	105
Dill pickle	1 large	15
Frozen popsicle (all fruit/no-sugar)	1	25
Fruit puree butter and oil replacement used for baking (like "Lighter Bake")	1 TBS	35
Hoison sauce	1 TBS	35
Honey	1 TBS	65
Low-fat graham cracker, double square	1	110
Low-fat ice cream	check labels	
Low-fat ice cream bars and ice cream sandwiches	check labels	
Molasses, blackstrap	1 TBS	47
Molasses, blackstrap	1 cup	480
Non-fat fruit Newtons	2	70-90
Non-fat hot chocolate mix	1 package	25-50
Non-fat whipped topping	1 TBS	25
Non-fat, no-sugar fruit flavored gelatin mix, prepared	1 cup	20
Non-fat, no-sugar instant pudding (made with non-fat milk), prepared	½ cup	80
No-sugar added jams and jellies	1 TBS	30

(MISCELLANEOUS LITTLE "EXTRAS" CONT.)

	SERVING SIZE	CALORIES
No-sugar maple syrup	1 TBS	10
Onion soup mix, dehydrated	1 ½ ounce package	150
Parmesan cheese, grated	1 TBS	45
Pesto	1 TBS	80
Pickle relish, sweet	1 TBS	20
Real bacon bits (Hormel, refrigerate after opening)	1 TBS	30
Salsa	2 TBS	10
Sugar (brown sugar, packed)	2 TBS (⅛ cup)	104
Sugar (white table sugar)	1 teaspoon	15
Unsweetened applesauce	½ cup	55
Vanilla wafers	4	75

COMMON HIGH FAT-HIGH CALORIE FOODS
Beware of these foods!!!!
They can really add up the fat and calories fast!!!!

Beer (domestic)	12 ounces	150
Beer (microbrew)	12 ounces	170
Beer (light)	12 ounces	90
Red wine	5 ounces	95
Spirits: gin, rum, vodka, whiskey, etc (94 proof)	1 ounce	50
Spirits: gin, rum, vodka, whiskey, etc. (100 proof)	1 ½ ounces	125
Sugary mixers: tonic water, ginger ale, etc.	6 ounces	75
White wine, dry	5 ounces	95
White wine, sweet	5 ounces	135
Wine cooler	10 ounces	165
2% milk	1 cup	100
Bacon, crisp, well done	3 slices	110
Beef brisket	each 1 ounce	50
Beef ribs	each 1 ounce	100
Blue cheese salad dressing (full fat)	1 TBS	75
Butter	2 TBS	185
Corned beef	each 1 ounce	71
Cream - light whipping	¼ cup	150
Dark meat chicken - thigh, leg, wing	each 1 ounce	55
Duck, roasted (meat and skin)	each 1 ounce	62
Edam cheese	2 ounces	167
French salad dressing (full fat)	1 TBS	65
Full-fat cheddar cheese	2 ounces	206
Full-fat cream cheese	2 TBS	110
Full-fat mozzarella	2 ounces	59
Full-fat Swiss	2 ounces	188
Ground beef - regular	each 1 ounce	80
Half and half (cream)	¼ cup	68

COMMON HIGH FAT & HIGH CALORIE FOODS (CONT.)

	SERVING SIZE	CALORIES
Italian salad dressing (full fat)	1 TBS	70
Margarine	2 TBS	180
Mayonnaise (full-fat)	1 TBS	104
Pie: apple, cherry, lemon, pumpkin,	⅛ of the pie	300
Pie: pecan (1 crust)	⅛ of the pie	440
Piecrust	1 shell	900
Porterhouse steak	each 1 ounce	62
Roquefort	2 ounces	185
Salami	1 ounce	109
Sausage links, pork (broiled)	2 large	255
Sausage links, turkey (broiled)	2	90
Sausage, pepperoni	1 ounce	157
Tartar sauce	1 TBS	75
Thousand Island salad dressing (full fat)	1 TBS	60
Whole milk	1 cup	125

NOTES

NOTES

NOTES

NOTES

NOTES

NOTES

NOTES

APPETIZERS, DIPS AND SAUCES

BAKED ONION DIP

Preheat oven to 350 degrees.

2 cups sweet white onion, peeled and chopped
1 cup non-fat mayonnaise
8 ounces non-fat sour cream
8 ounces non-fat cream cheese
2 cups grated Parmesan cheese

In a large mixing bowl, combine all ingredients and mix until smooth.
Pour the mixture into a baking dish that has been sprayed with non-fat cooking spray.

Bake 45 minutes, until top is slightly browned.

Serve with baked tortilla chips, crackers, vegetable crudités, etc.

Recipe, Dip only = approximately 1,240 calories.

BAKED WHITE BEAN DIP

Preheat oven to 350 degrees.

1 tablespoon extra-virgin olive oil
1 cup onion, chopped
3 to 4 cloves garlic, minced
2 to 3 teaspoons dried rosemary
2 (15 ounces each) cans great northern beans, rinsed and drained
2 tablespoons grated Parmesan or Romano cheese
1 ⅓ tablespoons white-wine vinegar
½ teaspoon red pepper flakes
½ teaspoon garlic salt

Heat olive oil in a small frying pan over medium heat.
Cook and stir the onions, garlic and rosemary over medium heat until softened.
Next, blend the onion mixture in a food processor with the beans, vinegar, red pepper and salt until smooth.

Place the mixture into a baking dish that has been sprayed with two seconds of non-fat cooking spray. Bake at 350 degrees for 25-30 minutes until hot and bubbly.

Recipe, Basic dip only = approximately 1,170 calories.

Remove from the oven and stir in any or all of the following additions, if desired:

2 tablespoons sun-dried tomatoes, chopped (oil-packed, drained with a slotted spoon before chopping)
2 tablespoons black olives, chopped
2 tablespoons Kalamata olives, chopped

Use as a dip for all types of cut vegetables, warmed pita chips or whole-grain crackers.

HUMMUS

1 can (15 ½ ounces) garbanzo beans
2 to 3 cloves garlic, peeled
2 tablespoons lemon juice, freshly squeezed
4 tablespoons Tahini (sesame seed paste)
2 tablespoons extra-virgin olive oil
1 ½ teaspoons ground cumin

Drain garbanzo beans, reserving liquid.
Place beans into the food processor, fitted with the metal blade and blend until chunky.
Add all other ingredients and blend until smooth, adding a little of the liquid from the garbanzo beans if needed to make a nice smooth consistency.

Hummus makes a great dip for cut up vegetables. It's also good with warmed whole-wheat pita triangles.
This dip is filled with heart-healthy goodness, but it is somewhat calorie-dense, so be careful of your serving size!

Entire recipe = approximately 1,075 calories.

OLIVE TAMPONADE

20 pitted Kalamata olives
15 pitted black olives
1 teaspoon lemon juice
1 small clove garlic
1 teaspoon capers
2 teaspoons extra-virgin olive oil
Ground black pepper, to taste

Pulse all ingredients in the food processor until blended. The mixture should still be a little chunky.

Use as a dip for vegetable crudités, a spread for low-fat crackers or for pita chips.
Also good when tossed with pasta or cooked vegetables.

Entire recipe = approximately 335 calories.

SALMON APPETIZER DIP

4 ounces canned salmon, drained
½ cup non-fat sour cream
2 tablespoons black olives, finely chopped
1 ½ tablespoons green onions, finely chopped
1 tablespoon fresh parsley, chopped (or may used dried)
1 ½ teaspoons freshly-squeezed lemon juice
½ teaspoon fresh lemon zest

Mix all ingredients together and chill for 1 to 2 hours.

Serve with crackers or raw vegetables.

Recipe, Dip only = approximately 420 calories.

SPINACH-ARTICHOKE DIP

Preheat oven to 350 degrees.

⅔ cup grated Parmesan
½ cup non-fat mayonnaise
½ cup non-fat cream cheese
2 cloves garlic
3 ounces part-skim mozzarella cheese
1 cup artichoke hearts
1 package (10 ounces) frozen spinach, thawed and squeezed dry

Place the first four ingredients into a food processor and blend.
Add artichoke hearts and briefly pulse together, leaving a few "chunks."

Spray a baking dish with two seconds of non-fat cooking spray.
Place the entire mixture into the baking dish and fold the spinach into the mixture until blended.

Bake at 350 degrees for approximately 20 to 25 minutes, until bubbly.

Entire recipe = approximately 875 calories.

WARM PARTY DIP

Preheat oven to 350 degrees.

8 ounces non-fat sour cream
8 ounces non-fat cream cheese
8 ounce package "Buddig" sliced beef, chopped into small pieces

Mix all ingredients together and place in an oven-safe baking dish that has been sprayed with two seconds of non-fat cooking spray.

Cover the top of the mixture with 3 tablespoons chopped pecans (approximately 20 halves, chopped).

Bake for 30-35 minutes.

Serve warm with an assortment of crackers, toasted bread, baked tortilla chips and cut up vegetables.

Recipe, Dip only = approximately 735 calories.

BAKED TORTILLA CHIPS

Preheat oven to 400 degrees.

Use 98% fat-free 7" whole-wheat tortillas. Read the label to make sure they do not contain lard.
Cut each tortilla into 12 wedges, like a pie.

Place a cooling rack used for baking on top of a cookie sheet.
Lay out all of the tortilla wedges in a single layer on top of the cooling rack.
Spray the tortilla wedges with 3 seconds of non-fat cooking spray.
Sprinkle with salt, if desired.

Bake in the hot oven for 3-5 minutes.
Set the oven timer and/or watch carefully so you'll know the correct baking time for your particular oven.
Make sure they don't burn, but get lightly browned and crispy.

Remove chips from the oven and enjoy with salsa, or make nachos by adding cheese, beans, and other items.
* Check your calorie level plan to determine proportions of other ingredients to use to make nachos.*

Each 7" tortilla = approximately 120 calories.

CRISPY CHICKEN WONTON APPETIZERS

Preheat oven to 375 degrees.

3 cups cooked chicken, finely chopped
½ cup carrot, shredded
¼ cup water chestnuts, finely chopped
2 teaspoons cornstarch
1 tablespoon water
1 tablespoon soy sauce
½ teaspoon ground ginger
1 package small-sized wonton wrappers (or spring roll wrappers)

Choose from the following prepared sauces for dipping:
teriyaki sauce, sweet and sour sauce, no-sugar jam or hoison sauce.

Combine chicken, carrot and water chestnuts in one bowl.
Combine cornstarch, water, soy sauce and ginger in a second bowl.
Add the cornstarch mixture to the chicken mixture and toss to coat.

Spoon one teaspoon of the mixture into the center of each wrapper.
Dip your finger in a bowl of water and moisten the edges of the wrapper.
Fold the wrapper over the chicken mixture to form a triangle.
Pinch the edges to seal.
Place triangles in a single layer, without touching each other, onto a baking sheet that has been sprayed with two seconds of non-fat cooking spray.
Once all are arranged on the tray, spray the tops of the triangles with another two-second spray of non-fat cooking spray.

Bake for 10 to 12 minutes, or until golden brown.

Serve the finished wontons with sauces for dipping, as desired.

Entire recipe (makes about 3 dozen triangles) = approximately 1,300 calories.

GUACAMOLE

Cut a ripe avocado in half and scoop out the insides into a bowl.
Smash the avocado with a fork.
Add a clove of garlic, mashed through a garlic press.
Add 1 teaspoon fresh squeezed lime juice.

Stir all ingredients together.

You may add salsa and minced onion to the guacamole mixture, if desired.

Recipe, Basic Guacamole only = approximately 250 calories.

NACHOS

Preheat oven to 400 degrees.

Use 98% fat-free 7" whole-wheat tortillas. Read the label to make sure they do not contain lard.

4 whole-wheat tortillas, cut into wedges and baked into tortilla chips.
Cut each tortilla into 12 wedges, like a pie.

Lay chips out in a shallow layer on a cookie sheet and top the chips with:

1 cup black beans
½ cup non-fat refried beans
⅔ cup onion, chopped
2 oz part-skim mozzarella cheese, shredded
3 tablespoons black olive, chopped
Sprinkle with ½ tsp cumin

Place the cookie sheet into the hot oven and bake for 3-5 minutes, until cheese is melted.

Remove from oven and top the nachos with:

2 tablespoons non-fat sour cream
6 tablespoons salsa

Entire recipe = approximately 1175 calories.

Top with Guacamole, if desired.

DILL SAUCE

½ cup non-fat mayonnaise
½ cup non-fat sour cream
3 tablespoons parsley, minced (fresh tastes best)
2 tablespoons Dijon mustard
2 tablespoons dill, minced (fresh tastes best)
2 teaspoons lemon juice
Salt and pepper to taste

Blend all ingredients together and place in the refrigerator.
Allow the flavors to meld for at least ½ hour before serving.

Use this sauce to make potato salad or to put on a baked potato.
It's also great as a dip for cut vegetables or as a sauce for grilled salmon.

Recipe, Sauce only = approximately 240 calories.

EASY MARINARA SAUCE

Heat 2 teaspoons extra-virgin olive oil in a non-stick pan on medium heat.
Add 2 cloves minced garlic and sauté for a minute or two.

Add 2 cans (14 ½ ounces each) Italian stewed tomatoes, including the juice.
Crush the tomatoes with a fork.

Add ½ packet of Splenda sweetener.

Add oregano or Italian Seasoning mix, either 2 teaspoons fresh or 1 teaspoon dried.
Reduce heat and simmer for ½ hour or so, until thickened.

Basic recipe = approximately 325 calories.

VARIATION TO EASY MARINARA SAUCE

Add to basic recipe:

2 tablespoons capers
2 tablespoons fresh basil
1 cup mushrooms, chopped
Sauté ½ of an onion, chopped, along with the garlic
2 cups chopped fresh spinach, add and simmer during the last 5 minutes or so before serving.
1 jar (drained) artichoke hearts, chopped

Variation recipe = approximately 530 calories.

PESTO SAUCE

Not particularly low in calories, but very rich and pungent in flavor so the quantity used can be small.

1 large bunch of fresh basil, rinsed and dried
1 large or 2 small cloves garlic
2 tablespoons grated Parmesan
½ cup chopped walnuts

Put all of these ingredients into the food processor and pulse together.

With the food processor running, slowly drizzle 3 tablespoons extra-virgin olive oil through the top feed of the processor. Continue to process until smooth.

Empty into an air-tight plastic storage container and refrigerate.
Pesto Sauce will keep nicely for one week in the refrigerator.

Use on pasta, in soups, on pizza, or as a flavor addition to salads or sandwiches.

Entire recipe = approximately 800 calories.

TOMATO RELISH

One large tomato, diced
2 tablespoons olives, chopped
2 cloves garlic, minced
1 teaspoon extra-virgin olive oil
½ cup sweet white onion, minced
⅛ cup crumbled low-fat feta OR part-skim mozzarella cheese
Freshly ground pepper, to taste

Blend all ingredients together.
Place in the refrigerator and allow flavors to meld for at least ½ hour.

This relish has many uses: It makes a great topping for green salads.
It can be used as a spread for crackers or for bruschetta.
It makes a nice topping for pita pizzas.
It can be used as a topping for grilled chicken or fish.

Double, triple, or quadruple the recipe and make a supply to keep on hand in the refrigerator.
This relish keeps well in the refrigerator for up to five days.

Entire recipe = approximately 200 calories.

MANGO SALSA

½ cup tomato
½ cup mango, chopped
⅛ cup sweet onion, chopped
⅛ cup red pepper, chopped
⅛ cup fresh cilantro, chopped
1 ½ tablespoons freshly squeezed lime juice
1 to 2 teaspoons jalapeno, chopped
Salt and pepper, to taste

Mix all ingredients together in a bowl and place in the refrigerator for a minimum of ½ hour, to allow flavors to meld.

Use as a relish on grilled white fish or chicken. Also makes a good dressing for green salad.

Entire recipe = approximately 120 calories.

CREAMY WHITE SAUCE

1 tablespoon trans-fat free butter spread (like Smart Balance)
1 tablespoon extra-virgin olive oil
1 teaspoon ginger, minced
2 cloves garlic, minced
1 teaspoon lime juice

1 teaspoon soy sauce
¾ cup evaporated non-fat milk
1 tablespoon cornstarch
⅛ teaspoon nutmeg
2 tablespoons grated Parmesan
Salt and pepper to taste

Melt butter spread and olive oil, along with garlic and ginger, over low heat.
Reserve ¼ cup of the milk, and blend it with the cornstarch until smooth.
Add all other ingredients to the sauté pan.
Add the thickened ¼ cup of milk and cornstarch and stir all together.

Heat the entire mixture to a simmer, stirring frequently to prevent sticking, until mixture is thickened.
Add Parmesan to the sauce just before serving.

This sauce is great with pasta, which can be topped with shrimp, crab, chicken or vegetables.
It is also very good as a topping for salmon, or any other fish.
Add chopped fresh parsley, cilantro, or basil for variety and flavor.

Entire recipe = approximately 450 calories.

MARINADES FOR BEEF

MARINADE #1

Combine all of the following into a plastic zip-top bag:

¼ cup onion, minced
2 tablespoons each: chopped parsley and white vinegar
1 tablespoon each: extra-virgin olive oil and Dijon mustard
1 clove garlic, minced
½ teaspoon dried thyme

Place the meat into the plastic bag along with all of the other ingredients.
Close the bag and place into a bowl.
Place bowl into the refrigerator and marinate for 6 to 8 hours.
Turn the meat at least twice while marinating.
Remove meat from the bag and discard the marinating liquid.

Broil or grill the meat, as desired.
Carve the meat into thin slices to serve.

Recipe, Marinade only = approximately 120 calories.

MARINADE #2
Combine all of the following into a plastic zip-top bag:

½ cup soy sauce
¼ cup red wine (or use non-fat beef broth instead of red wine)
2 green onions, sliced
3 tablespoons lemon juice
1 tablespoon extra-virgin olive oil
2 tablespoons Worcestershire sauce
3 cloves garlic, minced

Place the meat into the plastic bag along with all of the other ingredients.
Close the bag and place into a bowl.
Marinate in the refrigerator for 6 to 8 hours.
Turn the meat at least twice while marinating.
Remove meat form the bag and discard the marinating liquid.

Broil or grill the meat, as desired.
While the meat is grilling, brush both sides of the meat with 2 tablespoons Dijon mustard.

Carve the meat into thin slices to serve.

Recipe, Marinade only = approximately 120 calories.

SOUPS AND BEANS

TURKEY CHILI

¾ lb (12 ounces) lean ground turkey (white meat, no skin)
1 cup onion, chopped
½ cup green pepper, finely chopped
3 large cloves garlic, chopped
1 can (16 ounces) stewed tomatoes
1 can (16 ounces) red kidney beans, drained
1 can (16 ounces) white (cannellini) beans
1 can (8 ounces) tomato sauce
2 to 3 teaspoons chili powder
1 teaspoon dried basil
1 teaspoon cumin
A dash hot pepper flakes (if desired)
½ teaspoons salt, or to taste
½ teaspoons pepper, or to taste
½ cup frozen corn kernels

Sauté the turkey, onion, pepper and garlic together until meat is browned.
Stir in un-drained stewed tomatoes, beans, tomato sauce, and seasonings.
Bring to a boil and reduce to low heat.
Cover and simmer for 20 to 30 minutes.

Add the frozen corn and simmer another five minutes.

Entire recipe = approximately 1,400 calories.

SPLIT PEA SOUP

Place into a pot and simmer together for 1 hour, stirring occasionally:

1 cup dried split peas
4 cups water
1 small onion, chopped
10 small circles sliced Canadian bacon, cut into small pieces (optional)

After one hour, add to the pot:
1 stalk celery, chopped
1 carrot, chopped
1 small potato, diced
¼ teaspoon oregano
½ teaspoon thyme
½ teaspoon garlic salt
¼ teaspoon ground pepper
    (Adjust all seasonings to taste)

Simmer the entire mixture for an additional 30 minutes, until thickened.
You may add more water, if needed, to reach desired consistency.

Entire recipe = approximately 690 calories.

MINESTRONE SOUP

Place all of the following ingredients into a large stockpot:

1 can fat-free chicken broth, OR substitute the broth with three chicken, vegetable or beef bullion cubes plus 32 ounces of water
2 cans stewed tomatoes, including liquid
1 can great northern beans, garbanzo beans, or cannellini beans, including liquid
1 can kidney beans, including liquid
2 cans cut green beans, including liquid
1 can (12 ounces) vegetable juice (like V-8)
2 stalks celery, diced
3 carrots, cut into bite sized pieces

1 small onion, diced
1 whole bay leaf
2 cloves garlic, cut into fourths and placed into the broth
1 teaspoon oregano
1½ teaspoons dried thyme
2 dashes Worcestershire sauce
½ teaspoon red pepper flakes
Salt and pepper, to taste

Add salt only after the soup has been simmering for ½ hour or so, after you've tasted it, as the liquids already added contain salt.

Simmer for 1 to 2 hours until vegetables are tender.

During the last ½ hour or so of simmering, add ¼ cup (dry) tiny elbow pasta.

During the last 5 minutes of simmering, add ⅔ cup green peas.

Entire recipe = approximately 1,500 calories.

Sprinkle each serving with 2 teaspoons grated Parmesan cheese, if desired (adds 50 calories).

LENTIL SOUP

In a large saucepan, heat the following to boiling and then simmer for 30 minutes:

1 cup dried lentils
1 carrot, chopped
3 cups water
1 teaspoon dried thyme
1 bay leaf

After 30 minutes, add the following to the saucepan:

½ of a 10 ounce package frozen, chopped spinach
1 can diced tomatoes, including liquid
1 can great northern beans, including liquid
Add salt and pepper, to taste

Simmer for an additional 20 to 30 minutes.

Entire recipe = approximately 900 calories.

WHITE BEAN SOUP

2 teaspoons extra-virgin olive oil
1 onion, finely chopped
1 stalk celery, finely chopped
2 large cloves garlic, minced
2 (16 ounces each) cans great northern beans
1 (14 ounce) can non-fat chicken broth
¼ teaspoon ground black pepper
¼ teaspoon dried thyme
2 cups frozen spinach
1 tablespoon lemon juice

Heat the oil in a saucepan and cook the onion and celery until tender.
Add garlic and cook for an additional minute, while stirring.
Add beans, chicken broth, pepper, thyme and water.
Bring to a boil, reduce heat, and simmer for 15 to 20 minutes.

Remove 2 cups of the bean mixture from the pot with a slotted spoon and place into a bowl.
Mash the beans in the bowl with a fork or potato masher, until fairly smooth.

Return the mashed beans to the pot. Add the spinach to the pot and simmer for 3 to 5 more minutes.

Stir in lemon juice and remove from heat.

Entire recipe = approximately 1,000 calories.

Sprinkle each serving with 2 teaspoons grated Parmesan cheese, if desired (adds 50 calories).

BAKED BEANS

Preheat oven to 325 degrees.

2 cans (16 ounces each) of any combination: navy beans, great northern beans or kidney beans, including liquids.
4 large circles Canadian bacon cut into small pieces OR 3 tablespoons real bacon crumbles
½ cup no-sugar maple syrup
2 tablespoons molasses
2 packets Splenda sweetener
1 cup onion, chopped
1 teaspoon dry mustard
½ teaspoon salt
¼ teaspoon pepper

Mix all ingredients together and then place into a baking dish that has been sprayed with two seconds of non-fat cooking spray.
Place a cover on the baking dish.

Bake at 325 degrees for 1 hour.
After one hour, stir the mixture and place the cover back on.
Bake for 30-60 more minutes, until excess liquid has been absorbed.

Entire recipe = approximately 1,100 calories.

VEGETABLES AND SALADS

BAKED SWEET POTATO

Preheat oven to 400 degrees.

Clean and scrub the outside of one large sweet potato.
Puncture the skin with a small knife in two places, to allow steam to be released.
Pre-cook the sweet potato in the microwave for eight to ten minutes, until softened.
Cut the sweet potato in half, lengthwise, and place each half with cut-side up on a piece of foil.

Mash up the inside of the potato with a fork, leaving the skin intact (careful, it may be hot).

Top each potato half with:

1 tablespoon chopped pecans
1 tablespoon no trans-fat buttery spread (like Smart Balance)
2 tablespoons no-sugar maple syrup

Gently close foil around the potato to make a "packet," taking care to not have the top foil touch the toppings inside.

Place in a 400 degree oven for 5 to 7 minutes, allowing the toppings to melt and the flavors to blend.

Entire recipe = approximately 310 calories.

SPINACH WITH WALNUTS AND FETA

Heat 2 teaspoons extra-virgin olive oil in a large saucepan.
Add 2 minced garlic cloves to the pan and sauté for a couple of minutes.
Add 1 cup chopped sweet white onion to the garlic and continue to sauté until onions are slightly softened.

Add 5 cups (raw) spinach leaves which have been rinsed and dried.
Reduce heat, and let the spinach wilt, periodically folding the onion/garlic mixture and spinach together.

Add ¼ cup crumbled low-fat feta cheese.
Add 2 tablespoons chopped walnuts (any type of chopped nuts could be substituted).

Stir all ingredients together and serve immediately.

Entire recipe = approximately 350 calories.

ROASTED VEGETABLES

Preheat oven to 400 degrees.

Wash and cut into bite-sized pieces any combination of the following vegetables:

1 medium red potato
2 carrots
1 sweet white onion
1 medium sweet potato (peeled)

Pre-cook the cut carrots and potatoes (not the onions) in the microwave for approximately 8 minutes, until somewhat softened.

Place all of the vegetables (including the onions) in a single layer on a cookie sheet that has been sprayed with two seconds of non-fat cooking spray.

Spray the tops of the vegetables with an additional two second spray of the non-fat cooking spray. Sprinkle with a little garlic salt.

Bake in the hot oven until tender and browned, approximately 20 minutes.

Remove from the oven and place in a serving bowl.
Spray with one-second spray of non-fat cooking spray and serve.

You may toss the vegetables together with fresh herbs, as desired.

Entire recipe = approximately 350 calories.

BAKED SQUASH

Preheat oven to 350 degrees.

You may use either acorn or butternut squash for this recipe.
Cut the selected squash in half, lengthwise, and remove the seeds and pulp.

Place the squash, cut side down, into a shallow microwavable dish filled with 1" of water.
Microwave 6 to 8 minutes or until the squash is moderately softened.
Remove squash from the microwave and place cut-side up on a baking sheet.

Mix together in a small bowl:

1 apple, chopped
⅛ cup no-sugar maple syrup
2 tablespoons raisins
½ teaspoon cinnamon

Place this mixture into the center of each upturned half of the squash.
Bake for 8 to 12 minutes, until squash is thoroughly softened.

Entire recipe = approximately 375 calories.

BAKED HERBED TOMATOES

Preheat oven to 375 degrees.

6 large ripe tomatoes, halved
Remove the stem and core, then remove seeds and liquid with your fingers.
Place tomatoes onto a baking dish, cut side up.

Mix together:

1 cup bread crumbs (4 slices whole-grain bread made into fine crumbs in the food processor)
¼ cup green onions, minced (both the white and the green parts)
¼ cup fresh basil leaves, minced
2 tablespoons fresh parsley, minced
2 cloves garlic, minced
½ teaspoon fresh thyme, minced (or may use ¼ teaspoons dried)
Salt and pepper, to taste

Fill the tomatoes with the above mixture.

Spray the top of each tomato with one second of non-fat cooking spray.
Sprinkle the tops of each tomato with a total of 2 tablespoons grated Parmesan cheese.

Bake for about 15 minutes until tomatoes are tender.

Entire recipe = approximately 625 calories.

BAKED "FRIES"

Preheat oven to 400 degrees.

Use medium sized red potatoes or Yukon gold potatoes, for best results.
Scrub the potatoes well. Leave the skin on and cut into thin strips.

Place potato strips into a microwavable bowl.
Spray the potato strips in the bowl with two seconds of non-fat cooking spray.
Stir to coat.

Spray a cookie sheet with two seconds of non-fat cooking spray.

Spread the potato strips in a single layer on the cookie sheet.

Spray the potato strips with two seconds of non-fat cooking spray and sprinkle with a little salt, if desired.

Baking time will vary, depending on the type of potato used and the size of the strips.
Initially set the timer on the oven for 15 minutes.

About halfway through cooking, turn the potato strips with a spatula to allow both sides to brown.
Return them to the oven, and check them at 4 to 5 minute intervals, to avoid burning.

Bake until browned and crisp.

Calorie total will depend on how many and which variety of potato are used.
Refer to the calorie counts on the Healthy Foods List for details.

CAESAR SALAD DRESSING

CAESAR DRESSING #1

In a large serving bowl, blend the following:

2 cloves garlic, minced
¼ cup pasteurized real-egg product (like Egg Beaters)
1 tablespoon Dijon mustard
¼ teaspoon Worcestershire sauce
Juice of half a lemon, freshly squeezed
1 to 2 anchovy fillets, smashed
⅛ cup grated Parmesan

Rinse off one large head of romaine lettuce. Tear leaves and spin or pat dry. Place in a large salad bowl.
Pour dressing over lettuce. Add 2 tablespoons Parmesan to the bowl and toss.

Caesar Dressing #1 = approximately 100 calories.

If you add oil to this recipe: each 1 tablespoon extra-virgin olive oil added = approximately 120 calories.

CAESAR DRESSING #2

In a large serving bowl, blend the following:

1 ½ tablespoons lemon juice, freshly squeezed
2 tablespoons pasteurized real-egg product (like Egg Beaters)
2 cloves garlic, minced
2 teaspoons Dijon mustard
1 to 2 anchovy fillets, smashed
1 tablespoon red wine vinegar
1 tablespoon balsamic vinegar
¾ teaspoon Italian seasoning flakes
3 dashes Worcestershire sauce
⅛ cup grated Parmesan

Rinse off one large head of romaine lettuce. Tear leaves and spin or pat dry. Place in a large salad bowl.
Pour dressing over lettuce. Add 2 tablespoons Parmesan to the bowl and toss.
Caesar Dressing #2 = approximately 100 calories.

If you add oil to this recipe: each 1 tablespoon extra-virgin olive oil added = approximately 120 calories.

Both Caesar salad recipes yield FOUR salad portions or TWO main-course portions.

Top the salad with grilled chicken, salmon or shrimp to make into a meal.
Top with Skinny Homemade Croutons, if desired.

SKINNY HOMEMADE CROUTONS

Preheat oven to 425 degrees.

Cut three slices of whole-grain bread into 1 inch chunks.
Spray a baking sheet with two seconds of non-fat cooking spray.
Place bread chunks onto baking sheet.
Spray the bread with two seconds of non-fat cooking spray.
Sprinkle with a little garlic salt and fines herbs.

Place the baking pan into the hot oven and bake for 3-6 minutes, until croutons are lightly browned.
Watch carefully to make sure they don't burn.
When browned, turn off the oven and leave the pan inside to further crisp them up.

Entire recipe = approximately 300 calories.

SPINACH SALAD WITH SWEET ORANGE VINAIGRETTE

½ cup orange juice
2 tablespoons rice vinegar
2 tablespoons balsamic vinegar
1 tablespoon raspberry vinegar
1 teaspoon honey
3 packages Splenda sweetener

Stir all ingredients together and heat on low power in the microwave for a couple of minutes, just until honey is melted and the liquid is heated through.

Use the vinaigrette to dress 4 cups baby spinach leaves, washed and thoroughly dried.

Top the spinach leaves with:

2 tablespoons Craisins
2 tablespoons chopped almonds, pecans or walnuts
½ apple, chopped OR may substitute 1 orange, peeled and chopped
¼ purple onion, chopped fine

Entire recipe = approximately 340 calories.

POTATO SALAD

2 cups boiled red potatoes, diced
½ cup celery, diced
¼ cup onion, diced
1 hard cooked egg, chopped into small pieces
One small pinch each, dried thyme and celery salt
Salt and pepper to taste

Mix these ingredients with one recipe of Dill Sauce and gently stir to coat. Refrigerate for at least ½ hour before serving.

Total recipe (Potato Salad with Dill Sauce) = approximately 615 calories.

THAI CHICKEN SALAD

4 cooked boneless, skinless chicken breasts (4 ounces, each)

For the salad:

4 large carrots
2 sweet red peppers
2 teaspoons toasted sesame oil

221

3 green onions, chopped
2 heads red-leaf lettuce
2 cups bean sprouts
¾ cup fresh cilantro
1 can (11 ounces) mandarin orange slices

For the dressing:

4 cloves garlic
⅔ cup water
⅓ cup rice wine vinegar
3 tablespoons Spicy Thai Peanut Satay Sauce (Thai Kitchen brand)
1 tablespoon soy sauce
3 packets Splenda
½ teaspoon crushed red pepper flakes

Bake, broil or grill the chicken breasts, and chop into bite-sized pieces.

Using a vegetable peeler, peel carrots into long, thin strips.
Core and thinly slice the red peppers.
In a non-stick skillet, heat sesame oil over medium heat and then cook the carrots and peppers for 3 to 5 minutes, until tender.
Remove from heat.

On each plate, place a layer of lettuce, topped with bean sprouts.
Then top with the chicken, carrots, peppers, water chestnuts, onion, and orange sections.

In a blender or food processor, mix all of the ingredients for the dressing, until smooth.

Drizzle the salad with dressing, and garnish with fresh cilantro.

Entire recipe = approximately 1,420 calories.
Dressing = approximately 140 calories.
Total amount of chicken (16 ounces, cooked) = approximately 750 calories.
Salad = approximately 530 calories.

If desired, may top the salad with chopped peanuts (50 calories per tablespoon).

DINNERS AND CASSEROLES

BEEF STROGANOFF

12 ounces no-yolk egg noodles prepared as package directs. Drain and place into a warmed serving bowl.

¾ lb lean beef tenderloin or top round steak, all fat trimmed, cut cross-wise into very thin strips
1 onion, thinly sliced and quartered
½ lb mushrooms, stems removed and thinly sliced
2 tablespoons whole-wheat flour
1 can non-fat beef broth
2 teaspoons Worcestershire sauce
½ cup non-fat sour cream
Salt and pepper, to taste
Chopped parsley to garnish

Spray a non-stick pan with two seconds of non-fat cooking spray.
Sauté beef slices over medium heat and cook until browned.
Remove beef from heat and set aside.

Spray the pan again with two seconds of non-fat cooking spray.
Sauté the onion for 2 to 3 minutes, over medium heat.
Add mushrooms, cook and stir for an additional 3 minutes.
When some liquid is released, sprinkle with flour and continue to cook, stirring constantly for 1 additional minute.

Add the beef broth and Worcestershire sauce.
Continue to cook for 3 minutes, while stirring.
When the mixture is slightly thickened, remove from the heat.
Add non-fat sour cream and parsley.

Place beef back into the pan and then place the entire mixture on low heat.
Cook for 3 to 4 minutes until heated through.

Entire Recipe, not including noodles = approximately 1,155 calories.

CHICKEN ARTICHOKE CASSEROLE

Preheat oven to 350 degrees.

3 boneless, skinless chicken breasts, 4 ounces each, cut into bite sized pieces
1 small jar artichoke hearts, drained and chopped
⅔ cup non-fat sour cream
2 tablespoons grated Parmesan
2 tablespoons bread crumbs (½ slice of whole-grain bread made into fine crumbs in the food processor)

Spray a casserole dish with two seconds of non-fat cooking spray.
Place chicken pieces in baking dish and stir together with sour cream.
Gently stir in artichoke pieces.

Spread Parmesan and bread crumbs evenly on top.
Bake at 350 degrees for 45 minutes until bubbly and nicely browned on top.

Entire recipe = approximately 900 calories.

CHICKEN CORDON BLEU

Preheat oven to 400 degrees.

4 boneless, skinless chicken breasts, 4 ounces each
8 slices, thinly-sliced deli-style ham
4 tablespoons non-fat cream cheese
4 tablespoons non-fat mayonnaise
2 teaspoons mustard
1 cup crushed corn flakes

Pound each chicken breast to ¼ thick.
Spread each with 1 tablespoon of cream cheese.
Top each chicken breast with 2 slices ham.
Roll up and secure with toothpicks.

Place cornflakes in a plastic bag.

Mix mustard and mayonnaise together in a bowl and roll each chicken breast to coat.
Place one chicken breast at a time into the bag with cornflakes.
Toss to coat.

Spray a cookie sheet with two seconds of non-fat cooking spray.
Place chicken onto the sheet.
Bake at 400 degrees for 35-40 minutes.

Entire recipe = approximately 1,150 calories.

CHICKEN PARMESAN

Preheat oven to 350 degrees.

2 boneless, skinless chicken breasts, approximately 4 ounces each
Place each chicken breast into a large zip-lock baggie and place onto a solid surface.
Pound with a mallet until chicken breasts are approximately ½ inch thick.
Place ½ cup pasteurized real-egg product (like Egg Beaters) into a bowl.

Into another large zip-lock baggie, place:

½ cup fine bread crumbs
2 tablespoons parsley flakes
2 tablespoons grated Parmesan cheese
Salt and pepper, to taste

Holding the chicken breast with tongs, dredge it into the egg mixture and shake off the excess. Place the chicken breasts into the baggie with crumbs and spices and shake to coat well.

Set aside on a wire rack to dry for a few minutes.

Place coated chicken breasts onto a piece of foil.
Bake in a 350 degree oven until completely cooked through.

Entire recipe = approximately 560 calories.

Top the cooked chicken with Easy Marinara Sauce, or may use canned or jarred pasta sauce.

PASTA WITH CLAM SAUCE

Cooked whole-wheat pasta noodles, enough for 2 servings.
Cook pasta noodles according to package directions in salted water that has been brought to a rolling boil.

1 tablespoon extra-virgin olive oil
1 large clove garlic, chopped
2 tablespoons whole-wheat flour
2 (6 ½ ounces each) cans minced clams
4 tablespoons fresh (or 3 tablespoons dried) chopped parsley
¾ teaspoon dried thyme (or 1 teaspoon fresh)
¾ teaspoon dried basil (or 1 teaspoon fresh)
Cracked black pepper, to taste

Sauté chopped garlic in olive oil.
Add flour and clams, including liquid.
Add herbs and spices and simmer for a few minutes.
Because the clams are so salty, hold off on adding salt until you've tasted the sauce.

Drain the noodles with a colander and divide onto plates.
Top noodles with the clam sauce.
Top each serving with 1 tablespoon grated Parmesan cheese.

Recipe, sauce only = approximately 700 calories.

HERB MARINATED BEEF STEAK

1 lb very lean beef steak, cut to be 1 inch thick

Combine all of the following into a plastic zip-top bag:

¼ cup onion, minced
2 tablespoons parsley, chopped
2 tablespoons white vinegar
1 tablespoon extra-virgin olive oil
1 tablespoon Dijon mustard
1 clove garlic, minced
½ teaspoon dried thyme

Place the meat into the plastic bag along with all the other ingredients.
Close the bag and place into a bowl.
Marinate in the refrigerator for 6 to 8 hours.
Turn the meat over at least once while marinating.

Remove meat from the bag and discard marinating liquid.
Broil or grill meat, as desired.

Carve the meat into thin slices to serve.

Entire recipe = approximately 1,600 calories.

MEXICAN SAUTÉ

Thinly slice and sauté together, without oil:
1 large onion
1 green pepper
1 sweet red pepper
2 cups cabbage (if desired)

Season the mixture with cumin, chili powder, garlic powder, oregano, and lime juice, as desired.
Add ¼-⅓ cup water and continue to stir and cook until vegetables are tender.

Entire recipe = approximately 120 calories.

QUICK and EASY TACO SALAD

Rinse, spin and cut up 1 head of romaine and place into a large serving bowl.
Shave 1 carrot over the lettuce.
Cut up 2 ripe tomatoes and place in the bowl.
Cut up 1 small onion, either sweet or purple, and place in the bowl.

Divide the above salad mixture into two portions.

Top each salad with the following, in the amounts that fit your own calorie needs:

Mexican Sauté mixture
Salsa with chopped cilantro
1 to 2 tablespoons non-fat sour cream
½ cup black beans (rinsed and drained)
½ cup non-fat refried beans
Grilled chicken breast, seasoned with cumin, chili powder, lime, etc. and cut into bite-sized pieces

SPINACH EGG PIE

Preheat oven to 375 degrees.

1 cup pasteurized real-egg product (like Egg Beaters)
½ cup non-fat milk
2 tablespoons whole-wheat flour
1 (10 ounce) package frozen spinach, thawed, drained and pressed dry
½ cup part-skim mozzarella cheese, shredded
½ cup sweet onion, minced
3 tablespoons grated Parmesan cheese

Mix all ingredients together and pour into a glass baking dish that has been sprayed with two seconds of non-fat cooking spray.

Bake at 375 degrees for 45 minutes.

Entire recipe = approximately 500 calories.

ORIENTAL STIR-FRY

Stir-fry one of the following protein foods in a non-stick pan, using a little non-fat chicken broth or water to moisten, some minced ginger, and a little bit of low-sodium soy sauce.

Use the appropriate amount to meet your own calorie needs:

Grilled chicken breast chunks: 47 calories per ounce
Edamame: 120 calories per 1/2 cup
Tofu, any variety: 25 calories per ounce
Shrimp: 35 calories per ounce
Prawns: 35 calories per ounce

When cooked through, remove from pan and set aside.

Then add to the pan:
3 cups mixed vegetables (can buy frozen Oriental mixed vegetables).
Stir-fry together with a little low-sodium soy sauce, ginger and non-fat chicken broth.

When vegetables are done, add the cooked protein food back into the pan and reheat.
Add 1 tablespoon chopped almonds, cashews, walnuts or peanuts.

Vegetables and nuts mixture = approximately 175 calories.

Place the entire mixture on top of a portion of cooked brown rice (120 calories per ½ cup cooked rice).

STUFFED CHICKEN BREASTS

Preheat oven to 350 degrees.

4 cooked boneless, skinless chicken breasts, approximately 4 ounces each
¾ cup bread crumbs (3 slices whole-grain bread, made into fine crumbs in the food processor)

Toast bread crumbs under the broiler (or in a toaster oven) for a few minutes, until browned. Stir once or twice while browning, to make sure all surfaces get browned. Be careful not to burn!

Once browned, mix crumbs with:

2 teaspoons chopped basil
2 tablespoons grated Parmesan cheese
2 cloves garlic, minced
Freshly ground black pepper

Place chicken breasts one at a time in a plastic sandwich bag.
Pound each breast using the smooth edge of a meat mallet until about ½ inch in thickness.

Lay each chicken breast out flat and sprinkle each one with:

1 tablespoon part-skim mozzarella cheese, shredded
1 tablespoon sun-dried tomatoes, chopped

If using sun-dried tomatoes packed in oil, drain with a slotted spoon first, and then chop.
It is okay to use sun-dried tomatoes that are not packed in oil, just soften with a little hot water before chopping.
If this is done, subtract 150 calories from the calorie total for the entire recipe.

Roll up the chicken breast and secure with a couple of toothpicks.

In a shallow pan, whisk 1 egg white.
Brush the outsides of each chicken breast roll with the whisked egg white.
Gently press the bread crumb mixture onto each rolled breast until coated.

Bake at 350 degrees for approximately 35 minutes.

Entire recipe = approximately 1,650 calories.

GREEK OMELETTE

1 cup pasteurized real-egg product (like Egg Beaters)
8 Kalamata olives, pitted and cut into small pieces
2 tomatoes, diced
1 small sweet onion, diced
2 cups fresh spinach
¼ cup low-fat feta cheese chunks

Rinse the spinach thoroughly and spin or pat dry. Then wilt it in the microwave for 1 minute.

Heat 2 teaspoons extra-virgin olive oil in a medium-sized sauté pan set over medium heat.
Sauté the diced onions until soft, and then remove them from the pan.
Add the Egg Beaters to the pan.
Top the Egg Beaters with the olives, tomatoes, spinach, onion, and feta cheese and continue to cook over medium heat.
Lift the edges of the egg mixture a little and swirl the pan to allow the liquid to get underneath and cook.

Season the entire omelet with a pinch of nutmeg, and salt and pepper, to taste.

Remove from the heat when the egg mixture is set.
Gently fold the mixture in half.
Divide the mixture into two portions.

Entire recipe = approximately 575 calories.

PROTEIN-PACKED LASAGNA

Preheat oven to 375 degrees.

Sauce:
2 cans diced tomatoes, including liquid
2 cloves garlic, chopped
2 teaspoons Italian seasoning
2 teaspoons dried, minced onion

Filling:
1 (10 ounce) package chopped spinach, thawed and drained
1 cup non-fat cottage cheese
½ cup pasteurized real-egg product (like Egg Beaters)
⅛ cup grated Parmesan cheese
1 can garbanzo beans, drained
1 clove garlic

Simmer the sauce on the stovetop for 15-30 minutes, allowing flavors to meld.

Place the ingredients for the filling into the food processor and process until smooth.

To assemble the dish, first place a layer of sauce (approximately ⅓ of the sauce) in the bottom of a 9" x 13" baking pan.
On top of the sauce, place 4 lasagna noodles (uncooked) in a single lengthwise layer in the pan.
On top of the noodles, spread approximately ½ of the filling mixture.

Repeat each of these steps – sauce, then 4 noodles, then filling mixture.

Finally, place the last ⅓ of the sauce on top.
Sprinkle with ⅛ cup grated Parmesan and ½ cup shredded part-skim mozzarella cheese.

Cover the baking dish with foil and place it on a cookie sheet.
Place the baking dish into the oven.
Bake covered for 60 minutes.

After 60 minutes, remove the foil and bake for an additional 10-15 minutes.
Remove from the oven and allow lasagna to sit for 10-15 minutes before cutting into individual servings.

Entire recipe = approximately 2,000 calories.

BAKED CHIMICHANGAS

Preheat oven to 350 degrees.

12 ounces cooked boneless, skinless chicken breast.
8 ounces of your favorite salsa
1 (16 ounce) can non-fat refried beans
1 (16 ounce) can black beans, drained and rinsed
3 tablespoons green onions, chopped
4 ounces grated non-fat cheddar cheese
8 (7") whole-wheat tortillas

After cooking the chicken, use two forks to shred it.
Place the chicken, salsa, beans and onions into a large skillet.

Cook and stir the mixture over medium heat until it is warmed.

Add the cheese and stir it in.

For each chimichanga, place ½ cup of the chicken mixture in the center of a tortilla.

Fold in the sides and roll the tortilla.

Place each rolled tortilla seam-side down into a 13" x 9" x 2" baking pan that has been sprayed with a 2 second spray of non-fat cooking spray.

Place the pan into a 350 degree oven and bake for 15 to 20 minutes until the tortillas are crisp and browned.

During the last minute or two of baking, top each chimichanga with 1 tablespoon grated non-fat cheddar, and allow to melt.

To serve, top each chimichanga with 2 tablespoons each, of non-fat sour cream and salsa.

Makes 8 chimichangas.

Entire recipe = approximately 3,200 calories.

Additional non-fat sour cream, salsa, guacamole and grated cheese may be added, according to your preferences and calorie needs.

SWEET & SPICY CHICKEN

Mix the following ingredients together in a bowl:

⅔ cup all-fruit/no-sugar apricot jam
¼ cup orange juice
1 teaspoon cinnamon
½ teaspoon nutmeg
½ teaspoon ground ginger

In a glass bowl:

Spread the mixture onto 2 boneless, skinless chicken breasts, 4 ounces each.

Turn to coat both sides.

Cover tightly with plastic wrap and marinate in the refrigerator for a minimum of two hours, or even all night.

To cook:

Preheat the broiler or grill.

Spray grill with two seconds of non-fat cooking spray.

Lightly shake the chicken breasts to remove excess marinade.

Place chicken onto the grill or under the broiler.

Spread 1 tablespoon of the marinade onto each chicken breast.

While cooking, continue to spread 1 tablespoon of marinade onto each chicken breast every few minutes.

Turn chicken often and repeat the process of spreading the marinade until it has all been used.

Recipe, Marinade only = approximately 200 calories.

Total for marinade and 8 ounces of cooked boneless, skinless chicken breast = approximately 575 calories.

TURKEY MEATLOAF

Preheat oven to 400 degrees.

2 pounds ground white-meat turkey (no skin)
½ cup pasteurized real-egg product (like Egg Beaters)
1 small onion, minced
1 teaspoon pepper
½ cup non-fat milk
⅓ cup catsup
1 teaspoon salt
1 teaspoon garlic salt
½ teaspoon sage
½ cup oats (uncooked)
2 dashes Worcestershire sauce

Mix all ingredients together in a big bowl (use your hands to get it totally mixed together). Put the mixture into a loaf pan (or may use mini-loaf pans).

Bake for 30 minutes.
Reduce heat to 350 degrees and bake for an additional 45 minutes.

Entire recipe = approximately 1,575 calories.

TERIYAKI CHICKEN KABOBS

Marinade:

2 ½ tablespoons soy sauce
½ teaspoon ginger, minced
3 tablespoons honey
1 tablespoon balsamic vinegar
1 tablespoon white wine vinegar
1 garlic clove, minced
½ teaspoon salt

Cut two boneless, skinless chicken breasts (6 ounces each) into one inch chunks.
Marinate the chicken for a minimum of 20 minutes.

Reserve the marinade, placing ¾ of it into a saucepan, while keeping ¼ of it to brush on the skewers while they cook.
Place the saucepan on low heat and simmer the marinade until reduced and thickened.

Place the pieces of chicken onto skewers and grill for about 10 minutes, brushing with the 1/4 amount of reserved marinade.

Top chicken skewers with the reduced marinade sauce before serving.

Serve chicken skewers with grilled vegetable skewers: red, yellow, green and orange peppers, onions, and tomatoes.
Serve with cooked brown rice, according to your own calorie requirements.

Recipe, Marinade only = approximately 200 calories.
Total for marinade plus 12 ounces cooked boneless, skinless chicken breast = approximately 760 calories.

BREADS, SWEETS, AND DESSERTS

EASY APPLE CRISP

Preheat oven to 350 degrees.

Four apples, any variety, cut into thin slices and placed into a large mixing bowl.

In another bowl, mix together the following:

3 teaspoons cinnamon
1 teaspoon pumpkin pie spice
6 packets Splenda sweetener
⅔ cup oats, uncooked
2 tablespoons molasses
2 tablespoons chopped walnuts

Sprinkle the mixture over the apples.
Gently stir the apples until coated.
Place the entire mixture into a baking dish that has been sprayed with two seconds of non-fat cooking spray.

Bake for 1 hour, until bubbly.

Entire recipe = approximately 715 calories.

PUDDING CUPS

Preheat oven to 350 degrees.

Shells:
Into each compartment of a muffin tin place one spring roll wrapper.
Press the edges against the side of the cup, leaving the points sticking up.

Bake at 350 degrees for 8 to 12 minutes, until browned.

Filling:
Make one package non-fat pudding (any flavor), according to package directions.

Fill cooled shells with non-fat pudding.
Top the pudding with berries or chopped fruit, if desired.

Each shell = approximately 20 calories.
Each ½ cup non-fat pudding = approximately 80 calories.
Each ¼ cup berries or fruit = approximately 50 calories.

OATMEAL CHOCOLATE CHIP COOKIES

Preheat oven to 350 degrees.

Mix all of the following in a large mixing bowl:

½ cup no-sugar applesauce
½ teaspoon vanilla
2 egg whites
½ teaspoon baking soda
½ teaspoon cinnamon
¼ teaspoon salt
1 ¼ cup oats, uncooked
⅓ cup mini chocolate chips
6 packets Splenda sweetener (or may use 2 tablespoons Splenda for baking)
¼ cup no-sugar maple syrup
2 tablespoons extra-virgin olive oil

Next, add enough whole-wheat flour (⅓ to ⅔ cup), until dough is at the right consistency to form "balls" of dough.
Spray cookie sheets with two seconds of non-fat cooking spray.
Drop dough onto cookie sheets by rounded teaspoons, placed 2 inches apart.
Flatten each cookie slightly with a fork.

Bake for 7-10 minutes until golden brown.

Entire recipe = approximately 1,300 calories.

BLUEBERRY BARS

Preheat oven to 350 degrees.

Spray an 8" baking dish with a 5 second spray of non-fat cooking spray.

Batter:

¾ cup whole-wheat flour
4 packets Splenda sweetener
½ teaspoon baking soda
⅛ teaspoon salt
⅓ cup low-fat buttermilk
¾ teaspoon vanilla extract
1 ½ cups frozen or fresh blueberries

Mix together the flour, Splenda, baking soda and salt
Next, add the buttermilk and vanilla and gently mix all ingredients together.

Spread the mixture evenly into the prepared pan.
Sprinkle the berries evenly over the batter.

In a small bowl, combine:

4 Splenda packets
1 teaspoon cornstarch
1 teaspoon lemon peel, finely grated

Sprinkle this mixture evenly over the berries.

Bake on the top shelf of the oven for 30 minutes, or until golden brown and beginning to pull away from the edges of the pan.
Cool before cutting.

To serve, top with a dollop of non-fat, no-sugar whipped topping.

Entire recipe = approximately 530 calories.

CARROT RAISIN MUFFINS OR LOAVES

Preheat oven to 350 degrees.

¼ cup no-sugar maple syrup
9 packets Splenda sweetener (or 3 tablespoons powdered Splenda for baking)
½ cup no-sugar applesauce
¾ cup buttermilk
1 teaspoon vanilla

2 egg whites
¾ cup whole-wheat flour
1 ½ cup oats, uncooked
2 teaspoons baking powder
2 teaspoons cinnamon
¼ teaspoon baking soda
1 ⅓ cups carrots, shredded
½ cup raisins
3 teaspoons freshly grated orange rind
2 tablespoons walnuts, chopped

Place maple syrup, sweetener, applesauce, vanilla and egg whites into a food processor and mix together, briefly.
Add flour, oats, baking powder, baking soda, orange rind, and cinnamon and mix together until just blended.

Place the above mixture into a large mixing bowl and gently stir in carrots and raisins until just blended.
Spray non-stick muffin pans or loaf pans with two seconds of non-fat cooking spray.

Divide mixture evenly into muffin tins to make 12 large muffins OR place entire mixture into one large bread loaf pan.

Bake muffins for 30 minutes at 350 degrees, or until toothpick comes out clean.
Bake loaf for 55 minutes at 350 degrees, or until a knife inserted deep into the center comes out clean.

Entire recipe = approximately 1,050 calories.

MOLASSES OAT BREAD

Preheat oven to 350 degrees.

1 teaspoon baking soda
¼ cup molasses
½ cup no-sugar maple syrup
1 ½ cups plain, non-fat yogurt
1 ½ cups uncooked oats
1/2 cup raisins
1 ½ cups whole-wheat flour

Dissolve baking soda into molasses and maple syrup.
Add plain, non-fat yogurt and mix well.
Mix in the oats and raisins.
Gently fold in the flour.

Pour mixture into a loaf pan that has been sprayed with two seconds of non-fat cooking spray.

Bake 45 minutes in an oven preheated to 350 degrees.

Allow loaf to cool and cut into 12 slices.

Entire recipe = approximately 1550 calories.

TROPICAL OAT BRAN BREAD

Preheat oven to 350 degrees.

1 teaspoon baking soda
⅛ cup molasses
¾ cup no-sugar maple syrup
1 ½ cups plain, non-fat yogurt
1½ cups oat bran
½ cup dried tropical fruit (papaya, mango, pineapple)
1½ cups whole-wheat flour

Dissolve baking soda into molasses and maple syrup.
Add plain, non-fat yogurt and mix well.
Mix in the bran and fruits.
Gently fold in the flour.

Pour mixture into a loaf pan that has been sprayed with two seconds of non-fat cooking spray.

Bake 45 minutes in an oven preheated to 350 degrees.

Allow loaf to cool and cut into 12 slices.

Entire recipe = approximately 1550 calories.

REALLY GOOD MUFFINS OR BREAD

THE BASIC RECIPE

Place in a bowl and refrigerate overnight:
1 cup oats, uncooked
2 cups low-fat buttermilk

The next morning (or after 6 to 8 hours of soaking, when oats are softened) preheat oven to 350 degrees.

Mix together:

1 ⅔ cups whole-wheat flour
¼ cup packed brown sugar

¼ cup Splenda sweetener for baking
1 teaspoon baking powder
1 teaspoon baking soda
1 teaspoon salt

To the oats and buttermilk mixture, add:

1 tablespoon extra-virgin olive oil
¼ cup no-sugar maple syrup
½ cup pasteurized real-egg product (like Egg Beaters)

Beat the oats and buttermilk mixture with a mixer on medium speed.
Slowly add the flour mixture, while continuing to mix, until completely added and blended together.

VARIATION #1: Blueberry Muffins or Blueberry Loaf

To the basic mixture, fold in 1 cup dried blueberries after the entire mixture has been blended together.

VARIATION #2: Peanut Butter Muffins or Peanut Butter Loaf

Make the basic recipe with the following changes:
Delete the 1 tablespoon extra-virgin olive oil.
Instead, add 2 tablespoons (⅛ cup measure) all natural no-sugar peanut butter.
After the entire mixture has been blended together, fold in ¼ cup peanut butter chips and ¼ cup chopped peanuts.

VARIATION #3: Banana Muffins or Banana Bread

Make the basic recipe with the following changes:
Delete the 1 tablespoon extra-virgin olive oil.
Add 1 mashed ripe banana to the buttermilk and oats mixture before beginning to mix, and then continue as directed.
Fold in ¼ cup chopped walnuts, after mixing is completed.

VARIATION #4: Cinnamon Muffins or Cinnamon Bread

Make the basic recipe with the following additions:
Add 2 teaspoons ground cinnamon to the flour mixture.
Fold in ½ cup miniature cinnamon chips after the entire mixture has been blended together. (These may be difficult to find, but they're very good! Ask your store manager).

These recipes can either be made as muffins or can be baked into one large loaf.

Spray either 24 muffin cups or one large loaf pan with two seconds each of non-fat cooking spray.
Fill each muffin cup with ¼ cup of the batter or fill the loaf pan.

Bake at 350 degrees.

Bake muffins for 15 minutes, or until toothpick comes out clean.
Bake the loaves for 55 to 60 minutes, or until a knife inserted deep into the center of the loaf comes out clean.

Remove muffins or loaves from their containers and cool on a wire rack.
After cooling, cut the loaf into twelve slices, wrap and freeze.
Wrap muffins individually, and freeze.

Basic recipe = approximately 1,620 calories.

Variation #1 (Blueberry) = approximately 2020 calories.
Variation #2 (Peanut butter) = approximately 2100 calories
Variation #3 (Banana) = approximately 1920 calories.
Variation #4 (Cinnamon) = approximately 2180 calories.

PUMPKIN OATBRAN BREAD

Preheat oven to 350 degrees.

Mix these dry ingredients into a large bowl, and then make a well in the center of the mixture:

2 ½ cups whole-wheat flour
2 ½ cups oat bran
½ cup Splenda sweetener for baking
½ cup no-sugar maple syrup
1 banana, mashed
2 teaspoons cinnamon
½ teaspoon cloves
1 tablespoon baking soda

Add the following to the well in the dry ingredients and then stir everything together just until moistened:
4 egg whites
1 can (29 ounces) pumpkin
½ cup unsweetened applesauce

Stir into the mixture:
½ cup chopped walnuts
½ cup raisins

Spray two large bread loaf pans each with two seconds of non-fat cooking spray and pour in the batter.

Bake loaves in 350 degree oven for 55 minutes or until a knife inserted deep into the center of the loaf comes out clean.

After cooling, cut each loaf into twelve slices. Wrap slices individually and freeze.

Entire recipe = approximately 2,815 calories.

WHOLE-WHEAT PANCAKES or WAFFLES

⅔ cup whole-wheat flour
¼ teaspoon baking soda
½ teaspoon baking powder
2 packets Splenda sweetener
¼ teaspoon salt
½ cup buttermilk
1 tablespoon olive oil
¼ cup pasteurized real-egg product (like Egg Beaters)

Mix the first 5 ingredients in a bowl.
Combine the next 3 ingredients in another bowl and then stir into the dry mixture, mixing just until combined (don't over mix).

Heat a non-stick pan over medium-high heat (or pre-heat your waffle iron).
Spray with two seconds of non-fat cooking spray.

For pancakes: Ladle ⅓ of the batter onto the skillet for each pancake.
Cook 2 to 3 minutes or until small holes appear and the bottom is browned.
Turn them and cook for another minute or so, until browned.

For waffles: Experiment to determine how much batter to use to make each waffle.

Top with no-sugar maple syrup, or no-sugar jam.
Add non-fat yogurt and fruit to complete the meal.

Recipe, Pancakes or waffles only = approximately 475 calories.

Pancakes and waffles can be cooled, wrapped and frozen, if desired. At a later time they can then be popped into the toaster or toaster oven for a quick breakfast.

NOTES

NOTES

NOTES

NOTES

NOTES

BMR CHARTS

WOMEN'S CHART #1

AGE	18	19	20	21	22	23	24	25	26	27	28	29	30	31	32	33	34	35	36	37	38	39
HEIGHT																						
4'10"	836	831	826	821	817	812	807	803	798	793	789	784	779	775	770	765	760	756	751	746	742	737
4' 10½"	838	833	828	824	819	814	810	805	800	796	791	786	782	777	772	768	763	758	753	749	744	739
4'11"	840	835	830	826	821	816	812	807	802	799	793	788	784	779	774	770	765	760	755	751	746	741
4'11½"	842	837	832	828	823	818	814	809	804	801	795	790	786	781	776	772	767	762	757	753	748	743
5'	844	840	835	831	826	821	817	812	807	803	798	793	788	784	779	775	770	765	760	756	751	746
5' ½"	847	843	838	833	828	824	819	814	809	805	800	796	791	786	782	777	772	767	762	758	753	748
5'1"	849	845	840	835	831	826	821	816	812	807	802	798	793	788	784	779	774	769	764	760	755	750
5'1½"	852	847	842	837	833	828	823	818	814	809	804	800	795	790	786	781	776	771	766	762	757	753
5'2"	854	849	844	840	835	830	826	821	816	812	807	802	797	793	788	783	779	774	769	765	760	755
5' 2½"	856	851	846	842	837	832	828	823	818	814	809	804	799	795	790	785	781	776	772	767	762	757
5'3"	858	853	848	844	838	834	830	825	820	816	811	806	801	797	792	787	783	778	774	769	764	760
5' 3½"	861	856	851	847	841	836	833	827	823	818	813	809	804	799	794	789	785	780	776	771	766	762
5'4"	863	858	853	849	843	839	835	830	826	821	815	811	806	801	796	791	787	782	778	773	769	764
5' 4½"	865	860	855	851	846	842	838	833	828	823	818	813	808	804	799	794	789	786	781	776	771	767
5'5"	868	863	858	854	849	845	840	835	830	825	821	816	811	806	802	797	792	788	783	778	774	769
5' 5½"	870	865	860	856	851	846	842	837	833	828	823	818	813	808	804	799	794	790	785	780	776	771
5'6"	872	867	862	858	854	849	845	839	835	830	825	820	815	810	806	801	797	792	787	783	778	773
5' 6½"	874	869	864	860	856	851	847	842	838	832	828	822	818	813	808	803	799	795	790	785	781	776
5'7"	876	871	867	862	858	854	850	845	840	835	830	825	820	815	810	805	801	797	792	787	783	778
5' 7½"	878	873	870	865	861	857	852	847	842	837	832	827	822	817	812	807	803	799	794	789	785	780
5'8"	881	875	872	867	863	858	853	849	844	839	834	829	824	819	814	809	805	801	796	791	787	782
5' 8½"	884	879	874	869	865	860	854	850	846	842	837	832	826	821	816	812	807	803	799	794	789	784
5'9"	886	881	876	871	867	862	857	852	848	844	839	834	829	824	819	814	809	805	801	796	791	786
5' 9½"	888	883	879	873	869	864	859	854	850	846	841	836	831	826	821	817	812	807	803	798	792	788
5'10"	890	885	881	875	871	866	861	857	852	848	843	838	833	828	823	819	814	809	805	800	795	791
5' 10½"	893	888	883	878	873	868	864	859	854	850	845	840	835	830	825	820	816	811	807	803	798	794
5'11"	895	890	885	880	876	871	867	862	858	853	848	843	838	832	828	823	819	814	811	806	801	796

246

WOMEN'S CHART #1 (CONT.)

AGE	40	41	42	43	44	45	46	47	48	49	50	51	52	53	54	55	56	57	58	59	60
HEIGHT																					
4'10"	732	727	723	718	713	709	704	699	694	690	685	680	676	671	666	662	657	652	648	643	638
4'10½"	735	730	725	721	717	712	707	703	698	693	689	684	679	675	670	665	659	655	650	646	641
4'11"	737	732	727	723	719	714	709	705	700	695	691	686	681	677	672	667	663	657	652	648	643
4'11½"	739	734	729	725	721	716	711	707	702	697	693	688	683	679	674	669	665	659	654	650	645
5'0"	742	737	732	728	724	719	714	710	705	699	695	690	685	681	676	671	667	661	657	652	647
5'½"	744	739	734	730	726	721	716	712	707	701	697	692	687	683	678	673	669	663	659	654	650
5'1"	746	741	736	732	728	723	718	714	709	703	700	695	689	686	681	676	672	666	662	657	652
5'1½"	748	743	738	734	730	725	720	716	711	706	702	697	792	688	683	679	674	669	664	659	654
5'2"	751	746	741	737	732	727	723	718	713	709	704	699	695	690	685	681	676	671	667	661	656
5'2½"	753	748	743	739	734	729	725	720	715	711	706	701	697	692	687	683	678	674	669	664	658
5'3"	755	750	745	741	736	731	727	722	718	713	708	703	699	694	689	685	680	676	671	666	661
5'3½"	757	752	747	743	738	733	729	725	720	715	711	706	701	696	691	687	682	678	673	668	663
5'4"	759	754	749	745	740	735	731	727	722	717	713	708	703	698	693	689	684	680	675	670	665
5'4½"	762	757	752	747	743	738	733	729	724	719	715	710	705	700	695	691	686	682	677	673	668
5'5"	764	760	755	750	746	741	736	731	726	721	717	712	707	703	698	693	689	684	679	675	670
5'5½"	766	762	757	752	748	743	738	733	728	723	719	714	709	705	700	695	691	686	681	677	672
5'6"	768	764	759	754	750	745	740	735	730	725	721	716	711	707	702	697	693	688	683	679	674
5'6½"	771	766	761	756	752	747	742	737	732	727	723	718	713	709	704	699	695	690	685	681	676
5'7"	773	768	763	758	754	749	744	739	735	729	725	720	715	711	706	701	697	692	688	683	678
5'7½"	775	770	765	760	756	751	746	741	737	732	727	722	718	713	708	703	699	695	689	685	680
5'8"	777	772	767	762	758	753	748	744	739	734	730	725	720	715	710	706	701	697	692	688	683
5'8½"	779	774	768	764	760	755	750	746	741	736	732	727	722	717	712	708	703	699	694	690	685
5'9"	781	776	771	766	762	757	752	748	743	738	734	729	724	719	714	710	705	701	696	692	687
5'9½"	783	778	773	768	764	759	755	750	745	740	736	731	726	721	717	712	708	704	699	694	690
5'10"	786	781	776	771	766	761	757	753	748	743	738	733	728	723	719	721	712	707	701	697	692
5'10½"	789	784	779	774	769	763	759	755	750	745	740	736	731	726	722	718	713	708	703	699	694
5'11"	791	786	781	776	771	766	762	757	752	747	742	738	734	729	724	720	716	711	706	701	697

WOMEN'S CHART #1 (CONT.)

AGE	61	62	63	64	65	66	67	68	69	70	71	72	73	74	75	76	77	78	79	80
HEIGHT																				
4'10"	633	629	624	619	615	610	605	601	596	591	586	582	577	572	568	563	558	554	549	544
4' 10½"	636	632	627	622	618	613	608	604	599	594	590	585	580	576	571	566	561	556	551	545
4'11"	638	634	629	624	620	615	610	606	601	596	592	587	582	578	573	568	563	558	554	549
4'11½"	640	635	631	626	622	617	612	608	603	598	594	589	584	580	575	570	565	560	556	551
5'0"	643	638	633	629	624	619	614	610	605	600	596	591	586	582	577	572	567	562	558	553
5' ½"	645	640	635	631	626	621	617	612	607	602	598	593	588	584	579	574	569	564	560	556
5'1"	647	643	638	633	628	623	619	614	609	604	600	595	590	586	581	576	572	567	562	558
5'1½"	650	645	640	635	630	625	621	616	612	607	602	597	593	588	583	579	575	570	565	560
5'2"	652	647	642	638	633	628	624	619	614	610	605	600	596	591	586	582	577	572	568	563
5' 2½"	654	649	645	640	635	630	626	621	616	612	607	602	598	593	588	584	579	575	570	565
5'3"	656	651	647	642	638	633	628	623	618	614	609	604	600	595	590	586	581	577	572	567
5' 3½"	658	654	650	645	640	635	630	625	620	616	611	606	602	597	592	588	583	579	574	569
5'4"	660	657	652	647	642	637	632	627	622	618	613	608	604	599	595	590	585	581	576	572
5' 4½"	663	659	654	649	645	640	635	630	625	620	616	611	607	602	597	592	588	584	579	574
5'5"	665	661	656	651	647	642	637	633	628	623	619	614	610	605	600	595	591	587	582	577
5' 5½"	667	663	658	653	649	644	639	635	630	625	621	616	612	607	602	597	593	589	584	579
5'6"	670	665	660	655	651	646	641	637	632	627	623	618	614	609	604	599	595	591	586	582
5' 6½"	672	668	663	658	653	648	643	639	634	629	625	620	616	611	606	601	597	593	589	585
5'7"	674	670	665	660	655	650	645	641	636	631	627	622	618	613	608	604	599	595	591	587
5' 7½"	676	671	667	662	657	652	647	643	638	633	629	624	620	615	610	606	601	597	593	589
5'8"	678	673	669	664	659	654	649	645	640	635	631	626	622	617	612	608	603	599	595	591
5' 8½"	680	675	671	666	661	656	651	647	642	637	633	628	624	619	614	610	605	601	597	593
5'9"	683	678	673	668	663	658	653	649	644	639	635	630	626	622	617	612	607	603	599	595
5' 9½"	685	680	675	670	665	660	655	651	646	641	637	632	628	624	619	614	610	605	601	597
5'10"	688	683	678	673	668	663	658	653	648	643	639	634	630	626	621	617	612	608	603	599
5' 10½"	690	685	680	675	670	665	660	655	650	645	641	636	632	628	624	619	614	610	605	601
5'11"	692	687	682	678	673	668	663	658	653	648	644	640	636	631	626	621	617	612	607	603

MEN'S CHART #1

AGE	18	19	20	21	22	23	24	25	26	27	28	29	30	31	32	33	34	35	36	37	38	39
HEIGHT																						
5'	706	699	692	685	678	672	665	658	651	644	638	631	624	617	610	604	597	590	583	576	570	563
5' ½"	712	706	699	692	685	678	672	665	658	651	644	638	631	624	617	610	604	597	590	583	576	570
5'1"	718	712	705	698	691	684	677	671	665	657	650	643	637	630	623	616	609	603	596	590	582	575
5'1½"	725	718	711	705	698	691	684	677	671	664	657	650	643	637	630	623	616	609	603	596	589	582
5'2"	731	725	718	711	704	697	690	683	677	670	664	656	649	642	636	629	622	615	608	602	595	589
5'2½"	737	731	724	717	710	704	697	690	683	677	670	663	656	649	642	636	629	622	615	608	602	595
5'3"	744	737	730	724	717	710	703	696	689	682	676	669	663	655	648	641	635	628	621	614	607	601
5' 3½"	750	744	736	730	723	716	709	703	696	689	682	676	669	662	655	648	641	635	628	621	614	607
5'4"	757	750	743	736	729	723	716	709	702	696	689	681	676	669	662	655	647	640	634	627	620	613
5' 4½"	763	757	749	743	735	729	722	715	709	702	695	688	681	676	669	661	654	647	640	634	627	620
5' 5"	769	763	756	749	742	735	729	722	715	708	701	695	688	680	676	668	661	654	646	639	634	626
5'5½"	776	769	762	756	748	742	734	728	721	714	708	701	694	688	680	675	668	660	653	646	639	633
5'6"	782	776	768	762	755	748	741	734	728	721	714	707	700	694	687	679	675	667	660	653	646	638
5' 6½"	788	782	775	768	762	755	747	741	733	727	720	713	707	700	693	687	679	674	667	659	652	645
5'7"	795	788	781	775	767	761	754	747	740	733	727	720	713	706	699	693	686	678	674	666	659	652
5' 7½"	801	795	787	781	774	767	761	754	746	740	732	726	719	712	706	699	693	686	678	674	666	658
5'8"	807	801	794	787	780	774	766	760	753	746	739	732	726	719	712	705	698	692	685	677	674	666
5' 8½"	814	807	800	794	786	780	773	766	760	753	745	739	731	725	718	711	705	698	692	685	677	673
5'9"	820	814	806	800	793	786	779	773	765	759	752	745	738	731	725	718	711	704	697	692	684	676
5' 9½"	826	820	813	806	799	793	785	779	772	765	759	752	744	738	730	724	717	710	704	697	691	684
5'10"	833	826	819	813	805	799	792	785	778	772	764	758	751	744	737	730	724	717	710	704	696	691
5' 10½"	839	833	825	819	812	805	798	792	784	778	771	764	758	751	743	737	729	723	716	709	703	696
5'11"	846	839	832	825	818	812	804	798	791	784	777	771	763	758	750	743	736	729	723	716	709	703
5' 11½"	852	846	838	832	824	818	811	804	797	791	784	777	770	763	757	750	742	736	729	722	715	708
6'	858	852	845	838	831	824	817	811	803	797	790	783	776	770	762	757	749	742	735	728	722	715
6' ½"	864	858	851	845	837	831	823	817	810	803	796	790	783	776	769	762	756	749	741	735	728	721
6'1"	871	864	857	851	844	837	830	823	816	810	802	796	789	782	776	769	761	756	748	741	735	727
6' 1½"	877	871	863	857	850	844	836	830	822	816	809	802	796	789	782	775	768	761	755	748	740	734
6'2"	883	877	870	863	856	850	843	836	829	822	815	809	801	795	788	781	775	768	760	755	747	740
6' 2½"	890	883	876	870	862	856	849	843	835	829	821	815	808	801	795	788	781	774	767	760	754	747
6'3"	896	890	882	876	869	862	855	849	842	835	828	821	814	808	800	794	787	780	774	767	759	754
6' 3½"	903	896	889	882	875	869	861	855	848	842	834	828	820	814	807	800	794	787	780	773	766	759
6' 4"	909	903	895	889	881	875	868	861	854	848	841	834	827	820	813	807	799	793	786	779	773	766
6' 4½"	915	909	902	895	888	881	874	868	860	854	847	841	833	827	819	813	806	799	793	786	779	772
6'5"	922	915	908	902	894	888	880	874	867	860	853	847	840	833	826	819	812	806	798	792	785	778

MEN'S CHART #1 (CONT.)

AGE	40	41	42	43	44	45	46	47	48	49	50	51	52	53	54	55	56	57	58	59	60
HEIGHT																					
5'	556	549	542	536	529	522	515	508	502	495	488	481	474	467	461	454	447	440	434	427	420
5' ½"	563	556	549	542	536	529	522	515	508	502	495	488	481	474	467	461	454	447	440	434	427
5'1"	569	562	555	548	541	535	528	521	514	507	501	494	487	480	473	466	460	453	446	439	433
5'1½"	575	569	562	555	548	541	535	528	521	514	507	501	494	487	480	473	466	460	453	446	439
5'2"	581	574	568	561	554	548	540	534	527	520	513	506	500	493	486	479	472	465	459	452	445
5'2½"	588	581	574	568	561	554	547	540	534	527	520	513	506	500	493	486	479	472	465	459	452
5'3"	594	588	580	573	567	560	553	547	539	533	526	519	512	505	499	492	485	478	471	464	458
5'3½"	601	594	587	580	573	567	560	553	546	539	533	525	518	512	505	498	492	485	478	471	464
5'4"	606	600	593	587	579	572	567	559	552	546	538	532	525	518	511	504	498	491	484	477	470
5'4½"	613	606	600	593	586	579	572	566	559	552	545	538	532	524	517	511	504	497	491	484	477
5'5"	619	612	605	599	593	586	578	571	566	558	551	545	537	531	524	517	510	503	497	490	483
5'5½"	626	619	612	605	599	592	585	578	571	565	558	551	544	537	531	523	516	510	503	496	490
5'6"	633	625	618	611	604	598	592	585	577	570	565	557	550	544	536	530	523	516	509	502	496
5' 6½"	638	632	625	618	611	604	598	591	584	577	570	564	557	550	543	536	530	522	515	509	502
5'7"	645	637	632	624	617	610	603	597	591	584	576	569	564	556	549	543	535	529	522	515	508
5' 7½"	652	644	637	631	624	617	610	603	597	590	583	576	569	563	556	549	542	535	529	521	514
5'8"	658	651	644	636	631	623	616	609	602	596	590	583	575	568	563	555	548	542	534	528	521
5' 8½"	665	657	651	643	636	630	623	616	609	602	596	589	582	575	568	562	555	548	541	534	528
5'9"	673	665	657	650	643	635	630	622	615	608	601	595	589	582	574	567	562	554	547	541	533
5' 9½"	676	673	665	656	650	643	635	630	622	615	608	601	595	588	581	574	567	561	554	547	540
5'10"	683	675	673	665	656	649	642	634	629	621	614	607	600	594	588	581	573	566	561	553	546
5' 10½"	690	683	675	672	664	655	649	642	634	629	621	614	607	600	594	587	580	573	566	560	553
5'11"	695	690	682	674	672	664	655	648	641	633	628	620	613	606	599	593	587	580	572	565	560
5' 11½"	702	695	688	682	674	671	663	654	648	641	633	628	620	613	606	599	593	586	579	572	565
6'	708	702	694	688	681	673	671	663	654	647	640	632	627	619	612	605	598	592	586	579	571
6' ½"	714	707	701	694	686	681	673	670	662	653	647	640	632	627	619	612	605	598	592	585	578
6'1"	721	714	707	701	693	686	680	672	670	662	653	646	639	631	626	618	611	604	597	591	585
6' 1 ½"	727	720	713	707	700	693	685	680	672	669	661	652	646	639	631	626	618	611	604	597	591
6'2"	734	726	720	713	707	700	692	685	679	671	669	661	652	645	638	630	625	617	610	603	596
6' 2½"	739	733	726	719	712	706	699	692	684	679	671	668	660	651	645	638	630	625	617	610	603
6'3"	746	739	733	725	719	712	706	699	691	684	678	670	668	660	651	644	637	629	624	616	609
6' 3½"	753	746	738	732	725	718	711	705	698	691	683	678	670	667	659	650	644	637	629	624	616
6' 4"	758	753	745	738	732	724	718	711	705	698	690	683	677	669	667	659	650	643	636	628	623
6' 4½"	765	758	752	745	737	731	724	717	710	704	697	690	682	677	669	666	658	649	642	636	628
6' 5"	772	765	757	752	744	737	731	723	717	710	704	697	689	682	676	668	666	658	649	642	635

MEN'S CHART #1 (CONT.)

AGE	61	62	63	64	65	66	67	68	69	70	71	72	73	74	75	76	77	78	79	80
HEIGHT																				
5'	413	406	400	393	386	379	372	367	359	352	345	338	332	329	318	311	304	298	291	284
5' ½"	420	413	406	400	393	386	379	372	367	359	352	345	338	332	329	318	311	304	298	291
5'1"	426	419	412	405	399	392	385	378	371	366	358	351	344	337	331	328	317	310	303	297
5'1½"	433	426	419	412	405	399	392	385	378	371	366	358	351	344	337	331	328	317	310	303
5'2"	438	432	425	418	411	404	398	391	384	377	370	365	357	350	343	336	330	327	316	309
5'2½"	445	438	432	425	418	411	404	398	391	384	377	370	365	357	350	343	336	330	327	316
5'3"	451	444	437	431	424	417	410	403	397	390	383	376	369	364	356	349	342	335	329	326
5'3½"	458	451	444	437	431	424	417	410	403	397	390	383	376	369	364	356	349	342	335	329
5'4"	463	457	450	443	436	430	423	416	409	402	396	389	382	375	368	363	355	348	341	334
5'4½"	470	463	457	450	443	436	430	423	416	409	402	396	389	382	375	368	363	355	348	341
5'5"	476	469	462	456	449	442	435	429	422	415	408	401	395	388	381	374	367	362	354	347
5'5½"	483	476	469	462	456	449	442	435	429	422	415	408	401	395	388	381	374	367	362	354
5'6"	489	482	475	468	461	455	448	441	434	428	421	414	407	400	394	387	380	373	366	361
5'6½"	495	489	482	475	468	461	455	448	441	434	428	421	414	407	400	394	387	380	373	366
5'7"	501	495	488	481	474	467	460	454	447	440	433	427	420	413	406	399	393	386	379	372
5'7½"	508	501	494	488	481	474	467	460	454	447	440	433	427	420	413	406	399	393	386	379
5'8"	514	507	500	494	487	480	473	466	459	453	446	439	432	426	419	412	405	398	392	385
5'8½"	520	513	507	500	493	487	480	473	466	459	453	446	439	432	426	419	412	405	398	392
5'9"	527	520	513	506	499	493	486	479	472	465	458	452	445	438	431	425	418	411	404	397
5'9½"	533	527	519	512	506	499	492	486	479	472	465	458	452	445	438	431	425	418	411	404
5'10"	540	532	526	519	512	505	498	492	485	478	471	464	457	451	444	437	430	424	417	410
5'10½"	546	539	532	526	518	511	505	498	491	485	478	471	464	457	451	444	437	430	424	417
5'11"	552	545	539	531	525	518	511	504	497	491	484	477	470	463	456	450	443	436	429	423
5'11½"	559	552	545	538	531	525	517	510	504	497	490	484	477	470	463	456	450	443	436	429
6'	564	559	551	544	538	530	524	517	510	503	496	490	483	476	469	462	455	449	442	435
6' ½"	571	564	558	551	544	537	530	524	516	509	503	496	489	483	476	469	462	455	449	442
6'1"	578	570	563	558	550	543	537	529	523	516	509	502	495	489	482	475	468	461	454	448
6'1½"	584	577	570	563	557	550	543	536	529	523	515	508	502	495	488	482	475	468	461	454
6'2"	590	584	577	569	562	557	549	542	536	528	522	515	508	501	494	488	481	474	467	460
6'2½"	596	590	583	576	569	562	556	549	542	535	528	522	514	507	501	494	487	481	474	467
6'3"	602	595	589	583	576	568	561	556	548	541	535	527	521	514	507	500	493	487	480	473
6'3½"	609	602	595	589	582	575	568	561	555	548	541	534	527	521	513	506	500	493	486	480
6'4"	615	608	601	594	588	582	575	567	560	555	547	540	534	526	520	513	506	499	492	486
6'4½"	623	615	608	601	594	588	581	574	567	560	554	547	540	533	526	520	512	505	499	492
6'5"	627	622	614	607	600	593	587	581	574	566	559	554	546	539	533	525	519	512	505	498

WOMEN'S CHART #2

Target Body Weight in Pounds	Factor for Women	Target Body Weight in Pounds	Factor for Women
90	392.74	151	658.91
91	397.06	152	663.27
92	401.47	153	667.64
93	405.79	154	672
94	410.21	155	676.36
95	414.53	156	680.73
96	418.94	157	685.09
97	423.26	158	689.45
98	427.68	159	693.82
99	432	160	698.18
100	436.32	161	702.55
101	440.74	162	706.91
102	445.09	163	711.27
103	449.47	164	715.68
104	405.79	165	720
105	458.21	166	724.36
106	462.53	167	728.73
107	466.94	168	733.09
108	471.26	169	737.45
109	475.64	170	741.82
110	480	171	746.18
111	484.36	172	750.55
112	488.73	173	754.94
113	493.09	174	759.26
114	497.45	175	763.64
115	501.82	176	768
116	506.18	177	772.36
117	510.55	178	776.73
118	514.91	179	781.09
119	519.27	180	785.45
120	523.64	181	789.82
121	528	182	794.18
122	532.36	183	798.55
123	536.73	184	802.91
124	541.09	185	807.27
125	545.45	186	811.64
126	549.82	187	816
127	554.18	188	820.36
128	558.55	189	824.73
129	562.91	190	829.09
130	567.27	191	833.45
131	571.64	192	837.82
132	576	193	842.18
133	580.36	194	846.55
134	584.73	195	850.91
135	589.09	196	855.27
136	593.47	197	859.64
137	597.82	198	864
138	602.18	199	868.36
139	606.55	200	872.73
140	610.91	201	877.09
141	615.27	202	881.45
142	619.64	203	885.82
143	624	204	890.18
144	628.36	205	894.55
145	632.73	206	898.91
146	637.09	207	903.27
147	641.45	208	894.53
148	645.82	209	912
149	650.18	210	916.36
150	654.55		

MEN'S CHART #2

Target Body Weight in Pounds	Factor for Men	Target Body Weight in Pounds	Factor for Men
90	560.47	151	940.32
91	566.63	152	946.55
92	572.93	153	952.77
93	579.1	154	959
94	585.4	155	965.23
95	591.57	156	971.45
96	579.87	157	977.68
97	604.03	158	983.91
98	610.34	159	990.14
99	616.5	160	996.36
100	622.67	161	1002.59
101	628.97	162	1008.82
102	635.13	163	1015.05
103	641.43	164	1021.34
104	647.64	165	1027.5
105	653.9	166	1033.73
106	660.07	167	1039.95
107	666.37	168	1046.18
108	672.53	169	1052.41
109	678.77	170	1058.64
110	685	171	1064.86
111	691.23	172	1071.09
112	697.45	173	1077.37
113	703.68	174	1083.53
114	709.91	175	1089.77
115	716.14	176	1096
116	722.36	177	1102.23
117	728.59	178	1108.45
118	734.82	179	1114.68
119	741.03	180	1120.91
120	747.27	181	1127.14
121	753.5	182	1133.36
122	759.73	183	1139.59
123	765.95	184	1145.82
124	772.18	185	11 2.04
125	778.41	186	1158.27
126	784.64	187	1164.5
127	790.86	188	1170.73
128	797.09	189	1176.95
129	803.32	190	1183.18
130	809.55	191	1189.41
131	815.77	192	1195.64
132	822	193	1201.86
133	828.23	194	1208.09
134	834.45	195	1214.37
135	840.68	196	1220.55
136	846.93	197	1226.77
137	853.14	198	1233
138	859.36	199	1239.23
139	865.59	200	1245.45
140	871.82	201	1251.68
141	878.05	202	1257.91
142	884.27	203	1264.14
143	890.5	204	1270.36
144	896.73	205	1276.59
145	902.95	206	1282.82
146	909.18	207	1289.05
147	915.41	208	1295.27
148	921.64	209	1301.50
149	927.86	210	1307.73
150	934.09		

NOTES

NOTES

NOTES

NOTES

NOTES

NOTES

NOTES

APPENDIX E
STRENGTH-TRAINING PROGRAM

The following ten exercises comprise the Tortoise Diet strength-training program. These simple exercises will effectively challenge each major muscle group. The entire program should be performed twice each week (except for the first two weeks of the Tortoise Diet Training Assignments), allowing a minimum of 48 hours of rest between sessions. Begin each exercise session by performing a five minute aerobic warm-up. After your strength-training session is complete, cool down for five minutes by performing some long, slow stretches of all major muscle groups. When stretching, the key thing to remember is to do easy stretches that don't hurt. Once you have learned all of the exercises, your entire session won't take more than thirty minutes, including warm-up and cool-down.

Perform the exercises in the order shown. As you can see, the exercises are grouped into pairs. Two complete sets of each of the paired exercises will be completed before moving on to the next pair of exercises. For the first set of each exercise in a pairing, use a weight that allows you to complete a minimum of eight and a maximum of sixteen controlled full repetitions, while maintaining excellent form. To help keep the movement controlled, lift and lower the weight using a one-two-three-four count. Always breathe out when you are lifting the weight, and breathe in when you are lowering the weight.

After completing the first set of both exercises in the pair, immediately return again to the first exercise and begin set number two. The amount of weight you select for the second set of each exercise should be a heavier weight, one that allows you to only complete a minimum of four repetitions and a maximum of eight controlled full repetitions. Repeat the process described to complete two sets for each exercise in the program.

EXERCISE #1

Dumbbell Biceps Curls

1. Hold a dumbbell in each hand. Stand upright, keeping your back held straight.
2. Begin the exercise with your arms hanging down, elbows touching the sides of your abdomen, dumbbells resting near each thigh with palms forward.
3. With elbows kept at the sides, bend at the elbow and raise one dumbbell upward and slightly outward as far as you can go, until the palm is facing the shoulder.
4. Squeeze the bicep muscle at the top of the movement.
5. Lower the weight back to the starting position and repeat the same movement with the other arm.
6. One complete movement upward and then back downward of both arms equals one repetition.

Hint: The exercise may be done as described, with first one arm, and then the other lifting the weight OR both arms may be raised simultaneously.
Throughout the upward motion, keep elbows in, close to the abdomen. Lift an amount of weight that allows you to perform the exercise without swinging the weights or moving your torso around to help lift them up.

VARIATION: Standing Hammer Curls

Begin in standing position with a dumbbell in each hand, arms hanging in front of your thighs with palms facing inward. Keeping the hands in a position as though you were raising a hammer, curl up each arm simultaneously toward your shoulder, keeping your elbows held closely at your side. Keep the weights in front of you throughout the movement, not to the side. Lower the weights back to the starting position and repeat.

EXERCISE #2

Triceps Kickback

1. Stand with your right foot slightly in front of your left foot. Hold a dumbbell in your left hand. Lean forward from your hips and put your right hand on your right thigh. Avoid arching your back.
2. Press your left forearm straight back until it is straight. Squeeze the triceps muscle and then return the weight back to the starting position. Keep your elbow close to your side.
3. Repeat this motion with the left arm for the required number of repetitions.
4. When all reps have been completed, switch positions so your left foot is forward and the dumbbell is in your right hand. Repeat the movement for repetitions with this hand.

Return to Exercise #1 and Exercise #2 and perform a second set.

EXERCISE #3

Squats

1. Stand straight, feet slightly more than shoulder width apart. Hold a dumbbell in each hand, and place one on top of each shoulder.
2. Consciously place your body weight onto both heels. Keep your head up. Focus on a spot on the wall straight ahead just above eye level. Bend your knees to lower down into a squatting position, just as if you were going to sit on a chair. Your upper torso will lean forward slightly. Use a slow one-two-three-four count to complete the movement.
3. Lower your body until your thigh is as close to parallel to the floor as possible, without overly stressing your knees.
4. Press upward to return to starting position. Consciously squeeze your buttocks and push down into the floor with your heels during this upward motion.
5. Repeat for the required number of repetitions.

Hint: Maintaining control is very important with this exercise. Don't lean forward or bounce around. If you are not very limber, take it slow and easy.

VARIATION: Plie Squat

Place feet wider than shoulder width apart, one dumbbell held in both hands dangling between the legs. Once the dumbbell is in position, lift up your heels so you're standing on your toes and perform the squat.

EXERCISE #4

Bent-Over Lateral Raise

1. Sit on the edge of a chair, a flat bench, or an aerobic stepper while holding a dumbbell in each hand with palms facing inward.
2. Keeping your feet flat on the floor, lean forward until your chest nearly touches your thighs. Hold the dumbbells under your legs and behind your knees until they are almost touching each other.
3. Slowly raise each arm straight in an outward arc, until they are almost at shoulder level. Squeeze the shoulder blades together. During this motion your head and body will raise up a little.
4. Return the weights to the starting position.
5. Repeat for repetitions.

Hint: Maintain the position of your back throughout the exercise, without arching. Keep the weights under control at all times, without allowing them to drop and without "lurching" them into position.

Return to Exercise #3 and Exercise # 4 and perform a second set.

EXERCISE #5

Dumbbell Chest Press

1. Lie on your back on a flat bench or an aerobic stepper with feet flat on the floor and abdominal muscles contracted. Hold a dumbbell in each hand with arms extended directly upward over your chest, palms facing your feet.
2. Lower your elbows until dumbbells are near chest level.
3. Press the weights back upward and toward each other, so they almost touch at the top of the movement.
4. Repeat the lowering and raising motions for repetitions.

EXERCISE #6

Standing Lateral Raise

1. While standing, hold a dumbbell in each hand at sides with palms facing inward.
2. Keep your elbows straight and raise both arms straight outward until they are at a 90-degree extension on each side.
3. Keeping your elbows straight, lower both arms straight back down to your hips.
4. Repeat for additional repetitions.

Hint: Do not swing the dumbbells out and up. Remember to count to four as you raise the weight, and count to four as you lower the weight, maintaining complete control.

Return to Exercise #5 and Exercise #6 and perform a second set.

EXERCISE #7

Stiff-Legged Dead-lift

1. Stand with feet placed hip-width apart, holding a dumbbell in each hand. Find a point on a wall in front of you just above eye level. Keep your eyes fixed on that spot throughout the exercise.
2. With knees in a soft-locked position, and keeping legs and back straight, allow dumbbells to hang down in front of your legs.
3. Slowly bend your torso forward toward the floor, keeping your head up and eyes on that spot on the wall. Keep your chest out as you go down, abdominal muscles contracted and back straight throughout the motion.
4. Stop the forward movement when you feel a gentle stretch in your hamstring muscles. Do not go any farther than this gentle stretch!
5. Concentrate on squeezing your buttock muscles while straightening back up to starting position.
6. Repeat this motion for all repetitions.

EXERCISE #8

Standing Alternate Dumbbell Press

1. While standing, hold a dumbbell in each hand. Position dumbbells near the shoulders with elbows below the wrists, palms facing towards the front.
2. Extend one arm straight upward toward the ceiling. Palm should face the front.
3. Lower the dumbbell to the starting position, and repeat with the other arm.

Hint: Do not allow your body to sway from side to side as you are lifting the weight.

Return to Exercise #7 and Exercise #8 and perform a second set.

EXERCISE #9

Bent Leg Kick-up

1. This exercise does not require the use of weights. From a starting position on your hands and knees, raise your right leg up until your thigh is extended to hip height, parallel to the ground. Once in this position, bend the knee so your foot is aimed toward the ceiling.
2. While keeping your leg extended back in this position, drop the knee down a little bit (not all the way to the floor) and then squeeze the buttock muscles to press the foot back upward, toward the ceiling. Do not arch your back during this movement.
3. Do as many repetitions as you possibly can with the first leg, until you feel your buttock muscles "burning."
4. Repeat the exercise with your left leg.

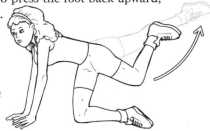

Hint: For best results, squeeze your buttocks as much as possible while you are raising your foot upward.

EXERCISE #10

Bicycle Crunch

1. This exercise does not require the use of weights.
Lie on your back with knees bent and feet on the floor.
2. Curl your head up while putting your hands behind your head.
3. Extend your left elbow forward while simultaneously raising both feet off the floor and extending left leg forward until straight.
4. Immediately, bring that leg back while extending the right leg, while at the same time bringing the left elbow back and bringing the right elbow forward.
5. Do as many repetitions as you possibly can, until you feel your abdominal muscles "burning."

Hint: Keep your hands lightly touching your head without pulling on your neck. **Also, the goal is not to do as many repetitions as you can in as short a time as possible. As with all the Tortoise Diet strength-training exercises, the goal is to take it slow and easy, flexing your muscles as much as possible, all the while maintaining absolute control.**

Return to Exercise #9 and Exercise #10 and perform a second set.

NOTES

NOTES

Activity Factor

In addition to the basic number of calories required each day (BMR), additional calories are needed for digestion and to fuel other activities. Just how much additional energy is needed will be influenced mostly by your usual level of activity, as determined primarily by your occupation.

Aerobic Exercise

Physical activity performed with the heart rate kept in the 60-85% range of maximum. At this level of activity, the muscles utilize large amounts of oxygen. This type of exercise can be tolerated for long periods of time.

Alcohol

Provides seven calories per gram, but contributes virtually nothing in terms of nutrition. Drinking alcoholic beverages stimulates the appetite and decreases willpower. It may also slow the metabolic rate and promote fat storage.

Anaerobic Exercise

Physical activity performed with a heart rate greater than 85% of maximum, preventing the muscles from utilizing oxygen. Because a different and very limited energy pathway is utilized by the muscles for this activity, this type of exercise can be tolerated for only very short periods of time.

Basal Metabolic Rate (BMR)

The number of calories required each day if all a person did was just "lie around on the couch all day." The Harris-Benedict Equation is the "gold standard" scientific calculation used to determine each individual's BMR.

Body Fat Percentage measurement, utilizing the YMCA method

Body fat percentage can be measured by using an individual's waist measurement. To measure, place a tape measure at the level of the naval (belly button). The tape should be held parallel to the floor and measured in inches. Use this measurement in the following calculation:

MEN
(-98.42)
Plus (4.15 x waist measurement at navel in inches)
Minus (.082 x current weight in pounds)
Divided by current weight
Equals Body Fat Percentage

WOMEN
(-76.76)
Plus (4.15 x waist measurement at navel in inches)
Minus (.082   x   current weight in pounds)
Divided by current weight
Equals Body Fat Percentage

Taking measurements and monitoring readings over a period of weeks will more accurately reveal changing body fat percentages.

Body Fat Percentage measurement, using the electronic body fat scale
Body fat percentage can be measured using an electronic scale which indicates both total body weight and body fat percentage. The accuracy of the reading may vary greatly, mostly depending on how hydrated (or dehydrated) a person is at the time. This tool is best utilized by recording weights and body fat percentage measurements once each week on the same day of the week, at the same time of day, and under similar conditions. As with the tape measure method, monitor readings over a period of time to more accurately gauge changing body fat percentages.

Calorie Deficit
Eating fewer calories than required to maintain current weight creates a calorie deficit, which is essential for weight loss to occur. When the calorie deficit is "just right", muscle tissue is preserved while body fat is utilized for energy to make up for the deficit. Thus, true fat loss is dependent on each person calculating their own personalized "just right" calorie deficit.

Calorie-Dense
Foods high in calories, but low in nutrition. These foods do not promote weight loss, and eating too many of them will not contribute to good health.

Carbohydrates (carbs)
Carbohydrate foods contain glucose, which is the primary fuel the body requires. Simple carbohydrates are quickly broken down into glucose. Complex carbohydrates, when eaten in their "whole foods" form, take longer to break down, and provide a more sustained energy.

Fat
The most calorie-dense nutrient, yielding nine calories per gram.

Fat Weight
The amount of the total body weight that is comprised of fat tissue.

Fiber
An indigestible component of complex carbohydrate foods. Fiber is removed from these foods when they are processed and "refined," (e.g. when made into white flour, white rice, and white sugar). The benefits of fiber range from providing a feeling of satiety while eating a low-calorie diet, to lowering the risks for heart disease and cancer.

"Fool Your Body"

Twice each week 400 calories should be added to your Weight Loss Calorie Plan. I recommend that these occasions be used for TGIW meals. Certainly, there is a lot of psychological benefit in being encouraged to enjoy a special meal once in awhile while losing weight. Additionally, there are true physiologic benefits for following this practice, as the body will be less likely to perceive "starvation" and slow the metabolic rate. It's a win/win situation, and it helps make the Tortoise Diet a plan that can be followed for a lifetime.

Glycemic Index

This scale rates foods according to how rapidly they are digested and broken down into glucose. The higher the Glycemic Index Number, the faster the breakdown into glucose occurs. This number is significant because the faster glucose enters the bloodstream, the more insulin is produced and the more likely excess energy will be stored as fat. The Tortoise Diet recommends that each meal containing high-glycemic foods should also include protein foods and a little heart-healthy fat if desired, so digestion and the subsequent release of glucose into the bloodstream will be slowed.

Habit

A behavior that you repeat so often that it becomes second nature and is done reflexively, without a single conscious thought.

Hara Hachi Bu

Making it a practice to stop eating when you feel 80% full.

"Hare-brained" Weight Loss Plan

The Tortoise Diet term for any weight loss plan that promotes "quick and easy" weight loss. Many of these lopsided plans do not promote good health and are not sustainable over the long term, causing muscle loss and weight rebound.

"How Low Can You Go?"

The technique of experimenting with favorite recipes to make them lower in fat, sugar and calories, yet still tasty and enjoyable. This is an important skill to develop to make the Tortoise Diet a livable, lifetime plan.

Lean Weight

The total body weight reflected on the scale is comprised of both lean weight and fat weight. Lean weight is comprised of everything in the body that is not fat: muscle, bone, organs, and water. For our purposes, lean weight is considered to be muscle tissue.

Low Intensity Fat Burning (LIFB)

Physical activity performed in the low-intensity aerobic zone, with the heart rate kept at 60-70% of maximum range. The Tortoise Diet recommends LIFB aerobic exercise because it promotes the use of body fat for energy, and doesn't cause the calorie deficit to become too large.

Lifetime Calorie Plan

This represents the total number of calories an individual will require each day to remain at their target body weight. This calorie total does not include additional energy requirements for purposeful exercise.

(BMR at Target Body Weight) x (Activity Factor) = Lifetime Calorie Plan.

Level of Perceived Exertion (LPE)
A scale which is utilized to help determine whether exercise is being performed in the proper aerobic range.

Metabolism
The process of breaking down the foods we eat and releasing energy. The higher the metabolic rate, the faster calories are burned. The more muscle a person has, the higher their metabolic rate will be.

Mono-unsaturated fats
These are the "good" unsaturated fats that should be part of any healthy diet. They are found primarily in cold-water fish, nuts, seeds, olives, and oils made from these foods.

Nutrient-Dense Foods
Foods low in calories but containing a lot of nutrition. These are the foods that promote weight loss and good health.

Personal Weight Loss Ratio (PWLR)
PWLR is a tool which is utilized to reveal how well an individual is preserving lean weight while they are losing fat weight. The PWLR is calculated by dividing the number of pounds of lean weight an individual can afford to lose, by the amount of fat weight to lose. Because of the expected large amount of initial water loss, the initial PWLR is not calculated until after the completion of week three of the Tortoise Diet. After that time, a current PWLR can be calculated each week. Strive to keep your current PWLR number higher than your initial PWLR, and strive to keep the number from "going negative."

Phytonutrients
Compounds found only in bright, colorful plant-origin foods that contribute to disease prevention. They act as anti-oxidants, protecting the cells of the body from excess aging and cellular breakdown. Eating a wide variety of colorful and fresh vegetables and fruits, either raw or lightly cooked to preserve their nutrition can help you to fight cancer, heart disease, and aging.

Protein
Protein-rich foods are essential to the body for tissue growth and repair. Complete proteins are found in animal-origin foods while incomplete proteins are found in a wide variety of plant foods. Soy foods are the exception, in that they are plant-based foods that provide complete protein. If necessary, protein foods can be broken down to provide glucose for energy, but they're a lot more expensive than carbohydrate foods and when they are used for energy the functions they usually perform are neglected, leaving the individual more prone to illness. The Tortoise Diet recommends that protein intake should be approximately 25% of the total daily calorie intake.

Saturated Fats
Dietary fats found primarily in animal-origin foods, like meats, eggs, butter, cheese and cream. These fats are implicated in contributing to heart disease. Intake of saturated fats should be very limited for any person who desires weight loss and good health.

Target Body Fat Percentage
Your "goal" amount of fat weight, expressed as a percentage of target body weight.

      Men <40 years old   12% Body Fat

      Men >40 years old   15% Body Fat

      Women <40 years old   18% Body Fat

      Women >40 years old   21% Body Fat

Target Body Weight
Your "goal" body weight based on a commonly used formula that takes into consideration your sex, height and frame size.

Target Fat Weight
The number of pounds of fat you should have when you reach your target body weight. (Target Body Weight) x (Target Body Fat Percentage, expressed as a decimal) = Target Fat Weight

Target Lean Weight
The number of pounds of lean weight you should have when you reach your target body weight. (Target Body Weight) - (Target Fat Weight) = Target Lean Weight

TGIW
The Tortoise Diet promotes the ongoing practice of enjoying two special meals each week. The additional calories included in these meals are useful to "Fool Your Body" into preventing metabolic slowdown. Successfully incorporating this habit helps to make the Tortoise Diet a livable plan to not only lose weight, but to keep it off for a lifetime. Care must be taken to limit these occasions to twice each week, and to not exceed the following calorie allotment:

    25% meal + 10% meal + 400 calories + any calories to be replaced for exercise = TGIW calorie allotment

"Top 40" List
A personalized list of foods that:
    1. you enjoy and that you will eat on a regular basis.
    2. provide good nutrition, containing low-fat protein, complex carbohydrates and heart-healthy fats.
    3. are quick and easy to prepare.
    4. everyone in your family will enjoy.

Trans-fats
Liquid fats which have been chemically altered in order to become solid or semi-solid (like shortening and margarine, for example). This substance is added to many packaged and processed foods to prolong shelf life and freshness. These should be avoided because they have been shown to cause increased LDL cholesterol, while, at the same time decreasing levels of "good" HDL cholesterol. The FDA will require that all trans-fats be listed on package labeling, beginning in 2006.

Weight Loss Calorie Plan

Because a "just right" calorie deficit is essential for fat loss to occur, the Lifetime Calorie Plan must be "adjusted" based on how many pounds a person currently is above their target body weight. To insure that the calorie deficit remains "just right", adjustments are made to the calorie level plans at 25 pound increments.

Whole-Foods

Fresh, colorful foods eaten as close to their natural state as possible, with minimal processing and refining. A primarily whole-foods diet is a healthy diet!

wintheracetolose.com

The Tortoise Diet web site, designed to help you succeed. Many services are available to members, for less than the price of one restaurant dinner per month. Members will have all of their calculations done for them to determine target body weight, target body fat percentage, target fat weight, target lean weight, Lifetime Calorie Plan, Weight Loss Calorie Plan and PWLR. Full color personalized graphs will be kept for each member, showing how goals of preserving lean weight and losing fat weight are being met. The site is filled with many helpful services that will help you "win the race to lose!"